P9-APA-452

15

Lippincott Williams & Wilkins'

Medical Assisting Exam Review for CMA, RMA & CMAS Certification

3rd Edition

Lippincott Williams & Wilkins' Medical Assisting Exam Review for CMA, RMA & CMAS Certification

Helen J. Houser, RN, MSHA, BS, RMA (AMT)

Faculty Medical Assisting
Phoenix College
Phoenix, Arizona

Janet R. Sesser, MS, BS, RMA (AMT), CMA (AAMA)

Director of Academic Operations
Anthem Education Group, Inc
Phoenix, Arizona

Wolters Kluwer Health | Lippincott Williams & Wilkins

Philadelphia • Baltimore • New York • London
Buenos Aires • Hong Kong • Sydney • Tokyo

Acquisitions Editor: Kelley Squazzo
Product Manager: Paula C. Williams
Marketing Manager: Shauna Kelley
Designer: Teresa Mallon
Compositor: Aptara, Inc.

351 West Camden Street
Baltimore, MD 21201

Two Commerce Square
2001 Market Street
Philadelphia, PA 19103

Printed in China

9 8 7 6 5 4 3 2 1

Library of Congress Cataloging-in-Publication Data

Houser, Helen J., author.
Lippincott Williams & Wilkins' medical assisting exam review for CMA, RMA & CMAS certification / Helen J. Houser, Janet R. Sesser. – Third edition.
p. ; cm.
Lippincott Williams and Wilkins' medical assisting exam review for CMA, RMA, and CMAS certification
Medical assisting exam review for CMA, RMA & CMAS certification
Includes bibliographical references and index.
ISBN 978-1-60913-368-9 (pbk. : alkaline paper)
1. Medical assistants–Examinations, questions, etc. 2. Physicians' assistants–Examinations, questions, etc. 3. Medical assistants–Licenses–United States–Examinations–Study guides. 4. Physicians' assistants–Licenses–United States–Examinations–Study guides. I. Sesser, Janet R., author. II. Title. III. Title: Lippincott Williams and Wilkins' medical assisting exam review for CMA, RMA, and CMAS certification. IV. Title: Medical assisting exam review for CMA, RMA & CMAS certification.
[DNLM: 1. Physician Assistants–Examination Questions. 2. Clinical Medicine–Examination Questions. 3. Practice Management, Medical–Examination Questions. W 18.2]
R728.8.H68 2012
610.737076–dc22

2010045361

DISCLAIMER

Care has been taken to confirm the accuracy of the information present and to describe generally accepted practices. However, the authors, editors, and publisher are not responsible for errors or omissions or for any consequences from application of the information in this book and make no warranty, expressed or implied, with respect to the currency, completeness, or accuracy of the contents of the publication. Application of this information in a particular situation remains the professional responsibility of the practitioner; the clinical treatments described and recommended may not be considered absolute and universal recommendations.

The authors, editors, and publisher have exerted every effort to ensure that drug selection and dosage set forth in this text are in accordance with the current recommendations and practice at the time of publication. However, in view of ongoing research, changes in government regulations, and the constant flow of information relating to drug therapy and drug reactions, the reader is urged to check the package insert for each drug for any change in indications and dosage and for added warnings and precautions. This is particularly important when the recommended agent is a new or infrequently employed drug.

Some drugs and medical devices presented in this publication have Food and Drug Administration (FDA) clearance for limited use in restricted research settings. It is the responsibility of the health care provider to ascertain the FDA status of each drug or device planned for use in their clinical practice.

To purchase additional copies of this book, call our customer service department at **(800) 638-3030** or fax orders to **(301) 223-2320**. International customers should call **(301) 223-2300**.

***Visit Lippincott Williams & Wilkins on the Internet*:** **http://www.lww.com.** Lippincott Williams & Wilkins customer service representatives are available from 8:30 am to 6:00 pm, EST.

RRS1011

To the hardworking medical assistants and administrative medical specialists in the health care community, and to students and their instructors who recognize certification as a pursuit of excellence and professionalism.

ABOUT THE AUTHORS

Helen J. Houser is a registered medical assistant and a registered nurse and holds a master of science in health care administration. For the past ten years she served as the Director of the Medical Assisting Program at Phoenix College. Her experience in health care spans over 30 years with various positions involving medical assisting, including Vice President of Phoenix General Hospital, Deer Valley, where she opened and administered medical practices in rural areas. She is a national speaker on such topics as "Immunization Education for Medical Assisting Students" and the recipient of several awards, including the National Institute of Staff and Organizational Development Excellence Award and two Arizona Governor's Awards for Excellence. Houser lived on a Navajo reservation for four years and has extensive experience working with diverse populations.

Janet R. Sesser, a Registered Medical Assistant and Certified Medical Assistant holds a Master of Science in Health Education and Bachelor of Science in Health Care Management. She is currently the Director of Academic Operations, Anthem Education Group, Inc, Phoenix, Arizona. Her background includes many years working as a practicing medical assistant for various types of practices and as a cardiopulmonary technician. For the past 25 years, she has worked in postsecondary education teaching and writing allied health curricula. Sesser is very involved with American Medical Technologists, serving as a member on the AMT Board of Directors. She is a recipient of the Medallion of Merit Award, the highest honor bestowed by AMT to a medical assistant, and a frequent presenter at national medical conferences.

PREFACE

LWW's Medical Assisting Exam Review for CMA, RMA, and CMAS Certifications provides a capstone review for recent graduates from medical assisting and medical administrative specialist programs, and working medical assistants and medical administrative specialists who are preparing to take a national certification exam. Medical assisting faculty find the text an invaluable tool to both validate learning and integrate topics. The decision to write it grew out of our frustrated attempts to find a review book that provided a simple yet effective approach to preparing for the national medical assisting and medical administrative specialist exams.

Yet *LWW's Medical Assisting Exam Review for CMA, RMA, and CMAS Certification* is more than a review: You can use the first three chapters to develop a unique study plan that is tailored to your individual strengths and weaknesses. Next, you can implement the plan, study the material included in the rest of the book, and finally test your knowledge and retention with the simulated exams.

The book's user-friendly design follows a simple outline format to make the information easy to digest, and we have sequenced topics so they build on each other. For example, medical terminology is one of the early chapters because it is necessary to understand anatomy, physiology, and additional content areas in subsequent chapters.

Other unique features of *LWW's Medical Assisting Exam Review for CMA, RMA, and CMAS Certification* include:

- Material that is succinct, focused, pertinent and truly up to date incorporating the national exams' topics.
- New and expanded information on emergency and disaster preparedness, the increasing role of the practice manager, facility management, the Electronic Health Record and more.
- A pretest with an analysis to help you determine your strong and weak study areas
- A method for creating your own study plan and a calendar to help you track it
- A design that incorporates *Bloom's Taxonomy* for teaching with questions answers and rationale on the same page to avoid flipping back and forth; also, a sturdy bookmark to cover answers
- 2,000 questions; research shows that probably the best way to prepare for a specific exam is to practice answering lots of questions with the content worded differently.
- Practice exams specific to the CMA (AAMA), RMA (AMT) and CMAS (AMT).
- Important review terms with definitions included in each chapter
- Review and study tips pertinent to each chapter
- Test preparation tips for students for whom English is their second language
- Important information for study groups
- Explanation of the major national exams
- Exam-taking strategies and exam-day preparation
- Six timed simulated exams: one for each of the three national exams appear in the back of the book, and one for each of the three national exams is on the Student Resources CD-ROM in the back of the book.

The following are reviewer comments that attest to the effectiveness and practicality of the book's approach:

- "I think that this is one of the best review texts that I have ever seen - very inclusive."
- "This text is excellent and will be recommended to our students to study for the certification exam."
- "The short chapter reviews are very well done and effectively organized."
- "The students need a little levity once in a while. The cartoons are good. Made me smile."
- "Excellent."
- " Invaluable."
- "I use a different book in my review class at this time, but after seeing your text, I will switch."

Our goal is to help you succeed by providing you with the tools and information you need to ace the national medical assisting exams—and to retain that information to ensure a successful career. We have incorporated our expertise, creativity, interest in student success, and even a little humor into this book, and believe we will achieve our goal while helping you achieve yours.

Helen J. Houser, RN, MSHA, BS, RMA
Janet R. Sesser, MS, BS, RMA, CMA

ADDITIONAL RESOURCES

Lippincott Williams & Wilkins' Medical Assisting Exam Review for CMA, RMA, and CMAS Certification includes additional resources for instructors that are available on the book's companion website at http://thePoint.lww.com/Houser3e and resources for students that are available on the CD-ROM packaged with the book and on the book's companion website at http://thePoint.lww.com/Houser3e.

INSTRUCTOR RESOURCES

Approved adopting instructors will be given access to the following additional resource:

- WebCT/Blackboard access

STUDENT RESOURCES

- Interactive Exam Simulator on CD-ROM and online with over 2,000 questions simulating the CMA, RMA, and CMAS national exams
- Electronic flashcards with audio pronunciation
- Audio Glossary

In addition, purchasers of the text can access the searchable Full Text On-line by going to the *Lippincott Williams & Wilkins' Medical Assisting Exam Review for CMA, RMA, and CMAS Certification* website at http://thePoint.lww.com/Houser3e. See the inside front cover of this text for more details, including the passcode you will need to gain access to the website.

ACKNOWLEDGMENTS

We would like to thank Pamela Rogers, Phoenix College 2003 Distinguished Teacher of the Year, for providing insight and for advising us on the challenges of students with limited English proficiency. We would also like to thank Daniel Celaya, Practice Manager Gregory Celaya MD, PC, for sharing his expertise in the role of the practice manager and the electronic health record and ellise hayden, Chief Operating Officer of Adelante Healthcare, Inc., for her emergency preparedness knowledge.

We are extremely grateful for the efforts of the exceptional, dedicated reviewers whose thoughts positively influenced the content of the book.

REVIEWERS

Gerry A. Brasin, AS, CMA (AAMA), CPC
Coordinator
Corporate Education
Premier Education Group
Springfield, MA

Christine Cusano, CMA (AAMA), CPhT, CHI
Senior Regional Director of Education
Lincoln Technical Institute
Brockton, MA

Donna Domanke-Nuytten
Professor
Health Science Technology
Macomb Community College
Clinton Township, MI

Anne Gailey, CMA (AAMA)
Instructor
Medical Assisting
Ogeechee Technical College
Statesboro, GA

Kari Williams, BS, DC
Director
Medical Office Technology
Front Range Community College
Longmont, CO

CONTENTS

Unit 1

The Starting Point

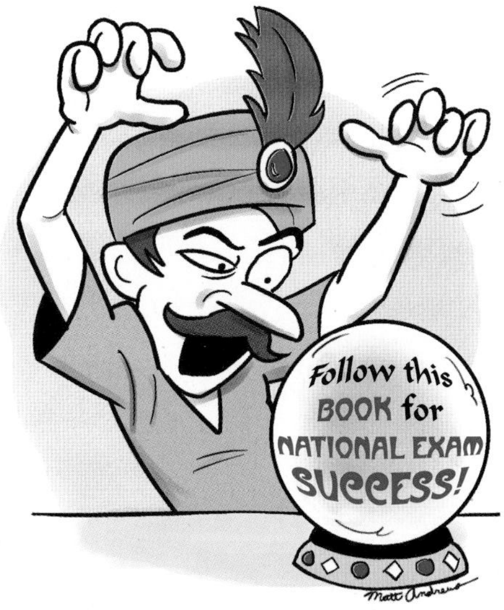

1 The Certification Process

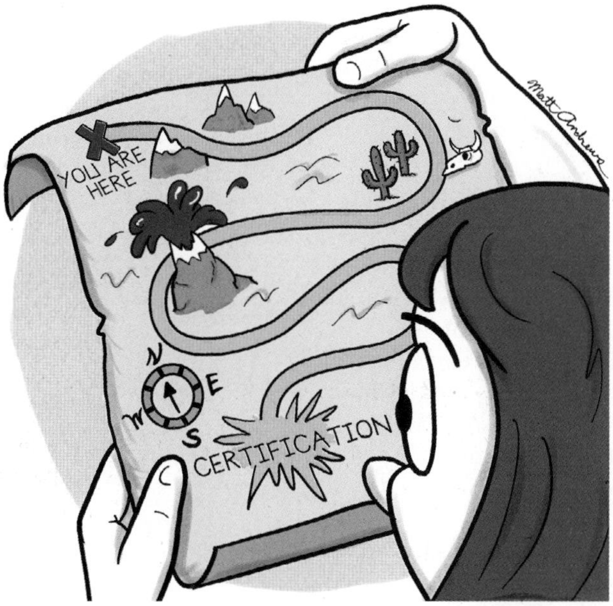

You opened this book, so you are probably preparing to take one of the national medical assisting exams or the medical administrative specialist exam. Good idea! If you are a recent graduate of a program, the best time to take the exam is now, while the knowledge is fresh in your mind and your information is up to date. If you are a practicing medical assistant, the best time is still now, and here's why:

- Holding a recognized national certification demonstrates to employers, potential employers (especially if you are moving to another state or changing jobs), patients, and others that you have a standardized body of knowledge. This is an important credential that is recognized and respected by the public.
- Medical assisting was traditionally guided by local informal standards. An increasing number of states now regulate the medical assistant role and credentials through legislation. The different training options and criteria required to be considered a valid medical assistant vary among states, but they all recognize medical assistants who have passed one of the two major national exams, the American Association of Medical Assistants (AAMA) and the American Medical Technologists (AMT) exams.
- Expanding administrative responsibilities now warrant specialization and validation of knowledge through a certification process such as the AMT Certified Medical Administrative Specialist (CMAS).
- Increasing numbers of medical offices are affiliated with health care organizations accredited by The Joint Commission (TJC) (formerly the Joint Commission on Accreditation of Healthcare Organizations [JCAHO]), the National Committee on Quality Assurance (NCQA), or other agencies. Staff credentials are always inspected, and national certifications are looked on favorably.
- Health care is ever-changing. Preparing for a national exam is a method to keep up with practice, to review the

latest standards, and to demonstrate your knowledge of entry-level competencies.

NATIONAL MEDICAL ASSISTING EXAMS

The two major organizations offering nationally recognized medical assisting examinations are the American Association of Medical Assistants (AAMA) and the American Medical Technologists (AMT), both of which are respected associations. The question content of both exams is similar, and both use a multiple choice format. The medical assisting certifications issued by the AAMA or AMT are equally accepted by employers. The eligibility criteria for each exam differ. Your choice of which exam to take may be contingent on these criteria.

THE CMA (AAMA)

The certification received after passing the AAMA exam is called Certified Medical Assistant (CMA [AAMA]). Those eligible to take the CMA (AAMA) exam are:

Figure 1-1 Insignia of the American Association of Medical Assistants (AAMA).

- Graduating students or recent graduates of a medical assisting program accredited by the Commission on Accreditation of Allied Health Education Programs (CAAHEP) or the Accrediting Bureau of Health Education Programs (ABHES)
- Nonrecent graduates (more than 12 months after graduation) of a CAAHEP or ABHES accredited medical assisting program [beginning January 1, 2010, candidates will have 60 months from the date of graduation to pass the exam; if a candidate does not pass within this time frame, the candidate will not be eligible for the CMA (AAMA) credential]
- CMAs (AAMA) recertifying their credential by way of examination

Beginning April 1, 2009, the examination became computerized and is available throughout the year at testing sites. Information on the application, testing locations, dates, and fees can be found at www.aama-ntl.org or by emailing certification@aama-ntl.org or calling or writing to:

AAMA Certification Department
20 North Wacker Drive, #1575
Chicago, IL 60606
1-800-228-2262

The CMA (AAMA) exam contains 200 multiple choice questions with five answer options. Twenty of the questions are for trial only and do not count toward your score. It is not indicated which questions are the trial questions. The questions are in no particular order. Refer to the tables at the end of this chapter for the content outline and corresponding study chapters. Exam review questions for Anatomy & Physiology and Medical Terminology are available on the AAMA website.

THE RMA (AMT)

The certification received after passing the AMT Medical Assisting exam is called Registered Medical Assistant (RMA, AMT). Those eligible to take the RMA exam are:

Figure 1-2 Insignia of the American Medical Technologists (AMT).

- Graduates of (or students scheduled to graduate from) a medical assistant program that holds programmatic accreditation by the ABHES or CAAHEP or students in a postsecondary school or college that holds institutional accreditation by the ABHES or CAAHEP
- Graduates of (or students scheduled to graduate from) a medical assisting program in a postsecondary school or college that has institutional accreditation by a regional accrediting commission or a national accrediting organization approved by the U.S. Department of Education; the program must include a minimum of 720 clock-hours (or equivalent) of training in medical assisting (including a clinical externship)
- Graduates of (or students scheduled to graduate from) a formal medical services training program of the U.S. Armed Forces
- Medical assistants employed in the profession for a minimum of 5 years, no more than 2 years of which may have been as an instructor in the postsecondary medical assistant program

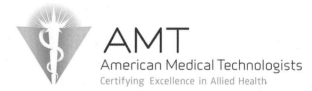

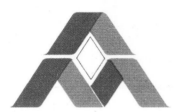

The exam is offered throughout the year at testing sites in two testing formats—a test booklet with answers written in pencil on a "bubble" answer sheet or a computer test. Information on the application, testing locations, dates, and fees can be found at www.amt1.com or by emailing rma@amt1.com or calling or writing to:

AMT
10700 W. Higgins Road, Suite 150
Rosemont, IL 60018
1-847-823-5169

The RMA exam consists of 200 to 210 multiple choice questions with four answer options. If there are 210 questions, 10 will be trial questions and, as with the AAMA, they do not count toward your score. You have 2 hours to take the exam. The questions are in no particular order. Refer to the tables at the end of this chapter for the content areas and corresponding study chapters. Exam review questions are located on the AMT website, and for a nominal fee, you may send for a practice exam.

NATIONAL MEDICAL ADMINISTRATIVE SPECIALIST EXAM

At the time of this writing, the AMT is the only nationally recognized organization offering the Medical Administrative Specialist examination. The credential received upon successful completion is the Certified Medical Administrative Specialist (CMAS). Those eligible to take the CMAS exam are:

- Graduating students or graduates of a medical office administrative program that holds programmatic accreditation or is part of a postsecondary school or college that holds institutional accreditation by the ABHES
- Graduating students or graduates of a medical office administrative program in a postsecondary school or college that holds institutional accreditation by a regional accrediting commission or a national accrediting organization approved by the U.S. Department of Education; the program must include a minimum of 720 clock-hours (or equivalent) of training in medical office administration skills (including a practical externship). The training must include at least:
  - Medical records management
  - Health care insurance processing, billing, and coding
  - Office financial responsibilities
  - Information processing
- RMAs or equivalent who possess a minimum of 2 years working as a medical office administrative specialists
- Medical office administrative specialists employed in the profession for a minimum of 5 years

The exam is offered throughout the year at testing sites in two testing formats—a test booklet with answers written in pencil on a "bubble" answer sheet or a computer test. Information on the application, testing locations, dates, and fees can be found at www.amt1.com or by emailing cmas@amt1.com or calling or writing to:

AMT
10700 W. Higgins Road, Suite 150
Rosemont, IL 60018
1-847-823-5169

The CMAS exam consists of 200 to 210 multiple choice questions with four answer options. If there are 210 questions, 10 will be trial questions, and as with the CMA (AAMA) and RMA, they do not count toward your score. You have 2 hours to complete the exam. The questions are in no particular order. Refer to the tables at the end of this chapter for the content areas and corresponding study chapters. Exam review questions are located on the AMT website.

MAINTAINING CERTIFICATION

Once you have received your certification, in order to maintain it, you must earn a specific number of continuing education units (CEUs) each year or in a designated number of years. The purpose is to stay current in your field by keeping up to date with changing or new standards and practices. Generally, one CEU is equivalent to 1 clock-hour. CEUs may be earned in various ways. The most common are:

- Attending seminars and conferences approved for CEUs by your certifying organization
- Completing online modules of appropriate topics approved for CEUs by your certifying organization
- Reading material in journals approved for CEUs by your certifying organization and answering related questions
- Listening to audio modules approved for CEUs by your certifying organization and completing required exercises or answering related questions

Not only is staying up to date important to maintain your certification, but you are also responsible for staying current in your field as a legal obligation. You will be held accountable for the standards in place at any given time.

STRATEGY ADVICE

A graduate, who recently took the certification examination, gives this advice: "Study this book, study the practice exam at the end, and then study this book again." If both the computerized and "bubble" answer sheet formats are available for the exam you are eligible to take, you should decide which option works best for you. The simulated computerized exam on the CD-ROM and the simulated written exam with an answer sheet are located in the back of the book.

STUDYING

This book is designed for simple, efficient study. The combination of narrative and an outline structure keeps the information succinct, emphasizes what is most likely to be on the exams, and decreases reading time. Material is presented in three areas: the body of the text, the review terms, and the questions with associated rationale. This method reinforces previous information and provides additional information. Be sure to study all content areas that are applicable to your exam. Refer to the tables at the end of this chapter. The material may be phrased differently throughout the text to ensure understanding because it is unlikely that the wording will appear exactly as it does on the actual exam. Some questions require critical thinking, but the necessary knowledge to formulate the correct answer is contained in the book. Use study techniques that have been successful for you in the past, and incorporate new strategies, as appropriate. Suggestions include the following:

- Inform your family, friends, employer, and fellow employees that you are preparing for the exam. Ask them to support you, and include them in the review process. Ask your family to allow you uninterrupted study time; determine when that time will be and stick to it.
- Read each chapter, and underline or highlight information that needs reinforcement. Reread those areas at different times until you believe you know them. Write down information you cannot remember; writing helps memorization.
- Write difficult information in your own words to assure understanding; ask your employer, a teacher, or a peer if you need assistance.
- Read the important review terms at the end of each chapter.
- Develop flashcards by writing the review term on the front of an index card and the definition on the back. Again, writing enhances the memorization process.
- Look for learning moments. These are times outside of your planned study regimen when you can sneak in some studying, such as during breaks; at lunch; while riding as a passenger in a car or bus, using exercise equipment, or walking the dog; or even during television commercials. Be creative!
- Have friends and family test you using your flashcards.
- Develop rhymes to assist memory (such as, for diabetic coma, "hot and dry, sugar high").
- Use alphabetical connections, for example, arteries (begins with an "a") carry blood away (also begins with an "a").
- Incorporate as much repetition as you can.
- Read the review tip boxes at the beginning of each chapter.
- Take lots of practice tests, using the tests in this book and the practice questions from the AAMA and AMT.
- Contact local programs—some offer national exam reviews.
- Cram only if you are confident of your overall knowledge and need only cursory last-minute review.
- Consider joining a study group as additional preparation, but not as your only preparation.

MULTIPLE CHOICE EXAMS

The national exams consist of multiple choice questions. The AMT exam has four answer choices for each question; the AAMA exam has five answer choices. The questions have various levels of difficulty. Do not think you will be able to recognize the correct answer without studying if you do not know the topic. The questions purposefully contain what are called decoys. These are words that look similar to the correct answer and can easily confuse you. Studying and preparedness are the only way to pass any exam. Use these strategies for solving multiple choice questions:

- Read the question and answer it in your head, and then look for the answer you think is correct in the choices, but do not mark it yet.
- Read the whole question with each of the choices. Some questions have more than one correct answer, but one answer is more correct than the others. Do not mark your answer before considering all of the alternatives. That last choice may be better than the first. A word that is similar but not correct may appear first and act as a decoy.
- Watch your time. Do not spend more than 45 seconds on one question. Come back to it after completing the questions you know.
- Eliminate choices you know are wrong. The more choices you eliminate, the better your chance of selecting the correct one.
- Watch for "all of the above" answers. If you eliminate one answer, "all of the above" cannot be correct.
- Watch for "none of the above." If one answer is correct, "none of the above" is not the answer.

- Use caution with questions that contain the word "except." The answer you are looking for is the opposite of the question. If the question says, "You would use sterile technique in all of the following situations, except," look for the opposite of when "you would use sterile technique," such as when taking a blood pressure. Read "except" questions extra carefully and be sure of what they are asking.
- Watch for words such as "always," "never," "all," and "none." If you can think of one exception to a choice, then that answer is not correct.
- Handle decoys. Some questions lead you to think another answer is correct when you are relatively sure it is not. Read the whole question with each alternative separately. Think about what each question with each answer means. Frequently, this helps confirm your original answer choice.

What about guessing? The scoring on some multiple choice examinations penalizes test takers for guessing by subtracting additional points for incorrect answers but not for blank answers. Neither the AAMA nor the AMT subtracts additional points for incorrect answers as opposed to blank answers, so use the strategies outlined previously, and if you are still not certain, give it your best guess. The most effective strategy for multiple choice tests is practice, practice, practice! Practice by trying ALL of the questions in this book.

ENGLISH LANGUAGE LEARNERS

ELL refers to English Language Learners. If English is not your primary language, the following are additional suggestions to assist you in preparing for a national certification exam.

- Do not rush into taking the exam; be prepared.
- Read and follow the previous strategies.
- Buy or borrow the textbook *Test of English as a Foreign Language* (TOEFL). It offers an effective method to evaluate your English. If you have difficulty with this text, consider first taking an English or ELL course at a community college or other school. Taking a course may also increase your employment opportunities.
- English tests called Combined English Language Skills Assessments (CELSA) are available at community colleges for non-English speakers to determine their level of English. A national exam will be difficult to pass if you score below the high school equivalent on the CELSA.
- Obtain an ELL medical terminology book and review it.
- Study with a native English speaker who is motivated and organized (see the next section on study groups).
- If a question on the exam does not seem to make sense to you, look closely at the verb. It may have another meaning different from the one you thought. An example is the word "pose," commonly meaning to assume a posture for a picture or artistic purposes (for example, "She posed for the picture"). Another meaning, more common in tests, is to present an idea for consideration, such as, "The doctor posed that the patient may not be taking his medication according to instructions." Consider other verb meanings before answering.
- Select only one answer—the best answer—for multiple choice questions. In some countries, you may select several correct answers. In the United States, if you select more than one answer, it is marked incorrect.
- Be sure you are familiar with the testing modality you select (computer or "bubble" answer sheet).

STUDY GROUPS

Study groups generally consist of three to six people meeting to study or to prepare for a course, test or exam, or project. A group may be more informal, such as a group of friends getting together to study on a Saturday afternoon, or more formal, such as staff members who work in the same medical complex and who have agreed to meet at designated times and places using an agreed-on structure. Study groups have advantages (pros) and disadvantages (cons).

Pros

- Study times and places are designated; people are more motivated to be prepared if others are relying on them.
- The work, such as researching or organizing a topic, is shared.
- One person's weak area may be another's strength, which sometimes makes studying easier.
- You can discuss issues related to the exam, relieve stress, and gain a fresh perspective.

Cons

- Participants must agree on study times and places, which is sometimes challenging.
- All members may not participate equally, resulting in more work for some.
- Everyone does not study at the same pace, leaving some behind and others frustrated with the slowness.
- Conversation and other distracters may interfere with study.

Should you organize or join a study group to prepare for a national exam? This is a personal decision. If you are a recent graduate and have a good study group from school, stick with it. If you study best alone, perhaps a group is not for you. If several colleagues that you know or work with are planning to take the exam, a study group could benefit all. The following are tips for working with study groups.

Study Group Advice

- Know the members and look at their performance in school or at work to determine whether they are committed and motivated before inviting them to join the group.
- Select a site and time conducive to study—for example, not the home of a friend who has active, small children.
- Allow only full-time members—coming to only some sessions should not be permitted because a part-time member requires time to catch up. An exception would be if a person only wants to participate for one or two subjects and the dates and times for those subjects are pre-established.
- Organize an overall study plan with topics, assignments, and a leader for each session. Do this at the first session. It is sometimes difficult but worth the time. There are many options for putting together a plan. One method is to plan an overall review of each topic or to concentrate on specific topics that most members of the group find difficult. Anatomy and Physiology is the most challenging area. The group may decide to concentrate on this and study other topics individually.
- Deal with disrupting or distracting members right away; sometimes humor works, for example, "Okay, time out for you until you stop gossiping and get down to work."
- Leave a study group if it is not working for you; simply say, "This is not working for me."
- Remember, the study group is only one tool; use the learning moments, flashcards, and other strategies previously mentioned. After you develop your study plan as described in Chapter 3, you will probably need more hours than the group provides, especially to cover difficult topics.

CONTENT OUTLINES FOR NATIONAL EXAMS AND CORRESPONDING CHAPTERS

Certified Medical Assistant–CMA (AAMA)

Work Area	Chapter Locations
I. *General*	
A. Medical Terminology	Chapters 5, 6, 18, 25
B. Anatomy & Physiology	Chapters 6, 18
C. Psychology	Chapter 7
D. Professionalism	Chapters 4, 7, 8, 9
E. Communication	Chapters 7, 10, 12
F. Medicolegal Guidelines & Requirements	Chapters 4, 11, 13, 14, 15
II. *Administrative*	
G. Data Entry	Chapters 9, 13, 14, 15
H. Equipment	Chapter 9, 16
I. Computer Concepts	Chapter 9
J. Records Management	Chapter 11
K. Screening & Processing Mail	Chapter 12
L. Scheduling & Monitoring Appointments	Chapter 10
M. Resources & Community Services	Chapters 8, 26
N. (At the time of this writing, there are no items for this category.)	Nonapplicable
O. Maintaining the Office	Chapters 4, 16, 26
P. Office Policies & Procedures	Chapter 16
Q. Practice Finances	Chapter 15
III. *Clinical*	
R. Principles of Infection Control	Chapters 17, 18,19, 21
S. Treatment Area	Chapters
T. Patient Preparation & Assisting the Physician	Chapters 18, 19
U. Patient History Interview	Chapters 18
V. Collecting & Processing Specimens; Diagnostic Testing	Chapter 18, 19, 20, 21, 22
W. Preparing & Administering Medications	Chapter 25
X. Emergencies	Chapter 26
Y. First Aid	Chapter 26
Z. Nutrition	Chapter 24

Registered Medical Assistant–RMA (AMT)

Work Area	Number of Questions	Percentage of Exam	Chapter Locations
I. *General Medical Assisting Knowledge*	82	41%	
A. Anatomy & Physiology			Chapters 6, 18
B. Medical Terminology			Chapters 5, 6, 18, 25
C. Medical Law			Chapters 4, 11, 13, 14, 15
D. Medical Ethics			Chapter 4
E. Human Relations			Chapters 7, 16
F. Patient Education			Chapters 8, 24
II. *Administrative Medical Assisting*	48	24%	
A. Insurance			Chapters 13, 14
B. Finance & Bookkeeping			Chapter 15
C. Medical Receptionist, Secretarial, Clerical			Chapters 9, 10, 11, 12
III. *Clinical Medical Assisting*	70	35%	
A. Asepsis			Chapters 17, 21
B. Sterilization			Chapter 17
C. Instruments			Chapters 18, 19
D. Vital Signs & Mensurations			Chapter 18
E. Physical Examinations			Chapter 18
F. Clinical Pharmacology			Chapter 25
G. Minor Surgery			Chapter 19
H. Therapeutic Modalities			Chapter 23
I. Laboratory Procedures			Chapter 21
J. Electrocardiography			Chapter 20
K. First Aid & Emergency Response			Chapter 26

Certified Medical Administrative Specialist–CMAS (AMT)

Work Area	Number of Questions	Percentage of Exam	Chapter Locations
I. *Medical Assisting Foundations*	26	13%	
A. Medical terminology			Chapters 5, 6, 18, 25
B. Anatomy & Physiology			Chapters 6, 18
C. Legal & Ethical Considerations			Chapters 4, 11, 13, 14, 15
D. Professionalism			Chapters 4, 7, 8, 9
II. *Basic Clinical Medical Assisting*	16	8%	
A. Basic Health History Interview			Chapters 7, 18
B. Basic Charting			Chapters 11, 18
C. Vital Signs & Measurements			Chapters 5, 6, 18
D. Asepsis in the Medical Office			Chapter 17
E. Examination Preparation			Chapters 5, 6, 18
F. Medical Office Emergencies			Chapter 26
G. Pharmacology			Chapters 5, 25
III. *Medical Office Clerical Assisting*	20	10%	
A. Appointment Management & Scheduling			Chapters 7, 10
B. Reception			Chapters 7, 10
C. Communication			Chapters 7, 10, 12
D. Patient Information & Community Resources			Chapters 8, 26
IV. *Medical Records Management*	28	14%	
A. Systems			Chapter 11
B. Procedures			Chapter 11
C. Confidentiality			Chapters 4, 11
V. *Health Care Insurance Processing, Coding, & Billing*	34	17%	
A. Insurance Processing			Chapter 13
B. Coding			Chapter 14
C. Insurance Billing & Finances			Chapters 4, 14, 15
VI. *Medical Office Financial Management*	34	17%	
A. Fundamentals of Financial Management			Chapter 15
B. Patient Accounts			Chapters 14, 15
C. Banking			Chapter 15
D. Payroll			Chapter 16

(*continued*)

VII. *Medical Office Information Processing*	14	7%	
A. Fundamentals of Computing			Chapter 9
B. Medical Office Computing Applications			Chapter 9
VIII. *Medical Office Management*	28	14%	
A. Office Communications			Chapters 7, 9, 12
B. Business Organization Management			Chapters 11, 14, 15, 16
C. Human Resources			Chapter 16
D. Safety			Chapters 4, 17, 21, 26
E. Supplies & Equipment			Chapter 16
F. Physical Office Plant			Chapter 16
G. Risk Management & Quality Assurance			Chapter 4

2

Pretest and Analysis

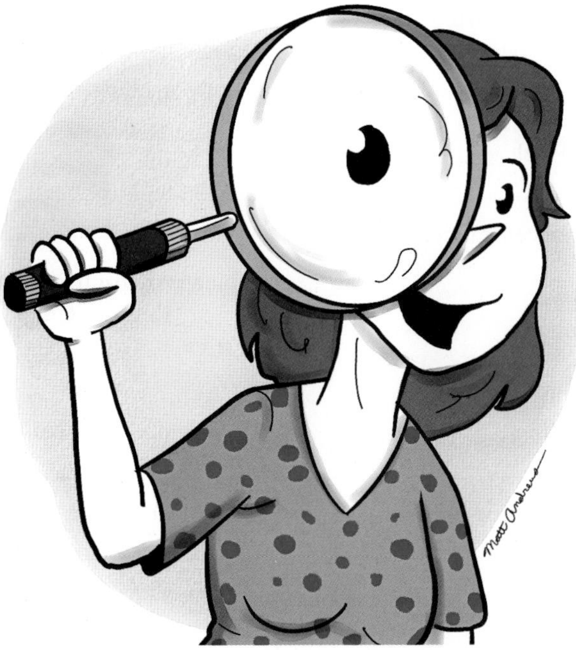

Relax and do not rush when taking the pretest. The purpose is to determine your strengths and weaknesses in the study subjects, not to produce a score. *Do not* time yourself. This test is designed to determine basic knowledge without intimidation. This also allows you to take the pretest in more than one sitting.

All questions are relevant for the CMA (AAMA) and RMA (AMT) exams. Questions 1 through 79 are relevant for the CMAS (AMT) exam. Answer the pretest questions by circling your answer or writing your answers on a separate sheet of paper. Use the special bookmark from the back of the book to cover the answers and work through *all* the questions without stopping to see if you are correct.

PRETEST

1. Which of the following positions is used for examination of the abdomen?
   A. Prone
   B. Supine
   C. Sims'
   D. Fowler's
   E. Semi-Fowler's

Answer: **B**

Subject: Patient Exams
Refer to Chapter 18

---

2. The two functions of the ear are hearing and:
   A. movement.
   B. equilibrium.
   C. sound production.
   D. maintaining upright position.

Answer: **B**

Subject: Anatomy and Physiology
Refer to Chapter 6

---

3. The two main divisions of the central nervous system are the:
   A. cerebrum and cerebellum.
   B. hypothalamus and medulla.
   C. spinal cord and brain.
   D. sympathetic and parasympathetic.
   E. endocrine and exocrine.

Answer: **C**

Subject: Anatomy and Physiology
Refer to Chapter 6

---

4. The portion of the eye that contains rods and cones is the:
   A. lens.
   B. sclera.
   C. conjunctiva.
   D. retina.

Answer: **D**

Subject: Anatomy and Physiology
Refer to Chapter 6

---

5. The term meaning **muscular pain** is:
   A. myosin.
   B. myoglobin.
   C. myalgia.
   D. myocardium.
   E. myomalacia.

Answer: **C**

Subject: Medical Terminology
Refer to Chapter 5

---

6. The reporting mechanism that goes from your direct supervisor to your supervisor's supervisor is called the:
   A. chain of infection.
   B. chain of authority.
   C. team administration.
   D. administrative management.

Answer: **B**

Subject: Practice Management
Refer to Chapter 16

7. Pathogens that thrive in oxygen are called:
   A. antitoxins.
   B. anaerobes.
   C. spores.
   D. aerobes.
   E. oxides.

Answer: **D**

Subject: Microorganisms and Asepsis
Refer to Chapter 17

---

8. The amount of money the medical office owes for supplies and equipment is considered:
   A. accounts payable.
   B. assets.
   C. accounts receivable.
   D. distributions.

Answer: **A**

Subject: Financial Practices
Refer to Chapter 15

---

9. Balancing a checkbook with the bank statement is called:
   A. tracking.
   B. reconciliation.
   C. disbursement.
   D. justification.
   E. endorsement.

Answer: **B**

Subject: Financial Practices
Refer to Chapter 15

---

10. The hiring process involves all of the following EXCEPT:
    A. recruiting
    B. interviewing
    C. verifying
    D. training

Answer: **D**

Subject: Practice Management
Refer to Chapter 16

---

11. The first aid procedure for a suspected fracture includes:
    A. immobilizing the part.
    B. applying an elastic bandage.
    C. straightening the bones involved.
    D. applying heat for pain control.
    E. preparing the patient for physical therapy

Answer: **A**

Subject: Emergency Preparedness
Refer to Chapter 26

---

12. Which condition is characterized by a deficiency in insulin production?
    A. Gouty arthritis
    B. Pancreatic cancer
    C. Diabetes mellitus
    D. Anemia
    E. Gastric reflux disease

Answer: **C**

Subject: Anatomy and Physiology
Refer to Chapter 6

---

13. When deciding whether to purchase or lease a piece of equipment, the manager would most likely decide to lease:
    A. an expensive piece of equipment.
    B. equipment with high utilization.
    C. equipment with a short guarantee.
    D. equipment that outdates rapidly.

Answer: **D**

Subject: Practice Management
Refer to Chapter 16

14. The heart is divided into right and left sides by the:
    A. aorta.
    B. atria.
    C. septum.
    D. valves.
    E. ventricles.

Answer: **C**

Subject: Anatomy and Physiology
Refer to Chapter 6

---

15. The cardiovascular system includes:
    A. heart and blood vessels.
    B. heart and lungs.
    C. lungs and capillaries.
    D. heart and kidneys.

Answer: **A**

Subject: Anatomy and Physiology
Refer to Chapter 6

---

16. A localized dilation of an artery is a(n):
    A. aneurysm.
    B. embolism.
    C. infarction.
    D. stenosis.
    E. thrombus.

Answer: **A**

Subject: Anatomy and Physiology
Refer to Chapter 6

---

17. One type of genetic bleeding disorder is:
    A. anemia.
    B. aneurysm.
    C. hemophilia.
    D. leukemia.

Answer: **C**

Subject: Anatomy and Physiology
Refer to Chapter 6

---

18. The measurement of height or length and weight is:
    A. auscultation.
    B. manipulation.
    C. palpation.
    D. mensuration.
    E. menstruation.

Answer: **D**

Subject: Patient Exams
Refer to Chapter 18

---

19. **Gastrectasia** means:
    A. inflammation of the stomach.
    B. ulceration of the stomach.
    C. stretching of the stomach.
    D. surgical repair of the stomach.

Answer: **C**

Subject: Medical Terminology
Refer to Chapter 5

---

20. The muscle that expands and contracts during respiration, allowing the lungs to fill and empty air, is the:
    A. pectoralis.
    B. deltoid.
    C. gastrocnemius.
    D. diaphragm.
    E. rectus abdominus.

Answer: **D**

Subject: Anatomy and Physiology
Refer to Chapter 6

21. The employee's performance appraisal should occur at least:
A. quarterly.
B. annually.
C. semi-annually.
D. bi-annually.

Answer: **B**

Subject: Practice Management
Chapter 16

---

22. The vocal cords are located in the:
A. bronchi.
B. epiglottis.
C. larynx.
D. pharynx.
E. trachea.

Answer: **C**

Subject: Anatomy and Physiology
Refer to Chapter 6

---

23. The most effective method of destroying spores is:
A. boiling.
B. disinfecting.
C. sanitizing.
D. autoclaving.

Answer: **D**

Subject: Microorganisms and Asepsis
Refer to Chapter 17

---

24. A sphygmomanometer is used to:
A. measure visual acuity.
B. listen to heart sounds.
C. record electrical activity of the heart.
D. measure blood pressure.
E. auscultate breath sounds.

Answer: **D**

Subject: Patient Exams
Refer to Chapter 18

---

25. When multiple patients are evaluated and prioritized for treatment, it is called:
A. screening.
B. triage.
C. referral.
D. scheduling.

Answer: **B**

Subject: Administrative Technologies
Refer to Chapter 9

---

26. During a job interview, the prospective employer may ask questions about all of the following EXCEPT:
A. certification.
B. citizenship.
C. job-related weaknesses.
D. reason for leaving previous employment.
E. marital status.

Answer: **E**

Subject: Practice Management
Refer to Chapter 16

---

27. The term **auscultation** means:
A. tapping.
B. feeling.
C. measuring.
D. listening.

Answer: **D**

Subject: Patient Exams
Refer to Chapter 18

28. The recommended temperature for effective sterilization in an autoclave is:
    A. 200°F.
    B. 212°F.
    C. 220°F.
    D. 250°F.

Answer: **D**

Subject: Microorganisms and Asepsis
Refer to Chapter 17

---

29. The organization that established guidelines for occupational exposure to blood is the:
    A. CDC.
    B. FDA.
    C. HCFA.
    D. CMS.
    E. OSHA.

Answer: **E**

Subject: Microorganisms and Asepsis
Refer to Chapter 17

---

30. Which manual identifies procedural codes for submitting insurance claims?
    A. PPO
    B. ICD
    C. CPT
    D. HMO

Answer: **C**

Subject: Medical Coding and Claims
Refer to Chapter 14

---

31. The "S" in SOAP charting means:
    A. symptoms.
    B. signs.
    C. source.
    D. subjective.
    E. signature.

Answer: **D**

Subject: Medical Records
Refer to Chapter 11

---

32. The pegboard system of accounting generates which of the following documents?
    A. Cashier's check
    B. Bank statement
    C. Collection letter
    D. Receipt

Answer: **D**

Subject: Financial Practices
Refer to Chapter 15

---

33. A business letter in which all lines start flush with the left margin is:
    A. simplified style.
    B. modified block style.
    C. modified indented style.
    D. formal.
    E. block style.

Answer: **E**

Subject: Correspondence
Refer to Chapter 12

---

34. Which of the following acts constitutes negligence?
    A. A patient and physician establishing a professional relationship
    B. Breach of the physician's duty of skill or care
    C. A patient who has a positive outcome as a result of treatment
    D. Revocation of the physician's license

Answer: **B**

Subject: Law and Ethics
Refer to Chapter 4

35. The Employee's Withholding Allowance Certificate is the:
   A. W-2.
   B. W-4.
   C. I-9.
   D. FICA.
   E. Social Security.

Answer: **B**

Subject: Financial Practices
Refer to Chapter 15

---

36. A file used as a reminder that something must be taken care of on a certain date is called a:
   A. matrix.
   B. tickler.
   C. triage.
   D. chronologic.

Answer: **B**

Subject: Appointment Scheduling
Refer to Chapter 10

---

37. A set of principles or values is called:
   A. ethics.
   B. legal rights.
   C. opinions.
   D. standards.

Answer: **A**

Subject: Law and Ethics
Refer to Chapter 4

---

38. An instrument used to test neurologic reflexes is a(n):
   A. tuning fork.
   B. audiometer.
   C. sphygmomanometer.
   D. goniometer.
   E. percussion hammer.

Answer: **E**

Subject: Patient Exams
Refer to Chapter 18

---

39. Slurred speech and one-sided paralysis are symptoms of:
   A. stroke.
   B. heart attack.
   C. syncope.
   D. epistaxis.

Answer: **A**

Subject: Emergency Preparedness
Refer to Chapter 26

---

40. The abbreviation "mL" means:
   A. microliter.
   B. megaliter.
   C. milliliter.
   D. macroliter.
   E. miniliter.

Answer: **C**

Subject: Pharmacology and Medication Administration
Refer to Chapter 25

---

41. Confirming that the message the listener received is the message you intended to send is called:
   A. observation.
   B. listening.
   C. empathy.
   D. feedback.

Answer: **D**

Subject: Professional Communication
Refer to Chapter 7

42. Insurance that provides protection for wage earners and pays for medical care resulting from an occupational accident is:
   A. disability.
   B. CHAMPUS.
   C. Medicare.
   D. workers' compensation.
   E. Medicaid.

Answer: **D**

Subject: Medical Insurance
Refer to Chapter 13

---

43. The type of appointment scheduling in which several patients are given the same appointment time is called:
   A. grouping.
   B. advance booking.
   C. wave scheduling.
   D. batching.

Answer: **C**

Subject: Appointment Scheduling
Refer to Chapter 10

---

44. A drug that relieves nausea and vomiting is classified as an:
   A. antispasmodic.
   B. anticoagulant.
   C. antiemetic.
   D. analgesic.
   E. antidiarrheal.

Answer: **C**

Subject: Pharmacology and Medication Administration
Refer to Chapter 25

---

45. Use of chemicals to clean infectious materials from items or surfaces is called:
   A. sterilization.
   B. disinfection.
   C. sanitation.
   D. cleansing.

Answer: **B**

Subject: Microorganisms and Asepsis
Refer to Chapter 17

---

46. Myopia is a condition of:
   A. blindness.
   B. farsightedness.
   C. nearsightedness.
   D. loss of peripheral vision.
   E. crossed eyes.

Answer: **C**

Subject: Anatomy and Physiology
Refer to Chapter 6

---

47. A fracture that causes the bone to break through the skin is called:
   A. greenstick.
   B. simple.
   C. spiral.
   D. compound.

Answer: **D**

Subject: Emergency Preparedness
Refer to Chapter 26

48. A document requiring a person to appear in court is a:
    A. subpoena.
    B. deposition.
    C. litigation.
    D. contract.
    E. transcript.

Answer: **A**

Subject: Law and Ethics
Refer to Chapter 4

---

49. The system used for classifying diseases to facilitate collection of health information is:
    A. RBRVS.
    B. CPT-4.
    C. ICD-9-CM.
    D. HCFA-1500.

Answer: **C**

Subject: Medical Coding and Claims
Refer to Chapter 14

---

50. An example of objective information in a patient chart is the:
    A. patient's statement of his or her medical history.
    B. patient's statement of the severity of the pain.
    C. medical professional's note of a red, swollen area.
    D. patient's statement of inability to perform tasks.
    E. medical professional's note that the patient complains of pain.

Answer: **C**

Subject: Medical Records
Refer to Chapter 11

---

51. In communication with patients, an example of an open-ended question would be:
    A. How much pain medication have you taken?
    B. During this illness, did you have an elevated temperature?
    C. What brings you to the doctor today?
    D. Are you allergic to any medications?

Answer: **C**

Subject: Professional Communication
Refer to Chapter 7

---

52. The predetermined amount of money paid by the insured party before the insurance company pays medical expenses is referred to as:
    A. capitation.
    B. premium.
    C. indemnity.
    D. deductible.
    E. coinsurance.

Answer: **D**

Subject: Medical Insurance
Refer to Chapter 13

---

53. When handling third-party requests for information over the telephone, you should ask the caller to:
    A. contact the physician's attorney.
    B. ask the patient to submit written permission.
    C. hang up and not call back.
    D. call back to speak with the physician only.

Answer: **B**

Subject: Administrative Technologies
Refer to Chapter 9

54. To ensure mail delivery the next day, you would send correspondence via:
A. first class.
B. registered mail.
C. certified mail.
D. express mail.
E. second-class mail.

Answer: **D**

Subject: Correspondence
Refer to Chapter 12

---

55. The agency that regulates controlled substances is the:
A. DEA.
B. FDA.
C. CDC.
D. OSHA.

Answer: **A**

Subject: Pharmacology and Medication Administration
Refer to Chapter 25

---

56. Orientation of a new staff member would include:
A. interview.
B. performance appraisal.
C. review of policies and procedures.
D. sending a W-2 form.
E. checking references.

Answer: **C**

Subject: Practice Management
Refer to Chapter 16

---

57. The pulse point located bilaterally in the groin is the:
A. apical.
B. dorsalis pedis.
C. femoral.
D. popliteal.

Answer: **C**

Subject: Patient Exams
Refer to Chapter 18

---

58. Following the indexing rules for filing, which name comes first?
A. McWilliams
B. McCally
C. Mahill
D. MacHall
E. McAllister

Answer: **D**

Subject: Medical Records
Refer to Chapter 11

---

59. When a patient authorizes an insurance company to make payment directly to the physician, it is called:
A. assignment of benefits.
B. direct billing.
C. claims submission.
D. reimbursement.

Answer: **A**

Subject: Medical Insurance
Refer to Chapter 13

---

60. A debt incurred but not yet paid is called:
A. account balance.
B. accounts payable.
C. accounts receivable.
D. credit balance.
E. adjustment.

Answer: **B**

Subject: Financial Practices
Refer to Chapter 15

61. An instrument used to examine the eyes is a(n):
  A. audiometer.
  B. otoscope.
  C. lensometer.
  D. ophthalmoscope.

Answer: D

Subject: Patient Exams
Refer to Chapter 18

---

62. The term **hematuria** means:
  A. infection in the blood.
  B. painful urination.
  C. protein in the urine.
  D. difficult urination.
  E. blood in the urine.

Answer: E

Subject: Medical Terminology
Refer to Chapter 5

---

63. The Centers for Disease Control and Prevention recommends universal precautions that include:
  A. recapping needles when finished using them.
  B. placing all soiled trash in the waste can.
  C. cleaning blood spills with soap and water.
  D. wearing personal protective equipment.

Answer: D

Subject: Microorganisms and Asepsis
Refer to Chapter 17

---

64. The signature on the back of a check is the:
  A. payer.
  B. endorser.
  C. disburser.
  D. check maker.
  E. bank.

Answer: B

Subject: Financial Practices
Refer to Chapter 15

---

65. Which pulse site is most commonly used?
  A. Radial artery
  B. Brachial artery
  C. Apical region
  D. Temporal artery

Answer: A

Subject: Patient Exams
Refer to Chapter 18

---

66. In the usual physical examination sequence, which area of the body does the physician examine first?
  A. Thorax and lungs
  B. Genital area
  C. Abdomen
  D. Head and neck
  E. Breasts

Answer: D

Subject: Patient Exams
Refer to Chapter 18

---

67. The attention line of a business letter is located:
  A. four lines below the date.
  B. three lines below the letterhead.
  C. two lines below the inside address.
  D. two lines below the salutation.

Answer: C

Subject: Correspondence
Refer to Chapter 12

68. When a physician's license from one state is accepted by another state, it is called:
    A. endorsement.
    B. acceptance.
    C. reciprocity.
    D. allowance.
    E. transfer.

Answer: **C**

Subject: Law and Ethics
Refer to Chapter 4

---

69. A patient with 20/30 vision in both eyes can see with:
    A. the right eye at 30 feet what the normal eye sees at 20 feet.
    B. both eyes at 20 feet what the normal eye sees at 30 feet.
    C. the left eye at 20 feet what the normal eye sees at 30 feet.
    D. both eyes at 30 feet what the normal eye sees at 20 feet.

Answer: **B**

Subject: Patient Exams
Refer to Chapter 18

---

70. Which structure is located in the RLQ?
    A. Appendix
    B. Liver
    C. Spleen
    D. Pancreas
    E. Gallbladder

Answer: **A**

Subject: Anatomy and Physiology
Refer to Chapter 6

---

71. CMS, formerly HCFA, regulates:
    A. prescriptions.
    B. Medicare insurance.
    C. banking institutions.
    D. clinical laboratories.

Answer: **B**

Subject: Medical Insurance
Refer to Chapter 13

---

72 A patient is placed in Sims' position to examine the:
    A. breasts.
    B. abdomen.
    C. rectum.
    D. heart.
    E. back.

Answer: **C**

Subject: Patient Exams
Refer to Chapter 18

---

73. The subdivisions of E&M insurance codes include:
    A. pathology and laboratory codes.
    B. diagnostic and treatment services.
    C. radiology codes.
    D. anesthesia codes.

Answer: **B**

Subject: Medical Claims and Coding
Refer to Chapter 14

---

74. Another term for a **living will** is:
    A. patient's release.
    B. implied contract.
    C. emancipation will.
    D. advance directive.
    E. power of attorney.

Answer: **D**

Subject: Law and Ethics
Refer to Chapter 4

75. A common charting abbreviation used during a complete physical examination is:
A. UTI.
B. BID.
C. HEENT.
D. NPO.

Answer: **C**

Subject: Patient Exams
Refer to Chapter 18

---

76. First aid treatment for someone experiencing syncope includes:
A. keeping the person sitting with head lowered to the knees.
B. inducing vomiting.
C. giving small amounts of water.
D. maintaining an open airway.
E.. using an external defibrillator.

Answer: **A**

Subject: Emergency Preparedness
Refer to Chapter 26

---

77. A drug classified as an antipyretic would be used to:
A. lower blood pressure.
B. decrease cholesterol.
C. improve breathing.
D. lower fever.

Answer: **D**

Subject: Pharmacology and Medication Administration
Refer to Chapter 25

---

78. Which statement is true about normal values for body temperature?
A. A rectal temperature is 2° higher than an oral temperature.
B. An axillary temperature is the most accurate method of determining temperature.
C. An oral temperature is 1° lower than a rectal temperature.
D. An oral temperature is the most accurate method of determining temperature.
E. An axillary temperature is 2° lower than an oral temperature.

Answer: **C**

Subject: Patient Exams
Refer to Chapter 18

---

79. Vaccines are an example of which kind of immunity?
A. Natural
B. Active
C. Genetic
D. Congenital

Answer: **B**

Subject: Pharmacology and Medication Administration
Refer to Chapter 25

---

80. A substance produced in the body in response to the presence of an antigen is:
A. atelectasis.
B. antibody.
C. inflammation.
D. allergen.
E. adrenalin.

Answer: **B**

Subject: Anatomy and Physiology
Refer to Chapter 6

81. Which of the following is a fat-soluble vitamin?
A. A
B. B_6
C. B_{12}
D. C

Answer: **A**

Subject: Nutrition
Refer to Chapter 24

---

82. A 12-lead electrocardiogram records:
A. four bipolar, four unipolar, and four precordial leads.
B. six precordial, two unipolar, and four bipolar leads.
C. three bipolar, three unipolar, and six precordial leads.
D. two bipolar, four unipolar, and six precordial leads.
E. six bipolar, three unipolar, and three precordial leads.

Answer: **C**

Subject: Electrocardiogram
Refer to Chapter 20

---

83. A normal male hematocrit reading would be acceptable within:
A. 12–18 g/dL.
B. 4,500–11,000/mm^3.
C. 43%–49%.
D. 300 g/dL.

Answer: **C**

Subject: Laboratory Procedures
Refer to Chapter 21

---

84. One (1) grain is equivalent to:
A. 100 mg.
B. 75 mg.
C. 60 mg.
D. 15 mg.
E. 10 mg.

Answer: **C**

Subject: Pharmacology and Medication Administration
Refer to Chapter 25

---

85. Which of the following is a normal specific gravity reading for urine?
A. 1.000
B. 1.010
C. 1.100
D. 1.115

Answer: **B**

Subject: Laboratory Procedures
Refer to Chapter 21

---

86. The device used to record cardiac activity of an ambulatory patient over a 24-hour period is a(n):
A. echocardiograph.
B. electrocardiograph.
C. cardiac ultrasound.
D. Doppler.
E. Holter monitor.

Answer: **E**

Subject: Electrocardiogram
Refer to Chapter 20

87. The treatment method that uses a tank with equipment that agitates the water for gentle massage is a(n):
A. paraffin bath.
B. infrared radiation.
C. diathermy.
D. whirlpool.

Answer: **D**

Subject: Physical Modalities
Refer to Chapter 23

---

88. When administering a 1-mL or greater amount of medication by injection, all of the following routes may be used EXCEPT:
A. intradermally.
B. subcutaneously.
C. intramuscularly.
D. intrathecally.
E. intravascularly.

Answer: **A**

Subject: Pharmacology and Medication Administration
Refer to Chapter 25

---

89. A radiographic technique that produces a film representing a detailed cross section of tissue structure is a(n):
A. angiogram.
B. barium enema.
C. computerized tomography.
D. myelogram.

Answer: **C**

Subject: Medical Imaging
Refer to Chapter 22

---

90. When requesting a clean-catch urine specimen from a female patient, you should instruct the patient to:
A. empty the bladder in the morning and then collect the second specimen of the day.
B. void most of the urine into the toilet before collecting the specimen.
C. cleanse each side of the urinary meatus from front to back.
D. avoid cleansing the urinary meatus to ensure all artifacts are collected in the urine.
E. increase fluid intake and then collect a late-day specimen.

Answer: **C**

Subject: Laboratory Procedures
Refer to Chapter 21

---

91. When performing venipuncture you should always:
A. enter the vein with the bevel of the needle placed downward.
B. enter the vein with the needle at a 45° angle.
C. recap used needles to avoid accidental needle punctures.
D. remove the tourniquet before removing the needle from the puncture site.

Answer: **D**

Subject: Laboratory Procedures
Refer to Chapter 21

92. In an electrocardiogram, the standardization mark is:
 A. 1 mm high.
 B. 5 mm high.
 C. 10 mm high.
 D. 20 mm high.
 E. 25 mm high.

Answer: **C**

Subject: Electrocardiogram
Refer to Chapter 20

---

93. A surgical instrument found on a suture removal tray is a:
 A. scalpel handle.
 B. towel forceps.
 C. needle holder.
 D. thumb forceps.

Answer: **D**

Subject: Minor Surgical Procedures
Refer to Chapter 19

---

94. Another term for the chest leads on an electrocardiogram (ECG) is:
 A. bipolar.
 B. unipolar.
 C. augmented.
 D. precordial.
 E. intercostal.

Answer: **D**

Subject: Electrocardiogram
Refer to Chapter 20

---

95. To obtain a capillary blood specimen, you should:
 A. squeeze the tip of the patient's finger.
 B. collect the first drop of blood.
 C. use the patient's index finger.
 D. wipe away the first drop of blood.

Answer: **D**

Subject: Laboratory Procedures
Refer to Chapter 21

---

96. The proper size needle for administering an intradermal injection is:
 A. 23 g–1".
 B. 20 g–$1\frac{1}{2}$".
 C. 27 g–$\frac{3}{8}$".
 D. 25 g–1".

Answer: **C**

Subject: Pharmacology and Medication Administration
Refer to Chapter 25

---

97. To obtain an anteroposterior (AP) x-ray view, the patient is positioned with the:
 A. anterior aspect of the body facing the x-ray tube.
 B. posterior aspect of the body facing the x-ray tube.
 C. left side of the body facing the film.
 D. right side of the body facing the film.
 E. right side of the body facing the x-ray tube.

Answer: **A**

Subject: Medical Imaging
Refer to Chapter 22

98. The best method to deliver deep heat to tissues is to use:
A. paraffin bath.
B. infrared radiation lamp.
C. whirlpool treatment.
D. ultrasound therapy.

Answer: **D**

Subject: Physical Modalities
Refer to Chapter 23

---

99. The muscle used for an intramuscular injection is the:
A. gluteus maximus.
B. rectus femoris.
C. triceps.
D. quadriceps.
E. deltoid.

Answer: **E**

Subject: Pharmacology and Medication Administration
Refer to Chapter 25

---

100. When preparing a sterile tray for a minor surgical procedure, remember to:
A. consider the 1-inch border around the perimeter of the tray nonsterile.
B. place the vial of local anesthetic on the sterile field.
C. prepare the tray in another location and carry it to the patient's location.
D. have a sharps container on the sterile field.

Answer: **A**

Subject: Minor Surgical Procedures
Refer to Chapter 19

---

101. A physician orders 125 mg of a drug; the available medication on hand is 500 mg/mL. How many mL of the drug would you give the patient?
A. 0.5 mL
B. 0.4 mL
C. 0.25 mL
D. 0.05 mL
E. 0.04 mL

Answer: **C**

Subject: Pharmacology and Medication Administration
Refer to Chapter 25

---

102. When performing an ECG, you should:
A. apply electrodes over bony prominences.
B. disregard artifacts.
C. ensure patient comfort.
D. place lead V1 on the left side of the sternum.

Answer: **C**

Subject: Electrocardiogram
Refer to Chapter 20

---

103. When instructing a patient about a low-cholesterol diet, you should tell the patient to decrease intake of which of the following foods?
A. Citrus fruit
B. Green vegetables
C. Cereal grains
D. Dairy products
E. Legumes

Answer: **D**

Subject: Patient Education
Refer to Chapter 8

104. Which of the following is a form of exercise therapy?
   A. Range of motion
   B. Hydrotherapy
   C. Ultrasound
   D. Massage

Answer: **A**

Subject: Physical Modalities
Refer to Chapter 23

---

105. In an ECG, aVR, aVL, and aVF represent:
   A. bipolar limb leads.
   B. augmented limb leads.
   C. precordial leads.
   D. standard limb leads.
   E. chest leads.

Answer: **B**

Subject: Electrocardiogram
Refer to Chapter 20

PRETEST ANALYSIS

The pretest analysis helps you determine which topics you need to study more or study less and how much study time you need. The analysis has three steps and takes approximately 15 minutes. This is important time to invest.

ANALYSIS STEP 1

Go back to each question in the pretest. Put a check mark by the answer if:

- Your answer was incorrect.
- Your answer was correct but you were unsure or you required more than 45 seconds to decide on an answer.

Table 2-1 Study Hours by Topic for CMA (AAMA) and RMA (AMT)

General Knowledge	Administrative Practice	Clinical Practice
Law and Ethics Suggested study time ____ hr. ☐	Administrative Technologies Suggested study time ____ hr. ☐	Microorganisms and Asepsis Suggested study time ____ hr. ☐
Medical Terminology Suggested study time ____ hr. ☐	Appointment Scheduling Suggested study time ____ hr. ☐	Patient Exams Suggested study time ____ hr. ☐
Anatomy and Physiology Suggested study time ____ hr. ☐	Medical Records Suggested study time ____ hr. ☐	Minor Surgical Procedures Suggested study time ____ hr. ☐
Professional Communication Suggested study time ____ hr. ☐	Correspondence Suggested study time ____ hr. ☐	Electrocardiogram Suggested study time ____ hr. ☐
Patient Education Suggested study time ____ hr. ☐	Medical Insurance Suggested study time ____ hr. ☐	Laboratory Procedures Suggested study time ____ hr. ☐
	Medical Coding and Claims Suggested study time ____ hr. ☐	Medical Imaging Suggested study time ____ hr. ☐
	Financial Practices Suggested study time ____ hr. ☐	Physical Modalities Suggested study time ____ hr. ☐
	Practice Management Suggested study time ____ hr. ☐	Nutrition Suggested study time ____ hr. ☐
		Pharmacology and Medication Administration Suggested study time ____ hr. ☐
		Emergency Preparedness Suggested study time ____ hr. ☐

Table 2-2 Study Hours by Topic for CMAS (AMT)

General Knowledge	Administrative Practice	Clinical Practice
Law and Ethics Suggested study time ____ hr. ☐	Administrative Technologies Suggested study time ____hr. ☐	Microorganisms and Asepsis Suggested study time ____ hr. ☐
Medical Terminology Suggested study time ____ hr. ☐	Appointment Scheduling Suggested study time ____ hr. ☐	Patient Exams Suggested study time ____ hr. ☐
Anatomy and Physiology Suggested study time ____ hr. ☐	Medical Records Suggested study time ____ hr. ☐	Pharmacology and Medication Administration Suggested study time ____ hr. ☐
Professional Communication Suggested study time ____ hr. ☐	Correspondence Suggested study time ____ hr. ☐	Emergency Preparedness Suggested study time ____ hr. ☐
Patient Education Suggested study time ____ hr. ☐	Medical Insurance Suggested study time ____ hr. ☐	
	Medical Coding and Claims Suggested study time ____ hr. ☐	
	Financial Practices Suggested study time ____ hr. ☐	
	Practice Management Suggested study time ____ hr. ☐	

ANALYSIS STEP 2

Each answer on the pretest has a subject that corresponds to one of the subjects in Table 2-1, for the CMA (AAMA) and RMA (AMT) exams, or Table 2-2, for the CMAS. (AMT) exam now count the total check marks for each subject. Place the total number of check marks for each subject in the corresponding box on the appropriate table for your exam. If you have no check marks for a subject, place a zero in the square.

You may, for example, have three answers checked for the subject "Law and Ethics." You would place a 3 in that box.

ANALYSIS STEP 3

The higher the number in each box, the more you need to study that subject. When all the boxes in Table 2-1 or Table 2-2 are completed, estimate your needed study time this way:

- 0 or 1 in the box suggests reasonable knowledge of the topic, minimum 1 hour per subject; write "1" on the line "suggested study time __ hr"
- 2 in the box suggests partial knowledge of the topic, minimum 2 hours per subject; write "2" on the line "suggested study time __ hr"
- 3 or higher in the box suggests limited knowledge of the topic, minimum 3 hours per subject; write "3" on the line "suggested study time __ hr"

Table 2-3 Study Hours Summary

Pretest suggested study hours	
Extra study hours added for Anatomy and Physiology	4
Timed exam and final prep hours	4
Total suggested minimum study hours	

ANALYSIS STEP 4

- Now count all the suggested study hours and place the total in Table 2-3.
- Add all hours in Table 2-3.

The pretest analysis is complete. Your results show you your likely areas of strength and weakness, suggested minimum study times for each subject, and a suggested total review time. Additional time is added in Table 2-3 for Anatomy and Physiology, which has the most content, and for the practice exam. Now you are ready to move on to make your plan using this information.

3

Making Your Study Plan

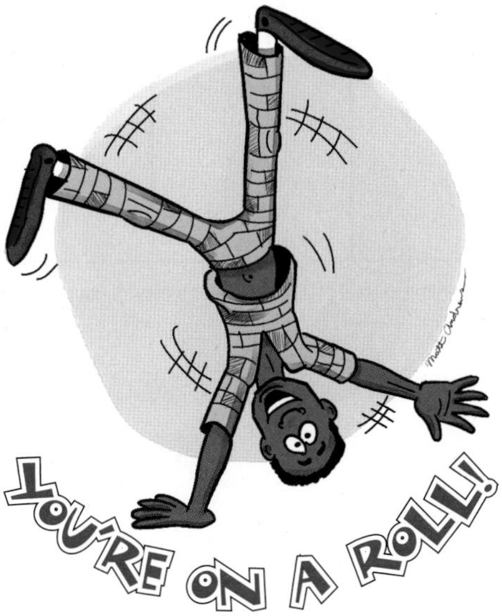

One of the common characteristics among those who pass the exam is that they had a study plan. It is a road map of where you are going and how to get there. Dedication and commitment are essential. They are like fuel for your vehicle—necessary to take you where you want to go.

An 8-week calendar is suggested to give you plenty of time to study. If your exam is already scheduled, you may modify the calendar based on that date. The following steps are guidelines only, and you should change them based on your individual learning needs. Planning is worth the time!

Remove the calendar from the back of the book or use a calendar you have. Work the following steps.

Sunday	Monday	Tuesday	Wednesday	Thursday	Friday	Saturday
4 total		1 total		1 total		2 total

Figure 3-1 Step 1. Fill in the total number of hours per day you will study. Here is an example week.

Sunday	Monday	Tuesday	Wednesday	Thursday	Friday	Saturday
4 total 1 hr (Correspondence) 2 hr (Patient Exam) 1 hr (Medical Terminology)		1 total (Medical Terminology)		1 total (Communication)		2 total Study Group (Anatomy & Physiology)

Figure 3-2 Step 2. Assign subjects to each of the days, according to level of difficulty and number of hours available. Here is an example week.

STEP 1

- Determine how many hours a week you can devote to study; be realistic.
- Refer to Table 2-3 in Chapter 2, which gives your total suggested minimum study hours.
- Use the Study Calendar to assign the study hours for each day.
- Refer to Figure 3-1 as an example.

STEP 2

- Refer to Table 2-1 or 2-2, which gives the total number of hours needed per subject.
- Plug these subjects into the assigned hours on the Study Calendar.
- Use Figure 3-2 as an example of a study week showing subjects assigned to the study hours.

Box 3-1

Staying Motivated

You've probably heard the slogan "Just do it!" Adopt this attitude for your exam preparation. Put all "nonessentials" on hold for 8 weeks and dedicate the time to study. Eight weeks go by very quickly. If you fall off your schedule, take a deep breath and jump back on. Let everyone know what you are doing and ask for their support. If you are in a study group, help—do not hinder—each other. Keep in mind the reason you chose to take the exam and stay focused.

Generally, keeping energized is related to physical well-being. Commit to eating healthy meals and snacks. Try to study in pleasant places. Outdoors is great if weather permits, and distractions are minimal.

Buy or borrow a little book of inspirational sayings and read one daily. Give yourself credit for milestones: When you complete each subject, you should feel a sense of accomplishment. When you complete the study hours for the week, reward yourself in small ways—buy a treat, watch a favorite television show, tell others, or plan a festive event to celebrate the completion of the exam. "Plan your work—then work your plan."

Unit 2

General Knowledge

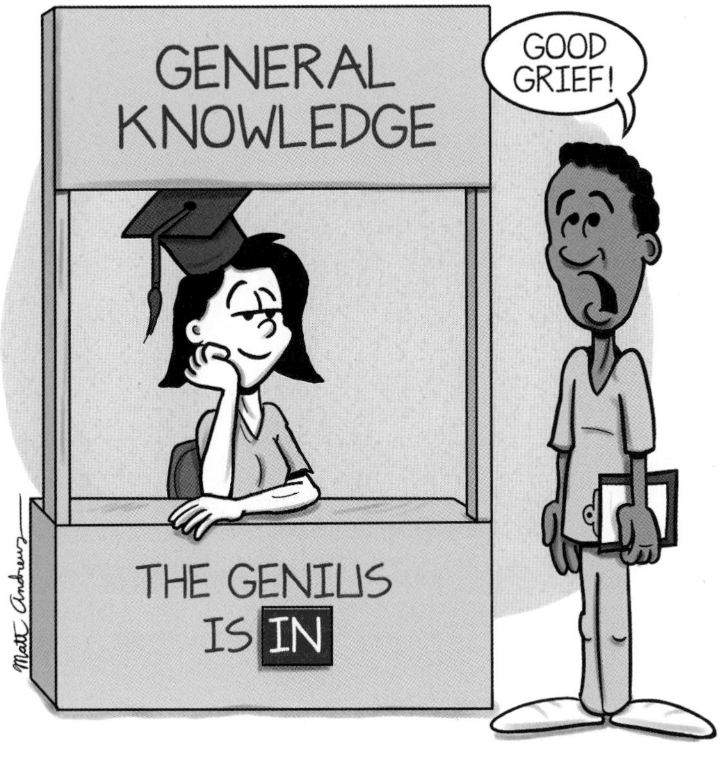

4

Law and Ethics

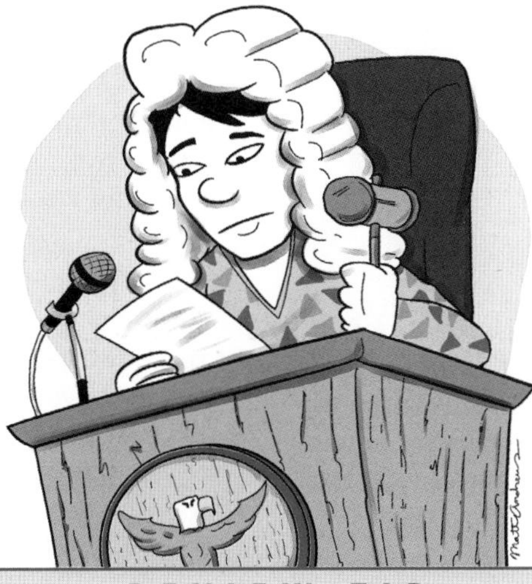

REVIEW TIP

Legal and ethical decisions arise in every aspect of medical assisting. Examples of legal and ethical practices include ensuring a patient has signed a consent form before releasing information and billing only for services actually performed.

Examples of illegal or unethical practices are knowingly using an incorrect insurance code, failing to report a medication error, or discussing patients with friends. Think about legal and ethical implications that occur in a routine day as you review each chapter.

LAW

Law is a set of rules governing conduct and action that are enforced by a recognized authority. The purposes of law are to:

- Regulate conduct
- Punish offenders
- Remedy wrongs
- Benefit society

The two main areas of law are:

1. Criminal—laws that govern crimes or wrongs committed against society, an individual, or property in violation of an ordinance; charges are brought forth by the government; a fine or imprisonment can occur. An example is Medicare fraud.
2. Civil—laws that govern crimes or wrongs committed against an individual or property; charges are brought forth by the individual or his representative; compensation (usually monetary) is sought.

The practice of medicine is generally regulated by civil law. Three types of civil law are most frequently involved:

1. Tort law—laws dealing with accidental or intentional harm to a person or property resulting from the wrongdoing of others
2. Contract law—laws dealing with the rights and obligations of enforceable promises
3. Administrative law—laws dealing with requirements and standards of governmental agencies

Box 4-1
The "Four Ds"

The "Four Ds" are used to determine whether a situation is malpractice:

1. Duty—the patient/physician relationship was established
2. Dereliction—the professional neglected a professional obligation to act or acted improperly
3. Direct cause—a negative outcome resulted directly from the professional's actions or failure to act
4. Damages—the patient sustained harm from the negligent act

TORT LAW

A **tort** is a wrongful civil act committed against an individual for which compensation is sought. **Negligence** is a common tort and is defined as failure to exercise the standard of care that a reasonable, comparably trained person would exercise in similar circumstances. The four forms of negligence are:

1. Nonfeasance—failure to act when duty is indicated, resulting in or causing harm
2. Misfeasance—improper performance of an act, resulting in or causing harm
3. Malfeasance—performance of an improper act, resulting in or causing harm
4. Malpractice—failure to act or improper performance of an act or performance of an improper act by a professional (professional negligence); Box 4-1 lists the "Four Ds," which help determine whether a situation is malpractice

A term used in obvious cases of negligence is ***res ipsa loquitur***, meaning "the thing speaks for itself." Another concept is ***respondeat superior***, which means "let the master answer." The employer is liable for the actions and conduct of employees while the employees are performing within the scope and job description of their position.

Good Samaritan Act as Tort Avoidance

The majority of states have a Good Samaritan Act, which is legislation enacted to encourage off-duty health care providers to render aid at the scenes of accidents. The Good Samaritan Act protects health care personnel from liability or tort claims. The care given must have been rendered in good faith and meet the standards of a reasonable and prudent person with similar training. You are *not* covered by the Good Samaritan Act if you are there as part of your health care position, no matter where the incident occurs. For instance, if you volunteer to give immunizations at a school or to provide first aid at a sporting event, you are volunteering as a health care professional and are not covered under the act. If you are attending a sporting event as a spectator or participant and render first aid, you are covered under the Good Samaritan Act. If money or other forms of compensation or gifts are accepted from the victim or the representative of the victim for administering help, the Good Samaritan Act no longer applies.

CONTRACT LAW

A **contract** is an obligation resulting from an agreement between two or more parties. Five components are required for a contract to be legal and binding:

1. An offer must be made.
2. The offer must be accepted.
3. An exchange of something of value between the parties must occur; this exchange is often referred to as *consideration*.
4. All parties must be legally capable of accepting the terms; this capability is often referred to as *capacity*.
5. The intent must be legal.

Contracts may be:

- Expressed—written or verbal and describing what each contractual party will do
- Implied—deduced by the actions of the contracting parties (for example, a patient coming to the physician's office seeking treatment)

Consents

Consent for medical care is voluntary permission given by a competent adult or legal agent of the patient (e.g., the parent of a minor child). Consents, as with contracts, may be **expressed** or **implied**. Except in life-threatening emergencies, consent must be **informed**, which requires the physician or an appropriately trained caregiver to explain the information necessary for the patient to make an educated decision regarding the procedure. The caregiver should provide the following information:

- An explanation of the procedure and the reason for the procedure
- The possible risks and side effects
- Alternative therapies and risks
- Prognosis with and without the procedure
- Any other information that may assist the patient in making an educated decision

Consentors

The following may consent for medical treatment:

- Competent adult for self or legal charge (e.g., his or her minor child)
- **Emancipated minor** (state-specific; generally, one who lives on his or her own and is self-supporting)
- Minors serving in the armed forces
- Minors seeking treatment for sexually transmitted diseases, birth control, or abortion (state-specific)
- Minor parent with custody of his or her minor child (*Note:* In some states, a minor not considered emancipated may consent for the treatment of his or her child *but* may not consent for his or her own medical treatment.)

Advance Directives

Advance directives are special documents signed by the patient, witnessed, and usually notarized that state the patient's wishes for medical decisions should the patient become incapable of making the decisions for himself or herself. Some advance directives are:

- Living will—document stating acceptable and unacceptable means to sustain the patient's life in case of terminal conditions
- Medical (durable) power of attorney—document stating whom the patient designates to make medical decisions regarding accepting and withholding treatment
- Designated anatomic donor—documentation or indication on an existing document (the driver's license in some states) expressing the patient's desire to donate all or specific anatomic organs

ADMINISTRATIVE LAW

Administrative law refers to regulations established and enforced by governmental agencies. Examples include the U.S. Drug Enforcement Agency (DEA), Food and Drug Administration (FDA), and various state-controlled licensing boards, such as nursing boards and boards of medical examiners. Some of the more common governmental regulators and regulations that affect the medical office are:

- Clinical Laboratory Improvement Amendments (CLIA)—issues laboratory testing standards for facilities performing specified tests.
- Occupational Safety and Health Administration (OSHA)—regulates safety in the workplace.
- Internal Revenue Service (IRS)—regulates federal payroll taxes.
- Equal Employment Opportunity Act (EEOA)—prohibits employment discrimination because of age, color, national origin, race, religion, or sex.

The Red Flags Rule (this comes under Administrative Law)

On August 1, 2009 the Federal Trade Commission enacted the **Red Flags Rule** to combat increasing **medical identity theft which** is when a person seeking healthcare uses another person's name or insurance. The law became effective June 1, 2010 and requires most medical offices to develop written programs to detect the warning signs or red flags of identity theft. The law defines two categories that determine if a business must comply:

- creditors—an entity that regularly defers payment for services or arranges the extension of credit; examples are billing patients after the service is rendered including fees that are billed after insurance payments are received
- **covered account**—a consumer (patient) account that allows multiple payments or transactions; most patient records fall in this category.

Not adhering to the law may result in financial penalties. The red flags include:

- suspicious documents:
  - altered or forged appearance
  - photo or description inconsistent with the patient's appearance
  - inconsistent information provided such as date of birth, chronic medical condition
- suspicious personal identifying information from other sources such as a social security number different then what is on file
- suspicious activities such as mail returned repeatedly but patient continues to keep appointments and maintain that address on file
- inconsistency with physical exam and past medical treatment
- notifications of identity theft from patients or staff

The law requires the implementation of a program that covers:

- prevention—implementing sound electronic and other security systems and HIPAA compliance
- detection—training staff and programming electronic "red flagging" such differences in dates of birth are automatically identified on the screen
- mitigation—assuring medical records of the perpetrator and the authentic patient are not commingled and knowing where and how to report suspicions or occurrences

Employment Law

Generally, employment law comes under administrative law because it involves administrative rulings that address the rights of employees and employers in the workplace. Medical offices must follow these laws:

- **Equal Employment Opportunity Commission (EEOC):** Prohibits job discrimination based on race, color, religion, sex, or national origin.
- **Equal Pay Act:** Prohibits sex-based pay discrimination for men and women performing the same jobs.
- **Age Discrimination in Employment Act:** Prohibits job discrimination for people age 40 years and older.
- **Americans with Disabilities Act (ADA):** Prohibits discrimination against people with disabilities in employment, transportation, public accommodation, communications, and governmental activities.
- **Family Medical Leave Act (FMLA):** Allows employees up to 12 job-protected weeks of leave without pay for family or medical needs.
- **Title VII of the Civil Rights Act of 1964:** Unwelcome sexual advances, requests for sexual favors, and other verbal or physical conduct of a sexual nature constitutes sexual harassment when submission to or rejection of this conduct explicitly or implicitly affects an individual's employment, unreasonably interferes with an individual's work performance or creates an intimidating, hostile or offensive work environment. (Definition from the U.S. Equal Employment Opportunity Commission.)

Licensure

Licensure, the strongest form of professional regulation, is a credential required to practice a profession and issued by an official state agency. This section discusses the physician's license to practice medicine, which is regulated by a state's **Medical Practice Act** and issued by the state's medical board. The license confirms that, after acceptable education and training, the doctor has met minimum standards as defined in the Medical Practice Act. Medical licensure may be obtained through:

- Examination—successful completion of a written or oral state examination
- Endorsement—acceptance by the state board of a passing score on a recognized national examination
- Reciprocity—acceptance by the state board of a valid medical license from another state

Renewal of medical licenses is mandatory, and failure to do so results in suspension or revocation. Other causes for suspension or revocation are:

- Conviction of a felony
- Unprofessional conduct
- Professional or personal incapacity

Certification, Registration, and Accreditation

Health care occupations that do not require a license may be subject to a credential called *certification or registration.* This process is often voluntary, with standards developed by a national organization that also administers a national exam. Although governmental agencies are usually not involved in the process, some states require certification or registration for many health care occupations. Examples are medical assisting, emergency medical technicians (EMTs), paramedics, laboratory technicians, and nursing assistants. These are state-specific.

Accreditation is another form of credentialing, usually involving a health care facility or organization. It is voluntary, with standards developed by a national organization, after a process including site visits and reports that determine whether the organization meets the standards. Accreditation is not issued by a governmental body. The Joint Commission (formerly the Joint Commission on Accreditation of Healthcare Organizations or JCAHO) is one example of an accreditation organization.

Schools and training programs may also become accredited, which implies that their graduates have met certain standards. Examples of agencies that accredit specific health care education schools and programs are:

- Commission on Accreditation of Allied Health Education Programs (CAAHEP)
- Accrediting Bureau of Health Education Schools (ABHES)

Scope of Practice

In addition to obtaining the appropriate and mandated licensing or certification, all health care staff is required to stay within their **scope of practice.** The scope of practice is the performance of duties and procedures allowed by law, standards, and educational preparation. As mentioned in Chapter 1, health care personnel are also responsible for staying current in their field as a legal obligation. The health care professional will be held accountable for the standards in place at any given time.

Public Duty and Mandatory Reporting

States require physicians and other health care personnel to report certain information to provide for the health, safety, and welfare of the public.

- Birth certificates must be completed and submitted to the designated local or state agency by the birth attendant.
- Death certificates must be completed by the physician in attendance.
- Deaths that must be reported to the medical examiner include:
  - Death resulting from violent or criminal activity
  - Death from an undetermined cause
  - Death without prior medical care
  - Death within 24 hours of admission to a health care facility
- Each occurrence of specified communicable diseases such as vaccine-preventable diseases, tuberculosis, and sexually transmitted diseases must be reported to the state or county health department. Each medical facility should have a list and reporting forms.
- Suspected abuse or criminal acts must be reported to specific governmental agencies. These acts include:
  - Child abuse
  - Elder abuse
  - Spousal abuse/domestic violence (most states)
  - Patient abuse
  - Injuries by weapons or assault
  - Injuries sustained in the commission of a crime
  - Suicides or attempted suicides
- Vaccine administration must be reported to the designated local or state agency in most states. The required information includes:
  - Date
  - Vaccine, lot number, manufacturer
  - Name, title of person administering the vaccine, and place administered
  - Any adverse reactions (also reportable to VAERS, the national Vaccine Adverse Events Reporting System)
- Specified medical surveillance, such as phenylketonuria (PKU) in newborns, must be reported to the designated local or state agency.

ETHICS

Ethics are moral principles, values, and duties. Whereas laws are enforceable regulations set forth by the government, ethics are moral guidelines set forth and formally or informally enforced by peers, professional organizations, and the community. Examples of enforcement for breeches in ethics are censorship of a writer, suspension from a hospital staff, or simply being left out by peers.

- Norm—behavior or conduct that is valued and usually expected
- Duties—commitment or obligations to act in a certain moral manner
  - Nonmalfeasance—an action that avoids harm
  - Beneficence—an action that creates benefit
  - Fidelity—practice of meeting patient's right to receive competent care and respect, adherence to laws and agreements
  - Veracity—truth
  - Justice—equitable distribution of benefits and burdens

CODE OF ETHICS

A **code of ethics** is a statement, usually from a professional group, listing the expected behaviors of its members. The code may also set standards and disciplinary actions for violations, including censure, suspension, fines, or expulsion. The following are examples of early codes of ethics that relate to health care:

- Code of Hammurabi—written 2500 BCE in Babylonia
- Hippocratic Oath—written 400 BCE in Greece by Hippocrates, a physician
- American Medical Association's (AMA) Code of Ethics—first written 1847 in Philadelphia and revised several times since then to remain current—refer to Box 4-2
- American Association of Medical Assistants (AAMA) Code of Ethics—refer to Box 4-3
- American Medical Technologists' Standards of Practice—refer to Box 4-4

PATIENT'S BILL OF RIGHTS

In 1973, the American Hospital Association was the first to publish the **Patient's Bill of Rights**. Several organizations, including health care insurers and providers, have followed suit. The bill outlines the courtesies and prerogatives to which the patient is entitled during all health care episodes and interactions.

The following is a condensed version of a typical Patient's Bill of Rights.

The patient has the right to:

- receive considerate and respectful care
- consult the physician of his choosing
- expect confidentiality and privacy
- receive all information regarding his condition, diagnosis, treatment, and prognosis

Box 4-2

AMA Principles of Medical Ethics (adopted June 2001)

I. A physician shall be dedicated to providing competent medical care, with compassion and respect for human dignity and rights.
II. A physician shall uphold the standards of professionalism, be honest in all professional interactions, and strive to report physicians deficient in character or competence, or engaging in fraud or deception, to appropriate entities.
III. A physician shall respect the law and also recognize a responsibility to seek changes in those requirements which are contrary to the best interests of the patient.
IV. A physician shall respect the rights of patients, colleagues, and other health professionals, and shall safeguard patient confidences and privacy within the constraints of the law.
V. A physician shall continue to study, apply, and advance scientific knowledge, maintain a commitment to medical education, make relevant information available to patients, colleagues, and the public, obtain consultation, and use the talents of other health professionals when indicated.
VI. A physician shall, in the provision of appropriate patient care, except in emergencies, be free to choose whom to serve, with whom to associate, and the environment in which to provide medical care.
VII. A physician shall recognize a responsibility to participate in activities contributing to the improvement of the community and the betterment of public health.
VIII. A physician shall, while caring for a patient, regard responsibility to the patient as paramount.
IX. A physician shall support access to medical care for all people.

- receive all necessary information to make an educated decision regarding the course of his care
- make his own decision if competent
- refuse treatment
- participate or not participate in research
- receive continuity of care
- obtain all lawful copies of his medical records

Box 4-3

Medical Assisting Code of Ethics

The Code of Ethics of the AAMA shall set forth principles of ethical and moral conduct as they relate to the medical profession and the particular practice of medical assisting.

Members of the AAMA dedicated to the conscientious pursuit of their profession, and thus desiring to merit the high regard of the entire medical profession and the respect of the general public which they serve, do pledge themselves to strive always to:

A. render service with full respect for the dignity of humanity;
B. respect confidential information obtained through employment unless legally authorized or required by responsible performance of duty to divulge such information;
C. uphold the honor and high principles of the profession and accept its disciplines;
D. seek to continually improve the knowledge and skills of medical assistants for the benefit of patients and professional colleagues;
E. participate in additional service activities aimed toward improving the health and well-being of the community.

Reprinted with permission from the American Association of Medical Assistants.

BIOETHICS

Bioethics is moral issues dealing with biologic studies, research, procedures, policies, and decisions. Some areas of bioethics are:

- Reproduction—artificial insemination, in vitro fertilization (IVF), surrogate parenthood, abortion, fetuses for research purposes
- Genetics—screening, engineering, testing, cloning, gene therapy
- Death and dying—euthanasia, do-not-resuscitate (DNR) orders, brain death, physician-assisted suicide, right to die
- Transplants—source of donations, financial compensation for donors, priority of recipients, recipients with diseases caused by unhealthy lifestyles
- Resource allocation—cost of health care; funds for research; rationing dependent on age, individual's value to society, and other socioeconomic factors; prolonging life

Box 4-4

AMT Standards of Practice

AMT seeks to encourage, establish, and maintain the highest standards, traditions and principles of the practices which constitute the profession of the Registry. Members of the AMT Registry must recognize their responsibilities, not only to their patients, but also to society, to other health care professionals, and to themselves. The following standards of practice are principles adopted by the AMT Board of Directors, which define the essence of honorable and ethical behavior for a health care professional:

1. While engaged in the Arts and Sciences, which constitute the practice of their profession, AMT professionals shall be dedicated to the provision of competent service.
2. The AMT professional shall place the welfare of the patient above all else.
3. The AMT professional understands the importance of thoroughness in the performance of duty, compassion with patients, and the importance of the tasks which may be performed.
4. The AMT professional shall always seek to respect the rights of patients and of health care providers, and shall safeguard patient confidences.
5. The AMT professional will strive to increase his/her technical knowledge, shall continue to study, and apply scientific advances in his/her specialty.
6. The AMT professional shall respect the law and will pledge to avoid dishonest, unethical or illegal practices.
7. The AMT professional understands that he/she is not to make or offer a diagnosis or interpretation unless he/she is a duly licensed physician/dentist or unless asked by the attending physician/dentist.
8. The AMT professional shall protect and value the judgment of the attending physician or dentist, providing this does not conflict with the behavior necessary to carry out Standard Number 2 above.
9. The AMT professional recognizes that any personal wrongdoing is his/her responsibility. It is also the professional health care provider's obligation to report to the proper authorities any knowledge of professional abuse.
10. The AMT professional pledges personal honor and integrity to cooperate in the advancement and expansion, by every lawful means, of American Medical Technologists.

CONFIDENTIALITY/HIPAA

A cornerstone of medical law and ethics, **confidentiality** has long been a standard and expectation in health care. In 1996, the federal government enacted the Health Insurance Portability and Accountability Act (HIPAA). A portion of the act was concerned with the security of the electronic medical record (EMR) and electronic submission of claims that contain sensitive information. In addition, HIPAA outlines what is considered confidential information:

- Names
- Geographic subdivisions smaller than a state
- Dates of birth, admission, discharge, death
- Telephone and fax numbers
- E-mail addresses
- Social Security numbers
- Medical records or account numbers
- Health plan beneficiary numbers
- Certificate/license numbers
- Vehicle or device numbers (for example, a pacemaker number)
- Biometric identifiers
- Full-face photos
- Any other unique identifying number, characteristic, or code
- Age older than 89

Patient information can only be released by written consent of the patient, by **subpoena**, or in cases of mandatory reporting, as listed previously. All medical personnel should be aware of the ordinary daily practices in the medical office that may inadvertently lead to breach of patient confidentiality, including the following examples:

- Computer screens, including personal digital assistants (PDAs), left in sight of unauthorized persons
- Telephone conversations in earshot of others
- Patient sign-in sheets
- Messages left on a patient's phone or answering machine with more information than simply to return the call
- Information given to callers who are not positively identified as authorized to receive information
- Information given to family members other than the legal caretaker
- Unattended fax machines and printers
- Unshredded patient material in open areas or trash baskets

- Patient issues discussed in unsecured areas
- Discussions with patients that can be overheard
- Appointment lists posted on exam room doors or other open areas

VULNERABLE POPULATIONS

Many states have enacted legislation protecting **vulnerable populations**, a group of people who may be physically or mentally at risk for harm or exploitation. Generally, infants and children, the elderly, and the disabled are considered vulnerable populations. The case is being made, in some areas, that all patients should be considered vulnerable. To decrease the risk of harm by convicted predators in certain workplace settings, including health care, the state and health care employers require employees to be screened and fingerprinted. The fingerprints are sent to a federal clearinghouse, where it is determined whether the person has been convicted of a crime. If a criminal record is determined to exist, the person may not be hired.

RISK MANAGEMENT, SAFETY, AND QUALITY IMPROVEMENT

As discussed earlier in this chapter, malpractice has the likelihood of resulting in lawsuits or torts. Other nonmedical areas of a practice, especially those involving safety, may also put the office at risk for lawsuits. These are called *risk factors* (e.g., patients tripping on an electrical cord or sustaining injury due to malfunctioning equipment). Avoiding malpractice and ensuring safety come under an umbrella called **risk management**, which is a process to routinely assess, identify, correct, and monitor any potential hazards or risks to prevent harm and loss. The office's malpractice/liability insurance company can be of assistance in the process and may offer reduced rates for reduced risk. Some common examples of risk management in the medical office are:

- Maintaining a daily temperature chart for refrigerators containing biopharmaceuticals
- Requiring and ensuring all employees are current in cardiopulmonary resuscitation (CPR)
- Reviewing drug expiration dates and removing all medications due to expire that month
- Replacing fire extinguishers once a year
- Ensuring a system is in place to review and report results of all diagnostic tests
- Using proper containers and techniques for disposal of biohazardous material

Many other examples are given throughout this book and can be found in the topics related to the chapters. The Joint Commission and the Occupational Safety and Health Administration (OSHA) have made safety a major emphasis in standards and surveys.

An **incident report**, sometimes called an *occurrence report*, is a form usually required when an event occurs in the health care facility that has the potential of resulting in harm or loss (lawsuits). The incident report may be one specific to that facility or one provided by the facility's insurance company or attorney. The report contains the following information:

- Names and contact information of persons involved in the event
- Date, time, and location of the event
- Brief but complete explanation of the event
- Names and contact information of witnesses
- Any treatment or other actions
- Name(s) of anyone who was notified

Quality improvement (QI), formerly called *quality assurance*, is measuring, improving, and remeasuring patient outcomes based on established criteria or indicators. The emphasis of quality improvement is improved outcomes for patients, whereas the emphasis of risk management is to avoid harm and loss. In some organizations, quality improvement is part of risk management, and in other organizations, quality improvement is a separate committee. Regardless of the organizational structure, the two are interrelated. For example, an insurance company, while reviewing financial losses, discovers that a large percentage of its asthma patients frequently visit the emergency department (ED), which is expensive. To reduce the loss, the insurance company creates a patient education program for its asthmatic patients and provides the medical practices with this program. The result is that the asthmatic patients use the ED less, reducing the company's financial loss. The outcome for the patient is that his or her asthma is better controlled and the quality of life is improved.

Some common indicators are patient immunization rates, percentage of female patients of recommended ages receiving mammograms, percentage of diabetic patients receiving eye exams, and rationale in prescribing specific antibiotics. The outcomes may be disease prevention, early diagnosis, or more rapid recovery.

TERMS

Law and Ethics Review

The following list reviews the terms discussed in this chapter and **provides other important terms that you may see on the exam.**

abandonment withdrawal by a physician from the care of a patient without reasonable notice or provisions for another equally or better qualified provider to assume care; the physician improperly terminates his or her contract with the patient

abuse wrong or improper use

advance directives documents signed by the patient and by witnesses stating the patient's wishes for medical care should he or she become incapacitated

Age Discrimination in Employment Act prohibits job discrimination for people age 40 years and older

age of majority age at which a person is considered an adult; this is state-dependent, but usually is 18 or 21 years old

Americans with Disabilities Act (ADA) prohibits discrimination against people with disabilities in employment, transportation, public accommodation, communications, and governmental activities

battery touching a person without his or her consent

beneficence actions that create benefit or good

bioethics moral issues dealing with biologic studies, research, procedures, and decisions

breach violation of a trust

civil law type of law governing crimes or wrongs committed against an individual or property, with charges brought forth by the individual or a representative; compensation (usually monetary) is sought

code of ethics a statement, usually from a professional group, stating the expected behaviors of its members

competent adult a person who has reached the age of majority and is considered of sound mind and not under the influence of drugs or other mind-altering substances

confidentiality protection of patient information from all but authorized persons

contract an agreement between two or more parties

covered account a patient account that allows multiple payments or transactions

criminal law laws that govern crimes or wrongs committed against society or an individual or property in violation of an ordinance, with charges brought forth by the government; fine or imprisonment can occur

defamation injury to a person's character or reputation by false or malicious statements

emancipated minor a person who has not reached the age of majority but is living on his or her own and is self-supporting; a minor serving in the armed forces is considered emancipated

endorsement a method of licensure through acceptance of a national examination score

Equal Employment Opportunity Commission (EEOC) prohibits job discrimination based on race, color, religion, sex, or national origin

Equal Pay Act prohibits sex-based pay discrimination for men and women performing the same jobs

ethics moral principles or values or duties

expressed consent verbal or written approval

Family Medical Leave Act (FMLA) allows employees up to 12 job-protected weeks of leave without pay for family or medical needs

fee splitting a fraudulent practice in which a physician receives money from another physician solely for referring patients to him or her

fidelity practice of meeting patients' rights to competent care, to respect, and to adherence to laws and agreements

fraud an act of deceiving or misrepresenting

implied consent a patient's permission in which his or her actions indirectly indicate approval

incident report a form that is usually required when an event occurs in a health care facility that has the potential to result in harm or loss (lawsuits); sometimes called an occurrence report

informed consent a patient's permission for a procedure, given after receiving all the information necessary to make an educated decision

invasion of privacy releasing patient information to unauthorized parties without the consent of the patient

justice equitable distribution of benefits and burdens

law a set of rules governing conduct and actions; enforced by a recognized authority

libel false or malicious writing against a person's character or reputation

malfeasance performance of an improper act, resulting in or causing harm

malpractice failure to act, improper performance of that act, or performance of an improper act by a professional, resulting in or causing harm

medical identity theft which is when a person seeking healthcare uses another person's name or insurance

Medical Practice Acts laws established by each state to define medical practice, establish educational requirements for physicians, describe licensing and renewal procedures and requirements, determine conditions for revoking or suspending licenses, and prohibit nonqualified individuals with or without a license from practicing medicine

misfeasance improper performance of an act, resulting in or causing harm

negligence commission or omission of an act that resulted in or caused harm

non compos mentis not of sound mind

nonfeasance failure to act when there was a duty to act, resulting in or causing harm

nonmalfeasance actions that avoid harm

Patient's Bill of Rights a list of reasonable expectations a patient should receive from health care professionals regarding treatment as a patient and as an individual; the lists are published by formal professional groups and health care institutions

quality improvement (QI) measuring, improving, and remeasuring patient outcomes based on established criteria or indicators; formerly called quality assurance

quid pro quo "something for something"; a term generally used in sexual harassment claims, suggesting that career-advancing favors (promotions, raises) would be exchanged for sexual favors

reciprocity the acceptance by one state of a license that is issued by another state

Red Flags Rule enacted August 1, 2009 by the Federal Trade Commission to combat medical identity theft

registration a process similar to certification in which an individual, after meeting the criteria of an organization (such as passing an exam), is listed on a state or national registry

release of medical records a form signed by a patient or his or her legal representative allowing a health care provider to give medical information to a person or agency

reportable incidents events or conditions that, by law, must be reported to a designated authority

res ipsa loquitur "the thing speaks for itself"; used to describe obvious cases of negligence

respondeat superior "let the master answer"; the employer is responsible for the actions of an employee if the employee followed policy and procedure and stayed within the scope of his or her position

risk management a process to routinely assess, identify, correct, and monitor any potential hazards or risks to prevent harm and loss

scope of practice performance of duties and procedures allowed by law, standards, and educational preparation

slander false or malicious verbal statement made against another

standard of care uniform criterion established by an authority to determine quality or measure of health care or that is recognized as acceptable by usage

statute of limitations a legal time limit in which a person may file suit or authorities may file charges for a violation

subpoena a court order requiring an individual to appear in court on a given date and at a specific time

subpoena duces tecum a court order requiring medical records to be brought to the court on or by a certain date and time

Title VII of the Civil Rights Act of 1964 Unwelcome sexual advances, requests for sexual favors, and other verbal or physical conduct of a sexual nature constitutes sexual harassment when submission to or rejection of this conduct explicitly or implicitly affects an individual's employment, unreasonably interferes with an individual's work performance or creates an intimidating, hostile or offensive work environment (definition from U.S. Equal Employment Opportunity Commission)

tort a wrongful civil act committed against an individual for which compensation is sought

unbundling collecting higher reimbursement by billing separately for individual components of a procedure rather than for the procedure as a whole

upcoding an illegal practice of billing more than indicated for a procedure by selecting a higher than appropriate code

veracity truth

vulnerable populations a group of people who may be physically or mentally at risk for harm or exploitation

REVIEW QUESTIONS

1. Informed consent requires that the:
   A. patient have a family member present when the consent form is signed.
   B. medical assistant inform the patient of all possible side effects of the procedure.
   C. attorney witness the signature.
   D. physician treat the patient if it is an emergency.
   E. information provided is enough for the patient to make an educated decision.

Answer: **E**

Why: E is the definition of informed consent. A family member or an attorney is not required to be present. The medical assistant may inform the patient of side effects, but side effects are only a portion of informed consent and not enough to make an educated decision.

Review: Yes ❑ No ❑

---

2. **Law** refers to the:
   A. recognized rule of conduct enforced by a legal authority.
   B. policy used to charge people fees.
   C. Patient's Bill of Rights.
   D. established standards of care.

Answer: **A**

Why: A is the definition of law. Charging a fee, the Patient's Bill of Rights, and standards of care are not law.

Review: Yes ❑ No ❑

---

3. The law requires a physician to report to the appropriate authorities:
   A. a person who has received a narcotic drug.
   B. a physician who participates in genetic research.
   C. a physician who conducts an abortion.
   D. a person suspected of elderly abuse.
   E. a person with cancer.

Answer: **D**

Why: Elderly abuse is against the law and must be reported to the proper authority. Under normal circumstances, it is not required to report the activities listed in A, B, C, or E.

Review: Yes ❑ No ❑

---

4. Consent for a person's own medical treatment may be given by a:
   A. 17-year-old university student whose parents are paying for school.
   B. 16-year-old who has a baby but is not married and lives at home.
   C. 21-year-old who has taken a narcotic pain medication.
   D. 17-year-old who is in the Navy.

Answer: **D**

Why: A person serving in the armed forces, even if a minor, is legally able to consent to his or her own medical treatment. In most states, a person 16 or 17 years old is considered a nonemancipated minor if still dependent on parents. Someone taking narcotic medication is not considered competent because of the narcotic's effects.

Review: Yes ❑ No ❑

---

5. A patient's implied consent usually covers a(n):
   A. organ donation.
   B. electrocardiogram.
   C. blood transfusion.
   D. appendectomy.
   E. release of medical information.

Answer: **B**

Why: An electrocardiogram is considered a common procedure in a medical practice and is generally understood to have little risk. Implied consent is sufficient for such procedures. The other procedures usually require expressed consent.

Review: Yes ❑ No ❑

6. A **tort** is:
   A. a type of criminal law.
   B. a type of civil law.
   C. exempt from the Good Samaritan Act.
   D. a standard of care.

Answer: **B**

Why: A tort is a type of civil law that deals with accidental or intentional harm to a person or property resulting from the wrongdoing of another. It is not criminal law or exempt from the Good Samaritan Act if malpractice is committed. A standard of care may be addressed in a tort but is not a tort itself.

Review: Yes ❑ No ❑

---

7. Malfeasance is one form of:
   A. misfeasance.
   B. nonfeasance.
   C. malpractice.
   D. malnutrition.
   E. malformation.

Answer: **C**

Why: Malfeasance is performance of an improper act that results in or causes harm. Malpractice is failure to act or an improper act that results in or causes harm. Malfeasance is a specific type of malpractice. Misfeasance and nonfeasance are different from malfeasance but are also forms of malpractice. Malnutrition and malformation are medical pathology.

Review: Yes ❑ No ❑

---

8. A physician may obtain his or her license by any of the following EXCEPT:
   A. endorsement.
   B. examination.
   C. reciprocity.
   D. registration.

Answer: **D**

Why: A physician may obtain a license through endorsement, examination, or reciprocity. Registration is not a process for obtaining a license to practice medicine.

Review: Yes ❑ No ❑

---

9. Advance directives include a:
   A. living memorial.
   B. medical power of attorney.
   C. notarized will.
   D. driver's license.
   E. medical examination.

Answer: **B**

Why: A medical power of attorney gives a designated person the legal authority to make medical decisions for the patient. This is done by the patient while he or she is still competent to make his or her own decisions.

Review: Yes ❑ No ❑

---

10. ***Respondeat superior*** refers to:
   A. a subpoena to come to court.
   B. a physician's responsibility for the actions of his or her staff.
   C. "something for something."
   D. "respond to your superiors."

Answer: **B**

Why: Respondeat superior means "let the master answer" and refers to the physician's responsibility for the actions of his or her staff.

Review: Yes ❑ No ❑

---

11. The Good Samaritan Act does not cover a health care provider who:
   A. renders first aid at the scene of an accident.
   B. volunteers to provide first aid at a charitable "fun run."
   C. helps a person who has fainted at a sporting event.
   D. provides care to a person having a seizure in a restaurant.
   E. provides first aid to a person who has a heart attack in the health care provider's home.

Answer: **B**

Why: The Good Samaritan Act only covers acts outside of the health care profession. If you volunteer as a professional, this is considered to be within the formal practice of your profession, and the Good Samaritan Act does not apply.

Review: Yes ❑ No ❑

12. A physician who accepts payment from another physician for the referral of a patient is guilty of:
A. fee splitting.
B. bundling.
C. battery.
D. abandonment.

Answer: **A**

Why: A physician who accepts money from another physician for referral of a patient is guilty of fee splitting. The physician paying for the referral is also guilty.

Review: Yes ❑ No ❑

---

13. Failure to act in a manner that a prudent and reasonable person would under similar circumstances is:
A. negligence.
B. implied consent.
C. breach of contract.
D. fraud.
E. abuse.

Answer: **A**

Why: Negligence is an omission or commission of an act that a prudent and reasonable person would or would not do in similar circumstances.

Review: Yes ❑ No ❑

---

14. The "Four Ds" are used to determine malpractice; the following are the "Ds" EXCEPT:
A. direct cause.
B. duty.
C. derelict.
D. defendant.

Answer: **D**

Why: A defendant is the person charged with an offense, not an element for determining malpractice. The "Four Ds" are duty, derelict, direct cause, and damage.

Review: Yes ❑ No ❑

---

15. A minor may consent for all of the following EXCEPT:
A. treatment of syphilis.
B. abortion.
C. birth control.
D. treatment of gonorrhea.
E. sterilization.

Answer: **E**

Why: A minor cannot consent for his or her sterilization. A minor 12 years of age and older, in most states, may consent for treatment of sexually transmitted diseases, birth control, and abortion.

Review: Yes ❑ No ❑

---

16. A communicable disease to be reported to the county health department is:
A. gastroenteritis.
B. streptococcus.
C. rubella.
D. tinnitus.

Answer: **C**

Why: Rubella, or German measles, is a reportable communicable disease. Gastroenteritis, infection of the stomach and small intestine; streptococcus, a bacterial infection; and tinnitus, ringing in the ears, are not required to be reported.

Review: Yes ❑ No ❑

---

17. Medical examiner cases involve:
A. deaths.
B. births.
C. communicable diseases.
D. professional misconduct.
E. *respondeat superior*.

Answer: **A**

Why: Medical examiner cases involve death caused by a criminal act or by violence, death without prior medical care, and death from an undetermined cause.

Review: Yes ❑ No ❑

18. A situation in which the very nature of the injury implicates malpractice is called:
    A. slander.
    B. assault.
    C. defamation.
    D. *res ipsa loquitur*.

Answer: **D**

Why: Res ipsa loquitur means "the thing speaks for itself" and is used in cases in which the malpractice is obvious.

Review: Yes ❑ No ❑

---

19. The strongest mandatory credential regulated by a state to practice a profession is a(n):
    A. declaration.
    B. licensure.
    C. matriculation.
    D. acceptance.
    E. warranty.

Answer: **B**

Why: Licensure is the strongest mandatory credential. The remaining items are voluntary and usually not issued by a governmental agency.

Review: Yes ❑ No ❑

---

20. Medical assistants may be:
    A. licensed.
    B. certified.
    C. accredited.
    D. reciprocated.

Answer: **B**

Why: Medical assistants may be certified. They are not licensed by any state; therefore, reciprocity does not apply. Organizations, not individuals, are accredited.

Review: Yes ❑ No ❑

---

21. Ethics deal with
    A. morals.
    B. *respondeat superior*.
    C. assault.
    D. customs.
    E. religion.

Answer: **A**

Why: Ethics are morals and values. *Respondeat superior* means the physician is responsible for his or her employees; assault is an attack or threat to a person; customs are traditions; religion is the worship of a deity.

Review: Yes ❑ No ❑

---

22. The Patient's Bill of Rights includes the right to:
    A. choose one's own housing.
    B. respect from employers.
    C. a fair wage.
    D. confidentiality.
    E. an education.

Answer: **D**

Why: The Patient's Bill of Rights includes the right to confidentiality. A, B, C, and E do not address health care.

Review: Yes ❑ No ❑

---

23. The first medical code of ethics was written by:
    A. Hippocrates.
    B. Socrates.
    C. the AMA.
    D. Hammurabi.

Answer: **D**

Why: The Code of Hammurabi was written in 2500 BCE. Hippocrates, Socrates, and the American Medical Association (AMA) wrote medical codes of ethics later.

Review: Yes ❑ No ❑

---

24. Which of the following is considered an ethical issue?
    A. Allocation of resources
    B. Childbirth
    C. Electrical engineering
    D. Appendectomies
    E. Long waits for patients in physician offices

Answer: **A**

Why: Allocation of resources refers to the distribution of funds (money), organs for transplants, needed medical procedures, or other resources, which are ethical issues. Childbirth is a medical or natural process; appendectomies are surgeries. Electrical engineering is a profession. (Long waits are an inconvenience!)

Review: Yes ❑ No ❑

25. A medical assistant publicly criticizes a physician's diagnostic skills. This is an example of:
A. slander.
B. veracity.
C. breach of confidentiality.
D. malpractice.

Answer: **A**

Why: The definition of slander is a false or malicious statement against another. Veracity means truth; breach of confidentiality refers to releasing protected information without consent; malpractice has to do with specific damages to a patient. Battery is touching a person without consent.

Review: Yes ❑ No ❑

---

26. Which of the following conditions must be reported?
A. Hypertension
B. Hepatitis B
C. Hemiplegia
D. Hemorrhage
E. Anemia

Answer: **B**

Why: Hepatitis B is a communicable disease that must be reported to the local or state health departments. The other choices are medical conditions that do not require reporting.

Review: Yes ❑ No ❑

---

27. A court order instructing the physician to report to court at a certain time and date is:
A. *quid pro quo*.
B. a contract.
C. a subpoena.
D. consent.

Answer: **C**

Why: A subpoena is a document that mandates a person to appear in court at a given time and date. *Quid pro quo* means "something for something," a favor. A contract is an agreement between parties; consent is permission to perform or do something.

Review: Yes ❑ No ❑

---

28. A living will:
A. names the beneficiaries of the estate.
B. is an advance directive stating the patient's decisions for medical care before an incapacitating event.
C. must be drawn up by an attorney.
D. is subject to estate taxes.
E. allows a person to give away his or her belongings while still alive.

Answer: **B**

Why: An advance directive is a set of instructions given while a person is fully capacitated. One type of advance directive is the living will, which states the health care desires of a patient. Advance directives have nothing to do with the estate or estate taxes and do not have to be drawn up by an attorney. No will is needed for selection E.

Review: Yes ❑ No ❑

---

29. Dr. Smith is no longer willing to take care of Mr. Watson. If Dr. Smith does not give Mr. Watson proper notification and appropriate time to find a new physician, Dr. Smith is guilty of:
A. violation of standard of care.
B. privacy.
C. failure to act.
D. abandonment.

Answer: **D**

Why: When a physician withdraws from the care of a patient without reasonable notice or provision for another equally or better qualified provider to assume care, the patient/physician contract is breached and the physician is guilty of abandonment.

Review: Yes ❑ No ❑

---

30. The patient puts out his or her arm to allow the physician to cleanse an abrasion. This type of consent is:
A. implied.
B. expressed.
C. contracted.
D. emergency.
E. positive.

Answer: **A**

Why: Consent is implied by the patient holding out his or her arm. Expressed consent is verbal or written. The only emergency consent is one that is "life or limb" threatening. The terms "positive" and "contracted" do not apply to consent.

Review: Yes ❑ No ❑

31. The physician performs an elective surgical procedure without a written consent. The physician is guilty of:
    A. a bioethic offense.
    B. breach of confidentiality.
    C. battery.
    D. endorsement.

Answer: **C**

Why: Battery is touching someone without his or her consent. There is no indication that bioethics are involved or that the patient's confidentiality has been breached. Endorsement is one method for a physician to obtain a license to practice medicine.

Review: Yes ❑ No ❑

---

32. The purpose of the Good Samaritan Act is to:
    A. reward health care providers for stopping at the scene of an accident.
    B. ensure physicians know first aid.
    C. protect health care workers from liability when rendering emergency care.
    D. avoid having to pay for first aid.
    E. encourage more people to go into health care professions.

Answer: **C**

Why: The Good Samaritan Act was designed to encourage health care workers to stop at the scene of emergencies by protecting them from liability for civil damages.

Review: Yes ❑ No ❑

---

33. Which of the following actions is governed by criminal law?
    A. Giving an incorrect medication
    B. Discounting
    C. Not reporting suspected measles
    D. Telling a family member the patient's diagnosis
    E. Purposefully overcharging on a Medicare claim

Answer: **E**

Why: Purposefully overcharging on a Medicare claim is considered fraud and is therefore covered under criminal law; the other choices are usually considered civil offenses if charges are made.

Review: Yes ❑ No ❑

---

34. A patient is treated for a minor gunshot wound that he states was sustained during a hunting accident. The physician is obligated to report this as part of:
    A. implied consent.
    B. public duty.
    C. mandatory counseling.
    D. standard of care.
    E. *respondeat superior*.

Answer: **B**

Why: It is the physician's public duty to report all gunshot wounds.

Review: Yes ❑ No ❑

---

35. A patient calls to make an appointment and states the symptoms for the office visit. The scheduler says, "That sounds like the flu." The health care worker violated the:
    A. code of ethics.
    B. Patient's Bill of Rights.
    C. Health Insurance Portability and Accountability Act.
    D. scope of practice.

Answer: **D**

Why: A person scheduling appointments has not been trained to diagnose. A diagnosis can only be made by a physician or mid-level provider such as a physician's assistant or nurse practitioner.

Review: Yes ❑ No ❑

---

36. Mandatory reporting is required in all of the following cases EXCEPT:
    A. child abuse.
    B. unknown cause of death.
    C. alcohol abuse.
    D. elder abuse.
    E. communicable disease.

Answer: **C**

Why: Alcohol abuse is not considered reportable, whereas child abuse, death from an unknown cause, and elder abuse must be reported.

Review: Yes ❑ No ❑

37. A form of malpractice is **nonfeasance**, which means:
   A. failure to act when duty is indicated, resulting in or causing harm.
   B. improper performance of an act, resulting in or causing harm.
   C. performance of an improper act, resulting in or causing harm.
   D. not charging a fee.

Answer: **A**

Why: The definition of nonfeasance is the failure to act when duty is indicated, resulting in or causing harm. B is misfeasance; C is malfeasance; D and E have nothing to do with malpractice.

Review: Yes ❑ No ❑

---

38. A physician casts a fracture of the ulna incorrectly. This results in malformation of the arm. The physician could be charged with:
   A. misadventure.
   B. malunion.
   C. tort.
   D. torticollis.
   E. battery.

Answer: **C**

Why: A tort is accidental or intentional harm to a person or property resulting from the wrongdoing of another. The other choices do not deal with medical wrongdoings.

Review: Yes ❑ No ❑

---

39. The medical office must comply with the regulations and standards of:
   A. AFL.
   B. AAMA.
   C. GOP.
   D. AARP.
   E. OSHA.

Answer: **E**

Why: The Occupational Safety and Health Administration (OSHA) is a regulatory governmental agency; its mandates must be followed or legal actions may be imposed. The American Federation of Labor (AFL), the American Association of Medical Assistants (AAMA), and the Republican Party (GOP) are voluntary special interest organizations.

Review: Yes ❑ No ❑

---

40. All of the following are governmental agencies setting standards and regulations that must be followed by medical offices EXCEPT:
   A. The Joint Commission.
   B. DEA.
   C. IRS.
   D. FDA.

Answer: **A**

Why: The Joint Commission is the only nongovernmental voluntary agency in this list. The Drug Enforcement Administration (DEA), Internal Revenue Service (IRS), and Food and Drug Administration (FDA) are all governmental agencies with regulations affecting the medical office.

Review: Yes ❑ No ❑

---

41. The physician's office shares a patient's medical information with an insurance company. The physician's office did not have the patient's written consent. The office is guilty of:
   A. breach of confidentiality.
   B. slander.
   C. abuse.
   D. breach of respect.

Answer: **A**

Why: Providing a patient's medical information to an outside party without the patient's written consent is a breach of confidentiality.

Review: Yes ❑ No ❑

42. A wheelchair patient could not use the medical office restroom because it was too small for the wheelchair. This office is in violation of:
    A. CLIA.
    B. FDA.
    C. OSHA.
    D. CDC.
    E. ADA.

Answer: **E**

Why: The Americans with Disabilities Act (ADA) mandates that certain workplaces, including medical offices, must provide accommodations for persons with special needs. CLIA is the Clinical Laboratory Improvement Amendments, FDA is the Food and Drug Administration, OSHA is the Occupational Safety and Health Administration, and CDC is the Centers for Disease Control and Prevention.

Review: Yes ❑ No ❑

---

43. A typical Patient's Bill of Rights includes the right to:
    A. request free treatment.
    B. report patient dissatisfaction with the doctor to the medical assistant.
    C. refuse treatment.
    D. sue the doctor for breach of contract.

Answer: **C**

Why: All Patient's Bills of Rights include the right to refuse treatment. A and B are not included in any Patient's Bill of Rights, and D involves tort law.

Review: Yes ❑ No ❑

---

44. A valid contract must:
    A. be paid in full at the beginning of the period covered.
    B. be entered into by competent parties.
    C. always be in writing.
    D. always cover the patient's family.
    E. always have a witness.

Answer: **B**

Why: One of the five components of a valid contract is that all parties must be legally capable of accepting the terms or be competent. The other four requirements are:

- an offer must be made,
- the offer must be accepted,
- an exchange of value between the parties must occur, and
- the intent must be legal.

Review: Yes ❑ No ❑

---

45. The purpose of law is to:
    A. legalize cardiopulmonary training.
    B. provide jobs.
    C. benefit special interest groups.
    D. remedy wrongs.

Answer: **D**

Why: The purposes of law are to regulate conduct, to punish offenders, to remedy wrongs, and to benefit society.

Review: Yes ❑ No ❑

---

46. An expressed contract is:
    A. written.
    B. implied.
    C. reportable.
    D. sent via FedEx.
    E. illegal.

Answer: **A**

Why: The definition of an expressed contract is one that is written or verbal and describes what each contractual party will do. A contract is implied when it is deduced by the parties' actions. Contracts are generally not reportable. How contracts are delivered is the decision of the consenting parties. An expressed contract is not illegal.

Review: Yes ❑ No ❑

47. Written consent for medical care must be:
   A. voluntary.
   B. uninformed.
   C. given for all procedures.
   D. done on a word processor.

Answer: **A**

Why: Consent for medical care is voluntary permission by the appropriate party. Consent should never be uninformed, and written consent is not given for all procedures; for noninvasive procedures with low risk, implied consent is sufficient. Written consent may be in many forms and can even be handwritten.

Review: Yes ❑ No ❑

---

48. Examples of ethical cases affected by the law are cases involving:
   A. the right to die.
   B. the use of synthetic drugs.
   C. endoscopy.
   D. licensure.

Answer: **A**

Why: The right to die is an ethical issue addressed by the law in cases such as assisted suicide or euthanasia. The use of synthetic drugs and endoscopy are common practices. Licensure is required by states and comes under administrative law.

Review: Yes ❑ No ❑

---

49. Ethical issues are addressed in:
   A. insurance codes.
   B. professional codes.
   C. billing codes.
   D. safety codes.
   E. tort law

Answer: **B**

Why: Professional codes, dating back to 2500 BCE, address moral behavior and ethics. The other codes listed involve medical office procedures.

Review: Yes ❑ No ❑

---

50. In cases of public safety:
   A. the laws protecting the general population usually take precedence over an individual's rights.
   B. the AMA is often consulted.
   C. a person cannot go in public with a communicable disease.
   D. the government must uphold all Patient's Bills of Rights.

Answer: **A**

Why: The laws protecting the public safety take precedence. In instances such as contamination and quarantine, the rights of patients are secondary to the public safety.

The AMA is not generally consulted in these cases, and very few communicable diseases mandate quarantine. The government is not obligated to uphold nongovernmental agencies' Patient's Bills of Rights.

Review: Yes ❑ No ❑

---

51. A medical assistant could be held liable for the actions of:
   A. a patient.
   B. the insurance company.
   C. a coworker.
   D. the court.
   E. the hospital

Answer: **C**

Why: A medical assistant who knowingly withholds information involving illegal and, in some cases, immoral actions of a coworker could be held liable. He or she is not responsible for the actions of the patient, insurance company, or court.

Review: Yes ❑ No ❑

52. A patient outcome resulting from the quality improvement process may be preventing:
 A. illness.
 B. an increase in insurance rates.
 C. financial loss.
 D. incident reports.

Answer: **A**

Why: Preventing illness is directly related to the patient and quality of care; preventing an increase in insurance rates, preventing financial loss, and preventing incident reports are components of risk management.

Review: Yes ❑ No ❑

---

53. All of the following are examples of risk management EXCEPT:
 A. ensuring the coffee pot is turned off at the end of the day.
 B. giving the patient an injection ordered by the physician.
 C. checking the emergency cart.
 D. reporting a frayed lamp wire.
 E. repairing a tear in the carpet to prevent tripping.

Answer: **B**

Why: Ensuring the coffee pot is turned off and reporting a frayed wire are intended to prevent fire (loss); checking the emergency cart is intended to provide an appropriate standard of care if an emergency occurs (prevent harm and loss). However, giving the patient an injection is part of the prescribed patient's treatment. It is not considered risk management.

Review: Yes ❑ No ❑

---

54. The AMA Principles of Medical Ethics require a physician to:
 A. belong to the AMA.
 B. treat patients on Medicare.
 C. contribute to political action campaigns (PAC).
 D. report other physicians deficient in character or competence.

Answer: **D**

Why: Article II of the AMA Principles of Medical Ethics states: "A physician shall uphold the standards of professionalism, be honest in all professional interactions, and strive to report physicians deficient in character or competence, or engaging in fraud or deception, to appropriate entities." The other answers may be implied but do not specifically deal with ethics.

Review: Yes ❑ No ❑

---

55. What prohibits job discrimination for race, color, religion, sex, or national origin?
 A. EEOC
 B. FMLA
 C. ADA
 D. Equal Pay Act
 E. HIPAA

Answer: **A**

Why: The Equal Employment Opportunity Commission is the agency that prohibits job discrimination for race, color, religion, sex, or national origin. The FMLA involves family leave; the ADA prohibits discrimination against people with disabilities; the Equal Pay Act requires equal pay for equal work; and HIPAA involves confidentiality in health care.

Review: Yes ❑ No ❑

---

56. Employment law is generally considered:
 A. criminal law.
 B. tort law.
 C. bioethics.
 D. contract law.
 E. administrative law.

Answer: **E**

Why: Employment law concerns administrative regulations for the workplace. Criminal law and tort law are not limited to a specific venue. Contract law concerns an agreement between two parties, and bioethics are not laws.

Review: Yes ❑ No ❑

57. The purpose of the Red Flags Rule is to:
   A. have national holidays off.
   B. watch for Medicare fraud.
   C. guard for medical identity theft.
   D. check references before hiring.

Answer: **C**

Why: The Red Flags Rule was enacted by the Federal Trade Commission August 2009 for the purpose of legislating certain businesses to implement a program to prevent, detect and mitigate medical identity theft.

Review: Yes ❑ No ❑

5

Medical Terminology

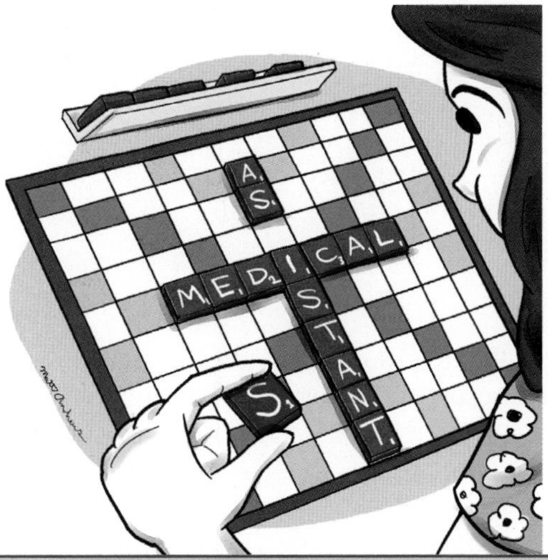

REVIEW TIP

Medical terminology is a good area for the "learning moments" strategies described in Chapter 1. Make flashcards and have people around you ask questions whenever there is an opportunity. Use the word list in this chapter. Continue to use flashcards as you study other chapters.

Caution: Be careful of terms that sound similar but have different meanings, such as "melanin" and "melatonin."

Medical terminology is a significant portion of the national exams. Questions in other chapters may be answered by knowing the meaning of the term. Medical terminology is comparable to a foreign language. You may pick up pieces and phrases just by being around those who speak it, but you could not expect to pass an exam in that language without some study. If you are a medical assistant or medical administrative specialist who received on-the-job training, this may apply to you, especially if you have been working in a specialty practice (e.g., obstetrics, where the terminology is basically limited to the female reproductive system). Certification exam questions may require you to select not only the meaning but also the correct spelling of a term.

WORD PARTS

A medical term may have three parts—the prefix, the root, and the suffix. The meaning is found by deciphering the clues.

1. Prefix = beginning of the word; it modifies the root (not all medical terms have a prefix)
   Example of a term with no prefix: TONSILLECTOMY (removal of tonsils)
   root: tonsil/o = tonsils
   suffix: -ectomy = removal of
2. Root = meaning or central part of the word; it often refers to a body part (nearly all medical terms have a root)

Box 5-1

Common Prefixes and Meanings

a/n-: absence of
ab-: away from
ad-: toward
ante-: before
anti-: against
auto-: self
bi-: both, two
bio-: life
circum-: around
con-: with, together
contra-: against, opposite
dis-: apart, separate
dys-: painful, difficult
ec-: out
ecto-: outside of
en-: in
endo-: within
epi-: on, attached to, over
ex-: out
hemi-: half
hemo-: pertaining to blood
hyper-: high, excessive
hypo-: below
inter-: between
intra-: within
iso-: equal
mal-: bad
mega-: large
meso-: middle
meta-: beyond
micro-: very small
milli-: one thousandth
mono-: one, single
multi-: many
neo-: new
para-: beside
per-: through
peri-: around, enclosing
poly-: many
post-: after
pre-: before
primi-: first
retro-: back, behind
semi-: half
sub-: under
super-: excessive
supra-: above
syn-: together, with

3. Suffix = ending of the word; it modifies the root and usually refers to a condition, procedure, or action (not all medical terms have a suffix)

   Example of a term with no suffix: TONSIL (lymphatic tissue in the pharynx)
   root: tonsil
   Example of a term with a prefix, root, and suffix: HYPERTHERMIC (abnormally high temperature)
   prefix: hyper- = high, above, super
   root: therm/o = related to temperature
   suffix: -ic = condition/state related to the root

Think of an example of a medical term for each of the prefixes (Box 5-1), suffixes (Box 5-2), and roots (Box 5-3). Medical terminology is difficult and may require more time. Use the Review Tip. Consider adding another week to your study plan if you are not comfortable with the material. Take a break, get some fresh air, and, as an unknown philosopher said, "Eat your elephant one bite at a time," which means that you should take it one step at a time.

MEDICAL TERMINOLOGY REVIEW AIDS

The following words and word parts will help with breaking down and building other medical terms and determining their meaning.

BODY PLANES

■ Median or midline plane—a lengthwise plane through the midline running front to back dividing the body into equal right and left halves

Box 5-2

Common Suffixes and Meanings

-ad: toward
-al: relating to
-ectomy: removal of
-emesis: vomiting
-genic: producing
-genetic: origin- related
-graph: recording instrument
-graphy: recording process
-iatric: treatment of
-iatry: field of medicine
-ic: relating to
-ism: condition of
-itis: inflammation
-logist: specialist in
-logy: study of
-lysis: destruction of
-megaly: enlargement
-meter: measurement instrument
-oma: tumor
-osis: condition of
-pathy: disease
-penia: abnormal decrease
-philia: abnormal attraction
-phobia: abnormal fear
-plasia: formation
-plasty: surgical repair
-ptosis: drooping
-rrhage: burst forth
-rrhea: discharge
-scope: viewing instrument
-scopy: procedure using a scope
-stomy: creating a surgical opening
-tomy: incision into

Box 5-3

Common Roots and Meanings

aden/o: gland	glyc/o: sugar, glucose
arteri/o: artery	hepat/o: liver
arthr/o: joint	hist/o: tissue
audi/o: hearing	ir/o: iris
blephar/o: eyelid	kal/i: potassium
bucc/o: cheek	lacrim/o: tear
burs/o: bursa	lamin/o: lamina
calc/i: stone	lapar/o: abdomen
cardi/o: heart	leuk/o: white
cervic/o: neck, neck of an organ	lip/o: fat
cholecyst/o: gallbladder	myel/o: spinal cord
conjunctiv/o: conjunctiva	my/o: muscle
cost/o: rib	nephr/o: kidney
crani/o: skull	neur/o: nerve
cutane/o: skin	onc/o: tumor
cyan/o: blue	opt/o: vision
cyst/o: bladder	oste/o: bone
cyt/o: cell	pector/o: chest
derm/o: skin	pneumon/o: lung
dors/o: back	psych/o: mind
encephal/o: brain	retin/o: retina
fasci/o: fibrous tissue	rhin/o: nose
fibr/o: connective tissue	synovi/o: lining the joint
gastr/o: stomach	tend/o: tendon
gingiv/o: gum	ven/o:- vein

- Sagittal plane—a lengthwise plane parallel to the midline running front to back dividing the body or any part of it into unequal right and left sides or parts
- Coronal or frontal plane—a lengthwise plane running side to side dividing the body into front and back parts
- Transverse or horizontal plane—a crosswise plane dividing the body into upper and lower parts

DIRECTIONAL TERMS

Directional terms make it possible to say that something is above, below, to the left or right of, behind or in front of, or nearer or farther from something else.

- Superior—toward the head end or toward the upper part of the body
- Inferior—farther away from the head or toward the lower part of the body
- Anterior or ventral—on the front or abdominal side of the body
- Posterior or dorsal—on the back side of the body
- Proximal—nearer a point of reference, usually the trunk or middle of the body
- Distal—farther away from a point of reference
- Medial—closer to the midline of the body
- Lateral—toward the side of the body or away from the midline
- Internal or deep—on the inside of the body
- External or superficial—on or close to the outside of the body

LOCATING TERMS

- Cephalic or cranial—referring to the head or head end
- Caudal—referring to the tail or tail end
- Palmar—referring to the front (while standing in anatomical position) or palm of the hand
- Plantar—referring to the sole or bottom of the foot

DIAGNOSTIC, SYMPTOMATIC, AND RELATED SUFFIXES

- -algia—pain
- -cele—hernia, swelling
- -genesis (-gen)—forming, producing
- -gram—record, a writing
- -graph—instrument for recording
- -iasis—abnormal condition
- -itis—inflammation
- -malacia—softening
- -oid—resembling
- -oma—tumor
- -osis—abnormal condition or increase (used primarily with blood cells)
- -pathy—disease
- -penia—decrease, deficiency
- -phagia—eating, swallowing
- -plegia—paralysis
- -rrhage—bursting forth
- -rrhea—discharge, flow
- -rrhexis—rupture
- -stasis—standing still
- -stenosis—narrowing, stricture

SURGICAL PROCEDURES

- -centesis—to puncture in order to aspirate
- -desis—binding or fixation

- -ectomy—excision, surgical removal of
- -lithotomy—incision for removal of stones
- -otomy—incision into
- -pexy—suspension or fixation
- -plasty—repair or surgical reconstruction of
- -scopy—inspection/examination through a lighted scope
- -stomy—creation of a new opening for drainage

TERMS

Medical Terminology Review

(*Suggestion:* use these terms to make flashcards.)

ab- away from, absent
abdominocentesis surgical puncture of the abdomen to remove fluid
acrocyanosis blue condition of the extremities
adenoma tumor of a gland
adrenomegaly enlargement of the adrenal gland(s)
-algesia pain, sensitivity to pain
analgesia take away pain, free from pain
anteroposterior passing from front to rear
antipyretic against fever; fever reducing
aplasia lack of formation or development; usually refers to an organ
arteriosclerosis thickening (hardening) of the arteries
arthritis inflammation of the joints
bradycardia slow heart rate (pulse)
cardiomegaly enlargement of the heart
cervicofacial pertaining to the face and neck
chiroplasty surgical repair of the hands
cholecystitis inflammation of the gallbladder
cyanosis bluish condition of the skin
cystitis bladder inflammation
cytology study of cells
cytoscopy microscopic examination of cells
dacryocystitis inflammation of a tear sac
dactyl/o digit, finger or toe
dermatosis any skin lesion or eruption
dextr/o right
duodenoscopy inspection of the duodenum with a scope
dyskinesia difficult or painful movement
dyspepsia indigestion or painful digestion
-emia pertaining to the blood
encephal/o pertaining to the brain
encephalitis inflammation of the brain
endocarditis inflammation of the inside lining of the heart
enteritis inflammation of the small intestine
gastrectasia stretching of the stomach
gastritis inflammation of the stomach
gingivoglossitis inflammation of the gums and tongue
gynecopathy any disease of the female reproductive system
hemiplegia paralysis of one half of the body
hemostasis to stop or control bleeding
hepatomegaly enlargement of the liver
hyperplasia excessive formation of cells or tissue
hypoglycemia less than normal blood sugar level
hypothermia below normal temperature
hysterorrhaphy suturing of the uterus
inter- between, in the midst
intracerebral within the main part of the brain
intravascular within a vessel
laparotomy incision of the abdominal wall
leukopenia decreased white cells
lipectomy excision of fatty tissue
litholysis destruction of a stone
-logy the study of
lymphadenitis inflammation of the lymph glands/nodes
-lysis destruction, destroy, dissolution
-malacia softening of tissue
mammoplasty surgical reconstruction of the breast
meningocele herniation of the meninges
menostasis suppression of menses
metrorrhexis rupture of the uterus
myc/o fungus or mold
nasopharyngeal pertaining to nose and throat
necrosis death of tissue or bone
nephrolysis destruction of kidney tissue
nephropathy disease of the kidney
neuralgia pain in the nerves
neuropathy disease of the nerves
neurotripsy surgical crushing of a nerve
onychocryptosis an ingrown (hidden) nail, finger or toe
onychomycosis condition of fungus of the nails
oophorectomy excision of an ovary
orchidectomy surgical removal of a testicle
osteoarthropathy disease of joints and bones
osteocyte bone cell
otalgia pain in the ear
-pepsis digestion
peri- around, about
phag/o to ingest or eat
phleborrhexis rupture of a vein
-phonia voice
pneum/o air
pneumon/o lung
posteromedial middle of the back, middle of back side
proctorrhagia hemorrhage from the rectum
pyeloplasty surgical repair of the renal pelvis
pyogenesis formation of pus
retinopathy disease of the retina
retroperitoneal behind the peritoneum

rhinorrhea flow or discharge from the nose
-rrhagia burst forth, hemorrhage
-rrhexis rupture of a vessel, organ, or tissue
splenomegaly enlargement of the spleen
-stasis to stop or control
sten/o narrowing
stomatomycosis condition of fungus in the mouth
-stomy forming a new opening
subpulmonary below the lungs
tachycardia increased heart rate (pulse)
tenodynia painful tendon
thrombectomy surgical removal of a blood clot
transthorax across the chest
tympan/o eardrum, drumlike
unilateral on one side
vas/o vessel or duct

REVIEW QUESTIONS

All questions are relevant for the CMA (AAMA), RMA (AMT), and CMAS (AMT) exams.

1. The word root **vas/o** means:
   A. vein.
   B. artery.
   C. vessel.
   D. capillary.

Answer: **C**

Why: vas/o = vessel or duct

Review: Yes ❑ No ❑

---

2. The word root **pneumon/o** means:
   A. air.
   B. breathing.
   C. bronchus.
   D. pleura.
   E. lung.

Answer: **E**

Why: pneumon/o = lung

Review: Yes ❑ No ❑

---

3. The suffix **-rrhexis** means:
   A. discharge.
   B. pain.
   C. flow.
   D. rupture.

Answer: **D**

Why: -rrhexis = rupture of a vessel, organ, or tissue

Review: Yes ❑ No ❑

---

4. The word root **myc/o** means:
   A. muscle.
   B. many.
   C. middle.
   D. mold.
   E. mucus.

Answer: **D**

Why: myc/o = fungus or mold

Review: Yes ❑ No ❑

---

5. The term **rhinorrhea** means:
   A. inflammation of the nose.
   B. suturing of the nostrils.
   C. discharge from the nose.
   D. enlargement of the nose.

Answer: **C**

Why: rhin/o = nose
-rrhea = flow or discharge

Review: Yes ❑ No ❑

---

6. The term **hepatomegaly** means:
   A. dysfunction of the kidneys.
   B. underdevelopment of the liver.
   C. increased production of blood cells.
   D. enlargement of the liver.
   E. hemorrhage from the liver.

Answer: **D**

Why: hepat/o = liver
-megaly = enlargement

Review: Yes ❑ No ❑

---

7. The suffix **-lysis** refers to:
   A. formation.
   B. hardening.
   C. abnormal.
   D. destruction.

Answer: **D**

Why: -lysis = dissolution or destruction

Review: Yes ❑ No ❑

8. The word root **phag/o** means:
   A. grow.
   B. chew.
   C. repair.
   D. narrow.
   E. ingest.

Answer: **E**

Why: phag/o = to ingest or eat

Review: Yes ❑ No ❑

---

9. The term for *voice* is:
   A. phobia.
   B. ptosis.
   C. phasia.
   D. phonia.

Answer: **D**

Why: -phonia, phon/o = voice

Review: Yes ❑ No ❑

---

10. The term **-malacia** means:
    A. accumulation.
    B. drooping.
    C. softening.
    D. constriction.
    E. hardening.

Answer: **C**

Why: -malacia = softening of tissues

Review: Yes ❑ No ❑

---

11. The term **neuropathy** means:
    A. inflammation of the nerves.
    B. hardening of the nerves.
    C. disease of the nerves.
    D. surgical removal of nerves.

Answer: **C**

Why: neur/o = nerves
-pathy = disease, disease process

Review: Yes ❑ No ❑

---

12. The suffix **-rrhagia** means:
    A. rupture.
    B. inflammation.
    C. painful.
    D. surgical suturing.
    E. burst forth.

Answer: **E**

Why: -rrhagia = bursting forth

Review: Yes ❑ No ❑

---

13. The term **gastritis** means:
    A. disease of the gallbladder.
    B. flow from the duodenum.
    C. inflammation of the stomach.
    D. rupture of the spleen.

Answer: **C**

Why: gastr/o = stomach
-itis = inflammation

Review: Yes ❑ No ❑

---

14. Inflammation of the joints is known as:
    A. tendonitis.
    B. bursitis.
    C. osteitis.
    D. arthritis.
    E. myositis.

Answer: **D**

Why: arthr/o = joints
-itis = inflammation

Review: Yes ❑ No ❑

---

15. The term **hypoglycemia** means:
    A. elevated blood sugar level.
    B. lower than normal blood sugar level.
    C. presence of sugar in the blood.
    D. elevated sodium level.

Answer: **B**

Why: hypo- = low, under normal level
glyc/o = sugar, glucose
-emia = pertaining to blood

Review: Yes ❑ No ❑

16. The term **otalgia** means:
   A. discharge from the ear.
   B. disease of the ear.
   C. pain in the ear.
   D. inflammation of the ear.
   E. opening in the ear.

Answer: **C**

Why: ot/o = ear
-algia = pain

Review: Yes ❑ No ❑

---

17. The medical term that means *to control bleeding* is:
   A. hemostasis.
   B. hemophilia.
   C. hematoma.
   D. hemoccult.

Answer: **A**

Why: hem/o = blood
-stasis = to stop or control

Review: Yes ❑ No ❑

---

18. The term **enteritis** means:
   A. inflammation of the colon.
   B. disease of the large intestine.
   C. inflammation of the small intestine.
   D. disease of the esophagus.
   E. inflammation of the mouth.

Answer: **C**

Why: enter/o = small intestine
-itis = inflammation

Review: Yes ❑ No ❑

---

19. The term meaning *indigestion* or *painful digestion* is:
   A. dyspnea.
   B. dysphagia.
   C. dysplasia.
   D. dyspepsia.

Answer: **D**

Why: dys- = painful or difficult
-pepsis = digestion

Review: Yes ❑ No ❑

---

20. The medical term used to describe any skin lesion or eruption is:
   A. dermatomycosis.
   B. dermatoplasty.
   C. dermatoid.
   D. dermatoma.
   E. dermatosis.

Answer: **E**

Why: dermat/o = skin
-osis = any condition, process

Review: Yes ❑ No ❑

---

21. The term meaning *bladder inflammation* is:
   A. cystorrhexis.
   B. cystocele.
   C. cystalgia.
   D. cystitis.

Answer: **D**

Why: cyst/o = bladder or sac
-itis = inflammation

Review: Yes ❑ No ❑

---

22. The term **bradycardia** means:
   A. slow blood pressure.
   B. increased blood flow.
   C. slow heart rate.
   D. increased heart rate.
   E. slow blood flow.

Answer: **C**

Why: brady- = slow
cardi/o = the heart
-a = pertaining to

Review: Yes ❑ No ❑

23. The word part **-algesia** means:
    A. against.
    B. pertaining to.
    C. pain.
    D. without.

Answer: **C**

Why: -algesia = sensation of pain

Review: Yes ❑ No ❑

---

24. The word part **dextr/o** means:
    A. sugar.
    B. glucose.
    C. left.
    D. back.
    E. right.

Answer: **E**

Why: dextr/o = right or on the right side

Review: Yes ❑ No ❑

---

25. The word part **encephal/o** means:
    A. brain.
    B. head.
    C. cerebrum.
    D. skull.

Answer: **A**

Why: encephal/o = inside the head (the brain)

Review: Yes ❑ No ❑

---

26. The term **osteocyte** means:
    A. compact bone.
    B. spongy bone.
    C. bone cell.
    D. bone cyst.
    E. bone infection.

Answer: **C**

Why: oste/o = pertaining to bone
-cyte = cell

Review: Yes ❑ No ❑

---

27. The word part meaning *eardrum* is:
    A. cochle/o.
    B. salping/o.
    C. myring/o.
    D. tympan/o.

Answer: **D**

Why: tympan/o = a structure that is drumlike

Review: Yes ❑ No ❑

---

28. The term **oophorectomy** means:
    A. formation of an ovum.
    B. repair of an ovary.
    C. rupture of the uterus.
    D. incision into the uterus.
    E. excision of an ovary.

Answer: **E**

Why: oophor/o = pertaining to the ovary
-ectomy = surgical removal, excision

Review: Yes ❑ No ❑

---

29. The term **nephropathy** means:
    A. distention of the bladder.
    B. infection in the kidney.
    C. inflammation of a nerve.
    D. disease of the kidney.

Answer: **D**

Why: nephr/o = kidney
-pathy = any disease

Review: Yes ❑ No ❑

---

30. The term **acrocyanosis** means a blue condition of the:
    A. extremities.
    B. neck.
    C. face.
    D. torso.
    E. head.

Answer: **A**

Why: acr/o = extremity
cyan/o = blue
-osis = any condition

Review: Yes ❑ No ❑

31. The term **splenomegaly** means:
    A. prolapse of the spleen.
    B. dysfunction of the spleen.
    C. pain in the spleen.
    D. enlargement of the spleen.

Answer: **D**

Why: splen/o = pertaining to the spleen
-megaly = great, enlarged

Review: Yes ❑ No ❑

---

32. The medical term meaning *within a vessel* is:
    A. intercellular.
    B. interarterial.
    C. intravascular.
    D. intravalvular.
    E. intra-articular.

Answer: **C**

Why: intra- = within
vascul/o = vessel
-ar = pertaining to

Review: Yes ❑ No ❑

---

33. The term **abdominocentesis** means:
    A. surgical puncture of the abdomen.
    B. swelling of the abdomen.
    C. dilation of the abdomen.
    D. suturing of the abdomen.

Answer: **A**

Why: abdomin/o = pertaining to the abdomen
-centesis = to puncture

Review: Yes ❑ No ❑

---

34. The suffix **-stomy** means:
    A. to cut into.
    B. surgical repair.
    C. surgical removal.
    D. to form a new opening.
    E. to suture an opening.

Answer: **D**

Why: -stomy = to make a new opening

Review: Yes ❑ No ❑

---

35. The term **stenosis** means:
    A. softening.
    B. dilation.
    C. spasm.
    D. narrowing.

Answer: **D**

Why: sten/o = narrow
-osis = condition

Review: Yes ❑ No ❑

---

36. **Cardiomegaly** is a term that means:
    A. rupture of the heart.
    B. hardening of the heart tissue.
    C. inflammation of the heart.
    D. occlusion of heart vessels.
    E. enlargement of the heart.

Answer: **E**

Why: cardi/o = heart
-megaly = large or enlargement

Review: Yes ❑ No ❑

---

37. The term **lymphadenitis** means:
    A. inflammation of lymph fluid.
    B. inflammation of adrenal glands.
    C. infection of the spleen.
    D. inflammation of the lymph glands/nodes.

Answer: **D**

Why: lymph/o = pertaining to lymph
aden/o = pertaining to a gland
-itis = inflammation

Review: Yes ❑ No ❑

---

38. A term meaning *rupture of the uterus* is:
    A. metrorrhea.
    B. metrorrhexis.
    C. menorrhagia.
    D. meatorrhaphy.
    E. metritis.

Answer: **B**

Why: metr/o = related to the uterus
-rrhexis = rupture of a body part

Review: Yes ❑ No ❑

39. The microscopic examination of cells is called:
    A. cytoscopy.
    B. cystoscope.
    C. cythemia.
    D. cystotomy.

Answer: **A**

Why: cyt/o = cell
-scopy = to study or examine

Review: Yes ❑ No ❑

---

40. The prefix meaning *between* is:
    A. extra-.
    B. intra-.
    C. inter-.
    D. supra-.
    E. infra-.

Answer: **C**

Why: inter- = between, in the midst

Review: Yes ❑ No ❑

---

41. The term used for surgical removal of a blood clot is:
    A. hematectomy.
    B. hemolysis.
    C. thrombolysis.
    D. thrombectomy.

Answer: **D**

Why: thromb/o = clot, blood clot
-ectomy = surgical removal, to excise

Review: Yes ❑ No ❑

---

42. The term meaning *hemorrhage from an artery* is:
    A. arteriosclerosis.
    B. arteriorrhagia.
    C. arteriorrhaphy.
    D. arteriolysis.
    E. arteriotomy.

Answer: **B**

Why: arteri/o = artery
-rrhagia = hemorrhage, to burst forth

Review: Yes ❑ No ❑

---

43. The term meaning *destruction of a stone* is:
    A. lithogenesis.
    B. litholysis.
    C. lithiasis.
    D. lithotomy.

Answer: **B**

Why: lith/o = stone, calculus
-lysis = destruction

Review: Yes ❑ No ❑

---

44. The term meaning *below the lungs* is:
    A. subpulmonary.
    B. infrapulmonary.
    C. interpulmonary.
    D. interthoracic.
    E. intercostal.

Answer: **A**

Why: sub- = beneath, under
pulmon/o = lungs
-ary = pertaining to

Review: Yes ❑ No ❑

---

45. The term **cholecystitis** means inflammation of the:
    A. gallbladder.
    B. liver.
    C. adrenal glands.
    D. kidneys.

Answer: **A**

Why: chol/e = bile (gall)
cyst/o = bladder, sac
-itis = inflammation

Review: Yes ❑ No ❑

46. The term **stomatomycosis** means a condition of:
   A. fungus in the mouth.
   B. mucus in the mouth.
   C. fungus in the stomach.
   D. mucus in the stomach.
   E. inflammation of the mouth.

Answer: **A**

Why: stomat/o = mouth, opening
myc/o = fungus
-osis = condition

Review: Yes ❑ No ❑

---

47. The term for inflammation of the gums and tongue is:
   A. gingivoglossitis.
   B. stomatitis.
   C. glossopharyngitis.
   D. glossostomatitis.

Answer: **A**

Why: gingiv/o = gum tissue
gloss/o = tongue
-itis = inflammation

Review: Yes ❑ No ❑

---

48. The term meaning *incision of the abdominal wall* is:
   A. abdominocentesis.
   B. laparectomy.
   C. laparotomy.
   D. peritonitis.
   E. gastrotomy.

Answer: **C**

Why: lapar/o = abdomen, abdominal wall
-tomy = incision into

Review: Yes ❑ No ❑

---

49. The term meaning *behind the peritoneum* is:
   A. subperitoneal.
   B. retroperitoneal.
   C. subabdominal.
   D. intraperitoneal.

Answer: **B**

Why: retro- = located behind, backward
peritone/o = pertaining to the peritoneum
-al = pertaining to

Review: Yes ❑ No ❑

---

50. The term meaning *surgical repair of the* hands is:
   A. chiromegaly.
   B. dactylomegaly.
   C. chiroplasty.
   D. dactyloplasty.
   E. dactylitis.

Answer: **C**

Why: chir/o = pertaining to the hand
-plasty = surgical repair, plastic surgery

Review: Yes ❑ No ❑

---

51. A term meaning *stretching of the stomach* is:
   A. gastrectasia.
   B. gastralgia.
   C. gastrorrhagia.
   D. gastroplasty.

Answer: **A**

Why: gastr/o = stomach
-ectasia = dilation, stretching

Review: Yes ❑ No ❑

---

52. The term meaning *take away pain, free from pain* is:
   A. algesia.
   B. analgesia.
   C. angina.
   D. anesthesia.
   E. dysplasia.

Answer: **B**

Why: an- = without
-algesia = sensation of pain

Review: Yes ❑ No ❑

53. The term meaning *inflammation of the brain* is:
   A. meningitis.
   B. cephalgesia.
   C. encephalitis.
   D. encephalomeningitis.

Answer: **C**

Why: en- = within
cephal/o = head
-itis = inflammation

Review: Yes ❑ No ❑

---

54. The word root **dactyl/o** means:
   A. ear.
   B. foot.
   C. hand.
   D. eye.
   E. finger.

Answer: **E**

Why: dactyl/o = digit, finger or toe

Review: Yes ❑ No ❑

---

55. The term **dyskinesia** means:
   A. painful knee.
   B. difficult movement.
   C. deformed spine.
   D. curved spine.

Answer: **B**

Why: dys- = difficult, painful
kinesi/o = movement, motion
-ia = pertaining to

Review: Yes ❑ No ❑

---

56. The term meaning *increased heart rate (pulse)* is:
   A. tachycardia.
   B. bradycardia.
   C. hyperpnea.
   D. hypoxia.
   E. arrhythmia

Answer: **A**

Why: tachy- = rapid, fast
cardi/o = pertaining to the heart
-ia = pertaining to

Review: Yes ❑ No ❑

---

57. The term meaning *on one side* is:
   A. medial.
   B. bilateral.
   C. transverse.
   D. unilateral.

Answer: **D**

Why: uni- = one
later/o = side
-al = pertaining to

Review: Yes ❑ No ❑

---

58. The term **cyanosis** means:
   A. lack of oxygen.
   B. swelling of the feet.
   C. bluish condition.
   D. condition of red cells.
   E. obstructed airway.

Answer: **C**

Why: cyan/o = blue, discoloration
-osis = condition of

Review: Yes ❑ No ❑

---

59. The term **antipyretic** means:
   A. increased temperature.
   B. bacteria-reducing.
   C. fever-reducing.
   D. decreased pus formation.

Answer: **C**

Why: anti- = against
pyret/o = relating to fever
-ic = pertaining to

Review: Yes ❑ No ❑

60. The suffix meaning *the study of* is:
   A. -logist.
   B. -graphy.
   C. -logy.
   D. -scopy.
   E. -osis.

Answer: C

Why: -logy = study of, knowledge

Review: Yes ❑ No ❑

---

61. The term **cytology** means:
   A. person who studies cells.
   B. study of the bladder.
   C. measuring bladder contents.
   D. study of cells.

Answer: D

Why: cyt/o = cell
-logy = study of

Review: Yes ❑ No ❑

---

62. The term **leukopenia** means:
   A. increased platelets.
   B. decreased white cells.
   C. enlarged red cells.
   D. increased thrombocytes.
   E. increased white count.

Answer: B

Why: leuk/o = white (cells)
-penia = decrease, lack of

Review: Yes ❑ No ❑

---

63. The term meaning *thickening (hardening) of the arteries* is:
   A. phlebectasia.
   B. arteriorrhagia.
   C. arteriosclerosis.
   D. phlebotomy.

Answer: C

Why: arteri/o = artery
scler/o = thickening, hardening
-osis = condition of

Review: Yes ❑ No ❑

---

64. The prefix **ab-** means:
   A. against.
   B. before.
   C. toward.
   D. uneven.
   E. away from.

Answer: E

Why: ab- = away from, absent

Review: Yes ❑ No ❑

---

65. The prefix **peri-** means:
   A. middle.
   B. side.
   C. below.
   D. around.

Answer: D

Why: peri- = around, about

Review: Yes ❑ No ❑

---

66. The term **neuralgia** means:
   A. tumor of nerve cells/fibers.
   B. surgical removal of nerve fibers.
   C. pain in the nerves.
   D. numbness of nerves.
   E. twitching of nerves.

Answer: C

Why: neur/o = nerve, nerve cell
-algia = pain

Review: Yes ❑ No ❑

67. The term **cervicofacial** pertains to the:
    A. neck and arm.
    B. face and neck.
    C. spine and pelvis.
    D. face and scalp.

Answer: **B**

Why: cervic/o = neck, neck of an organ
facial = pertaining to the face

Review: Yes ❑ No ❑

---

68. A term meaning *destruction of kidney tissue* is:
    A. renopathy.
    B. nephropexy.
    C. nephralgia.
    D. pyelitis.
    E. nephrolysis.

Answer: **E**

Why: nephr/o = kidney
-lysis = destruction, breakdown

Review: Yes ❑ No ❑

---

69. The term **posteromedial** pertains to:
    A. upper back.
    B. lower back.
    C. middle back.
    D. toward the back.

Answer: **C**

Why: poster/o = back, backside
medi/o = the middle
-al = pertaining to

Review: Yes ❑ No ❑

---

70. The term **osteoarthropathy** means:
    A. bone inflammation.
    B. inflammation of joints.
    C. condition of swollen joints.
    D. disease of joints and bones.
    E. infection of the bones.

Answer: **D**

Why: oste/o = bone
arthr/o = joint
-pathy = disease process, disease

Review: Yes ❑ No ❑

---

71. The term **orchidectomy** means:
    A. surgical removal of a testicle.
    B. incision into the scrotum.
    C. undescended testicle.
    D. excision of the scrotum.

Answer: **A**

Why: orchid/o = relating to the testicle
-ectomy = surgical removal

Review: Yes ❑ No ❑

---

72. The term **adenoma** means:
    A. benign tumor.
    B. malignant tumor.
    C. tumor of a gland.
    D. pituitary disease.
    E. abnormal growth.

Answer: **C**

Why: aden/o = gland
-oma = tumor

Review: Yes ❑ No ❑

---

73. The term **mammoplasty** means:
    A. surgical reconstruction of the breast.
    B. excision of breast tumor.
    C. x-ray exam of the breasts.
    D. biopsy of breast tissue.

Answer: **A**

Why: mamm/o = breast
-plasty = plastic surgery, surgical reconstruction

Review: Yes ❑ No ❑

74. The term **adrenomegaly** means:
    A. pathology of a gland.
    B. destruction of tissue.
    C. enlargement of the adrenal gland(s).
    D. condition of the thyroid.
    E. inflammation of a gland.

Answer: **C**

Why: adren/o = adrenal gland(s)
-megaly = enlargement

Review: Yes ❑ No ❑

---

75. The term **gynecopathy** means:
    A. study of female reproductive system.
    B. specialist who studies women's diseases.
    C. inflammation of female organs.
    D. any disease of the female reproductive system.

Answer: **D**

Why: gynec/o = female
-pathy = any disease process

Review: Yes ❑ No ❑

---

76. A term meaning *an ingrown nail* is:
    A. onychectomy.
    B. onychalgia.
    C. onychitis.
    D. onychocryptosis.
    E. onychorrhea.

Answer: **D**

Why: onych/o = fingernail or toenail
crypt/o = hidden, concealed (ingrown)
-osis = any condition of

Review: Yes ❑ No ❑

---

77. The term meaning *excision of fatty tissue* is:
    A. lipolysis.
    B. lipoma.
    C. lipectomy.
    D. lipoidosis.

Answer: **C**

Why: lip/o = fat, fatty tissue
-ectomy = surgical removal, excision

Review: Yes ❑ No ❑

---

78. The term meaning *rupture of a vein* is:
    A. phleborrhagia.
    B. phlebopexy.
    C. phlebectasia.
    D. phleborrhexis.
    E. phlebitis.

Answer: **D**

Why: phleb/o = vein
-rrhexis = rupture

Review: Yes ❑ No ❑

---

79. The term **duodenoscopy** means:
    A. examination of the colon.
    B. inspection of the duodenum with a scope.
    C. make a new opening into the duodenum.
    D. incision into the colon.

Answer: **B**

Why: duoden/o = duodenum, part of small intestine
-scopy = to examine or inspect using an endoscope

Review: Yes ❑ No ❑

---

80. A term meaning *a painful tendon* is:
    A. tendonitis.
    B. tenotomy.
    C. tenodynia.
    D. tendoplasty.
    E. tenorrhaphy.

Answer: **C**

Why: ten/o = tendon, connects muscle to bone
-dynia = pain

Review: Yes ❑ No ❑

81. The term **dacryocystitis** means:
A. excision of a tear sac.
B. protrusion of a lacrimal sac.
C. pain in a lacrimal sac.
D. inflammation of a tear sac.

Answer: **D**

Why: dacry/o = tear (lacrimal)
cyst/o = sac, bladder
-itis = inflammation of

Review: Yes ❑ No ❑

---

82. The term **intracerebral** means:
A. between the spine and brain.
B. within the spinal cord.
C. beneath the meninges.
D. within the main part of the brain.
E. between the meninges.

Answer: **D**

Why: intra- = within
cerebr/o = cerebrum, main part of the brain
-al = pertaining to

Review: Yes ❑ No ❑

---

83. The term meaning *condition of fungus of the nails* is:
A. dermatomycosis.
B. onychomycosis.
C. dermatosis.
D. onychitis.

Answer: **B**

Why: onych/o = finger or toe nail
myc/o = fungus
-osis = any condition

Review: Yes ❑ No ❑

---

84. The term meaning *death of tissue or bone* is:
A. necrosis.
B. necropsy.
C. necrophilia.
D. necrotomy.
E. necrectomy.

Answer: **A**

Why: necr/o = death, dead cells or tissue
-osis = any condition

Review: Yes ❑ No ❑

---

85. The term meaning *passing from front to rear* is:
A. anterosuperior.
B. anteroexternal.
C. anteroinferior.
D. anteroposterior.

Answer: **D**

Why: anter/o = anterior, front, before
poster/o = back, rear

Review: Yes ❑ No ❑

---

86. The term **aplasia** means:
A. decreased plasma.
B. lack of formation.
C. difficulty breathing.
D. without pulse.
E. painful breathing.

Answer: **B**

Why: a- = without, not
-plasia = development, formation

Review: Yes ❑ No ❑

---

87. The term **endocarditis** means:
A. infection of the heart valves.
B. heart attack.
C. inflammation of the inside lining of the heart.
D. aneurysm within the heart.

Answer: **C**

Why: endo- = inside, innermost
cardi/o = heart
-itis = inflammation of

Review: Yes ❑ No ❑

88. The term **pyeloplasty** means:
    A. surgical repair of the renal pelvis.
    B. plastic surgery of the kidney.
    C. incision into the kidney.
    D. excision of the renal pelvis.
    E. surgical repair of the pelvis.

Answer: **A**

Why: pyel/o = pelvis, renal pelvis
-plasty = surgical repair

Review: Yes ❑ No ❑

---

89. The term meaning *below normal temperature* is:
    A. hypoxia.
    B. hypotensive.
    C. hypothermia.
    D. hypotrophy.

Answer: **C**

Why: hypo- = below, sub, less than normal
therm/o = temperature
-ia = pertaining to

Review: Yes ❑ No ❑

---

90. The term **hysterorrhaphy** means:
    A. rupture of the uterus.
    B. removal of the cervix.
    C. suturing of the uterus.
    D. surgical fixation of the cervix.
    E. incision into the cervix.

Answer: **C**

Why: hyster/o = uterus
-rrhaphy = suturing, sewing

Review: Yes ❑ No ❑

---

91. The term **proctorrhagia** means
    A. rupture of the rectum.
    B. fissure of the anus.
    C. inflammation of the rectum.
    D. hemorrhage from the rectum.

Answer: **D**

Why: proct/o = rectum and anus
-rrhagia = hemorrhage, burst forth

Review: Yes ❑ No ❑

---

92. The term for *disease of the retina* is:
    A. renopathy.
    B. retinitis.
    C. retinoplasty.
    D. renography.
    E. retinopathy.

Answer: **E**

Why: retin/o = retina of the eye
-pathy = disease process

Review: Yes ❑ No ❑

---

93. The term meaning *herniation of the meninges* is:
    A. meningomyelocele.
    B. myelocele.
    C. meningocele.
    D. encephalocele.

Answer: **C**

Why: mening/o = meninges
-cele = herniation, protrusion

Review: Yes ❑ No ❑

---

94. The term meaning *suppression of menses* is:
    A. menstruation.
    B. menorrhagia.
    C. menorrhea.
    D. menostasis.
    E. dysmenorrhea.

Answer: **D**

Why: men/o = menstruation, menses
-stasis = control, suppress

Review: Yes ❑ No ❑

95. The term meaning *across the chest* is:
  A. anterolateral.
  B. transverse.
  C. transthorax.
  D. anterothoracic.

Answer: **C**

Why: trans- = across, cross over
thorax = pertaining to the chest

Review: Yes ❑ No ❑

---

96. The term meaning *excessive formation of cells or tissue* is:
  A. hyperphasia.
  B. hyperplasia.
  C. hypertonic.
  D. hyperopia.
  E. hypotonic.

Answer: **B**

Why: hyper- = excessive, more than normal
-plasia = formation

Review: Yes ❑ No ❑

---

97. The term **pyogenesis** means:
  A. growth of cells.
  B. formation of pus.
  C. production of bile.
  D. origin of a fever.

Answer: **B**

Why: py/o = pus
-genesis = beginning, formation

Review: Yes ❑ No ❑

---

98. The term **hemiplegia** means:
  A. inflammation of the lower legs.
  B. moving one half of the body.
  C. paralysis of upper body.
  D. paralysis of one half of the body.
  E. paralysis of one leg.

Answer: **D**

Why: hemi- = half, one half
-plegia = pertaining to paralysis

Review: Yes ❑ No ❑

---

99. The term **nasopharyngeal** means pertaining to:
  A. nose and sinuses.
  B. mouth and throat.
  C. nose and throat.
  D. mouth and sinuses.

Answer: **C**

Why: nas/o = nose
pharyng/o = pharynx, throat
-al = pertaining to

Review: Yes ❑ No ❑

---

100. The term **neurotripsy** means:
  A. removal of a nerve.
  B. surgical crushing of a nerve.
  C. suturing of a nerve.
  D. paralysis of a nerve.
  E. rupture of a nerve.

Answer: **B**

Why: neur/o = nerve, nerve cell
-tripsy = surgically crushing

Review: Yes ❑ No ❑

---

101. Select the correct spelling of the term:
  A. hemmorrhoid.
  B. hemorrhoid.
  C. hemmorhoid.
  D. hemorhoid.
  E. hemorroid.

Answer: **B**

Review: Yes ❑ No ❑

102. Scraping of a body cavity is:
   A. curretage.
   B. currettage.
   C. curetage.
   D. curettage.

Answer: **D**

Review: Yes ❑ No ❑

---

103. Inflammation of the tonsils is:
   A. tonsillitis.
   B. tonsilitis.
   C. tonsilittis.
   D. tonssilitis.
   E. tonsillittis.

Answer: **A**

Review: Yes ❑ No ❑

6

Anatomy and Physiology

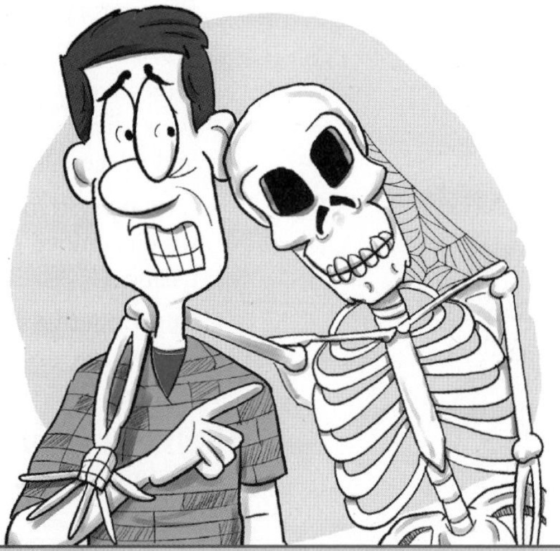

REVIEW TIP

Anatomy and Physiology is the most demanding chapter but one that provides a feeling of accomplishment when you have completed it. Study all the figures and tables. The national exams generally contain at least two questions on each body system. The endocrine system, with the glands and hormones, tends to be the most difficult. (Remember, during the exam, do not s pend too much time on any one question.) Schedule your study time by body system. Limit the number you tackle at each session. Reward yourself when you finish this chapter!

OVERVIEW

Knowledge of anatomy and physiology is a foundation for many areas of medical assisting and medical administrative specialization. It is used in both administrative (e.g., insurance billing and coding) and clinical practice (e.g., patient assessment). With a solid understanding of the structure and function of body parts, you will be able to analyze questions and to solve problems.

Anatomy—the study of body structure

Physiology—the study of body function

Pathology—the study of abnormal changes in body structure or function, usually caused by disease

BODY ORDERING

Living things are arranged from simple to complex. Figure 6-1 demonstrates the order of the structures that make up the human body.

- Chemicals—atoms and molecules
- Cells—structural and functional units of life
- Tissues—groups of cells with similar structures and functions (such as connective tissue)
- Organ—group of tissues working together to perform a function (e.g., kidney)
- Systems—group of organs working together to perform a set of related functions

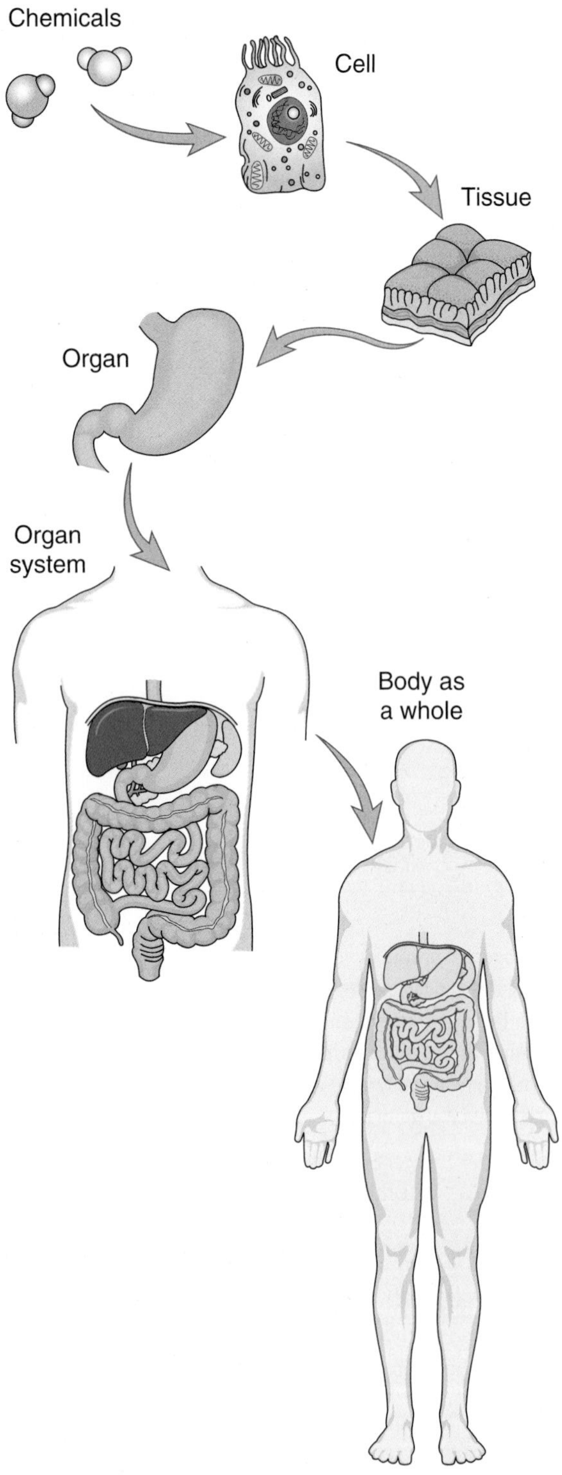

Figure 6-1 Body ordering. (Reprinted with permission from Cohen BJ, Wood DL. Memmler's The Human Body in Health and Disease. 9th Ed. Philadelphia: Lippincott Williams & Wilkins, 2000.)

- Integumentary system—skin and related structures that contain and protect
- Skeletal system—bones and related structures that support
- Muscular system—muscles and related structures that accommodate movement
- Nervous system—nerves and related structures that receive stimuli and initiate responses
- Sensory system—sensory neurons and special sense organs that detect the environment and changes
- Endocrine system—glands and related structures that produce hormones
- Cardiovascular system—heart and blood vessels that circulate blood to transport nutrients and remove waste from tissues
- Lymphatic system—lymph, lymph nodes, and related organs that protect against and fight disease
- Respiratory system—lungs and related structures that transport oxygen (O_2) and remove carbon dioxide (CO_2)
- Digestive system—mouth, esophagus, stomach, intestines, liver, gallbladder, and pancreas, which ingest and process food and eliminate solid waste products
- Urinary system—kidneys, ureters, bladder, and urethra, which remove nitrogen-type waste and regulate water balance
- Reproductive system—gonads (ovaries or testes) and related sex organs and structures that reproduce the species

■ Body (organism)—group of systems working together to maintain life

ANATOMIC DESCRIPTORS

The national exams contain several questions related to the location of specific organs and other anatomic structures. Directional terms of the body help describe and locate these structures.

Body Directions and Planes

Figure 6-2 shows the imaginary planes dividing the body: the **frontal** (or coronal) **plane**, the **sagittal plane**, and the **transverse** (or horizontal) **plane**. The body is in anatomic position—upright, face forward, and arms down and slightly away from the sides with palms forward and feet and legs parallel. Other important descriptors of body directions are as follows: **superior** (cranial or cephalic), **anterior** (ventral), **posterior** (dorsal), **inferior** (caudal), **proximal**, **distal**, **medial**, and **lateral**.

Body Cavities

The locations of organs are usually described as being in a specific body cavity or space. Directional terms (e.g., posterior, anterior, inferior) are used to determine the position in relation to other organs also found in that cavity. Figure 6-3 illustrates the following body cavities:

■ Cranial cavity—contains the brain

■ Spinal cavity—contains the spinal cord; runs continuously from the brainstem in the cranial cavity to the end of the spinal cord

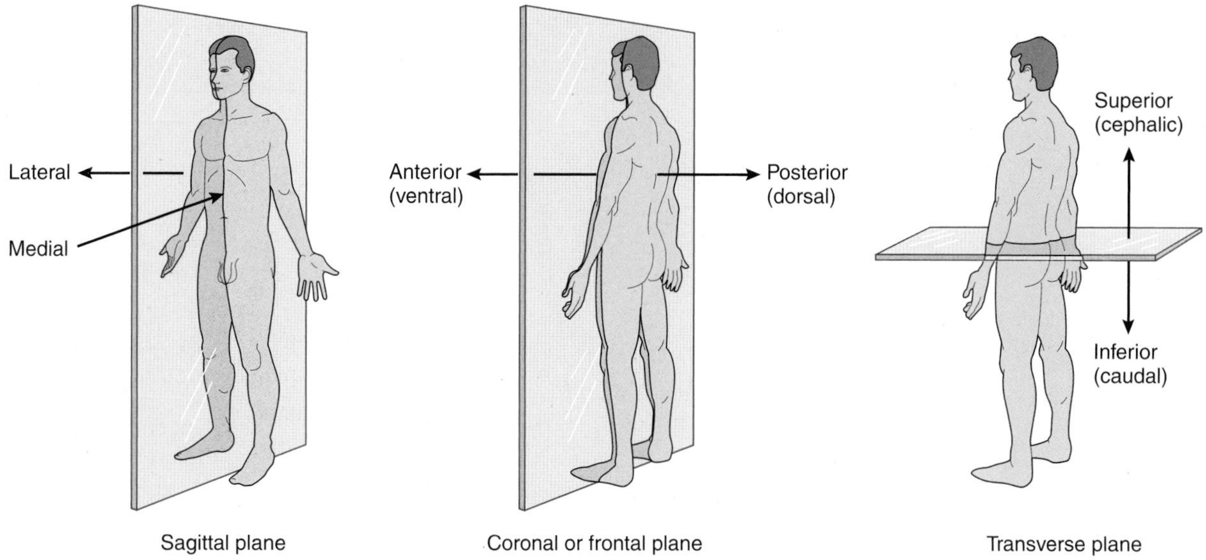

Figure 6-2 Body planes and directions. (Reprinted with permission from Willis MC, CMA-AC. Medical Terminology: A Programmed Learning Approach to the Language of Health Care. Baltimore: Lippincott Williams & Wilkins, 2002.)

- Thoracic cavity—contains the heart, lung, and large blood vessels; it is separated from the abdominal cavity by the diaphragm; within the thoracic cavity lies the mediastinum, a smaller cavity between the lungs that contains the heart and large blood vessels
- Abdominal cavity—contains the stomach, most of the intestines, the kidneys, liver, gallbladder, pancreas, and spleen; it is separated from the thoracic cavity (superior) by the diaphragm and from the pelvic cavity (inferior) by an imaginary line across the top of the hip bones
- Pelvic cavity—contains the urinary bladder, rectum, and internal organs of the male/female reproductive systems; it is separated from the abdominal cavity (superior) by an imaginary line between the hip bones

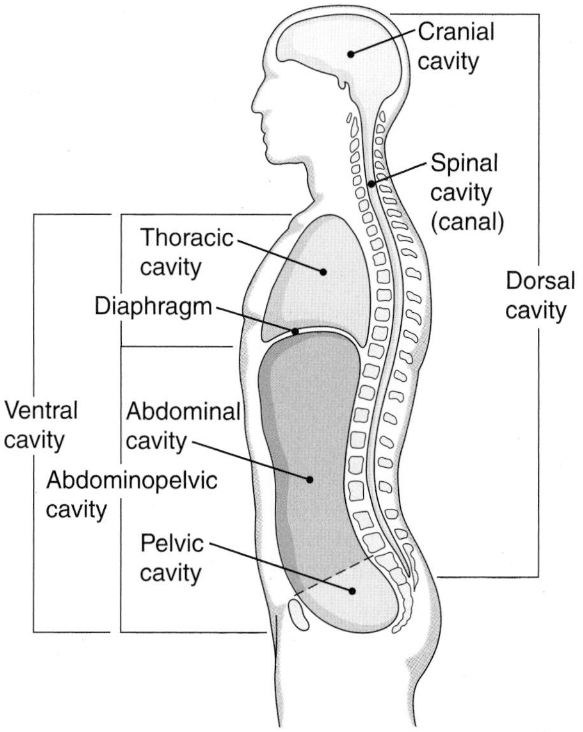

Figure 6-3 Body cavities. (Reprinted with permission from Cohen BJ, Wood DL. Memmler's The Human Body in Health and Disease. 9th Ed. Philadelphia: Lippincott Williams & Wilkins, 2000.)

Abdominal Quadrants and Regions

The abdomen is divided into four quadrants (right upper, left upper, right lower, and left lower) and nine regions (right hypochondriac, epigastric, left hypochondriac, right lumbar, umbilical, left lumbar, right iliac, hypogastric, and left iliac), as shown in Figure 6-4. Box 6-1 lists additional anatomic descriptors used to locate or describe the location of many body structures.

BASIC BODY PROCESSES

For the body to grow, repair itself, and maintain equilibrium, certain processes must occur. Metabolism, fluid balance, and homeostasis are basic processes that take place or begin at the cell level.

Metabolism

Metabolism is energy transformation in living cells. This transformation occurs in two metabolic processes:

- Anabolism—builds up and repairs cells
- Catabolism—breaks down cells

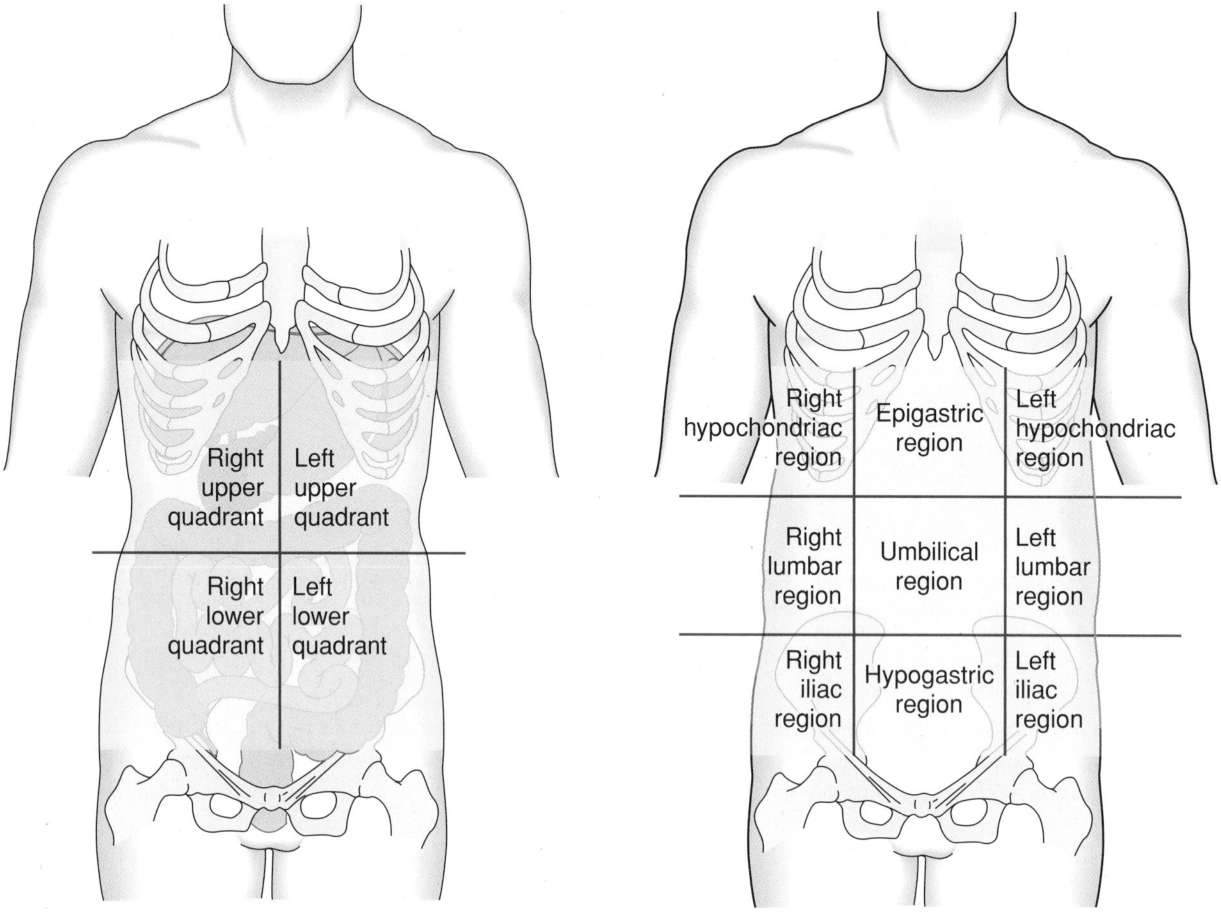

Figure 6-4 Abdominal divisions. **A.** Quadrants. **B.** Regions. (Reprinted with permission from Cohen BJ, Wood DL. Memmler's The Human Body in Health and Disease. 9th Ed. Philadelphia: Lippincott Williams & Wilkins, 2000.)

Box 6-1

Additional Anatomic Descriptors

Antebrachial: forearm
Axillary: armpit
Buccal: cheek
Celiac: abdominal
Cervical: neck or
Cranial: skull
Femoral: thigh
Inguinal: groin
Mammary: breast
Ophthalmic: eyes
Palmar: palm
Pectoral: chest
Plantar: sole of foot
Sacral: lower spine
Umbilical: navel
Antecubital: area anterior to elbow
Brachial: upper arm
Carpal: wrist
Cephalic: head
Costal: ribs female cervix
Cutaneous: skin
Gluteal: buttocks
Lumbar: lower back area
Occipital: lower posterior area of head
Otic: ears
Patellar: kneecap
Pedal: foot
Popliteal: back of knee
Tarsal: ankle
Vertebral: spine

Fluid Balance

Fluid balance is the regulation of the amount and composition of the body's fluids. The two major divisions of body fluid are:

- Extracellular fluid—body fluid outside the cell
- Intracellular fluid—body fluid inside the cell

The concentration of the fluid affects fluid movement and balance. The three basic solution concentrations are:

- Isotonic solution—this has the same concentration as intracellular fluid and moves in and out of the cell at the same rate; normal saline (0.9% salt) and 5% dextrose are examples of manufactured isotonic solutions
- Hypotonic solution—less concentrated than intracellular fluid, it results in excess fluid entering the cell and may cause the cell to rupture
- Hypertonic solution—more concentrated than intracellular fluid, it draws fluid away from the cell and causes the cell to shrink

Homeostasis

Homeostasis is the equilibrium or health of the body as measured by established norms for blood pressure, heart rate, temperature, respiratory rate, and other indicators.

BODY COMPOSITION

As previously noted, the body has an ordering of structures from simple to complex. Each type of structure (such as cells or tissues) has its own components or pieces, which are described in this section.

CELLS

Cells vary in size, shape, and function, but most cells contain the same basic components. Some of these components are shown in Figure 6-5.

- Cell (plasma) membrane—thin outermost layer of the cell; regulates what enters and leaves the cell
- Cytoplasm—colloidal substance (protoplasm) found in the cell; holds other structures in place
- Nuclear membrane—thin layer surrounding the nucleus
- Nucleus—located in the center of the cell; controls cell activity and contains genetic material (DNA)
- Nucleolus—small structure(s) in nucleus; holds ribonucleic acid (RNA) and ribosomes essential for protein formation

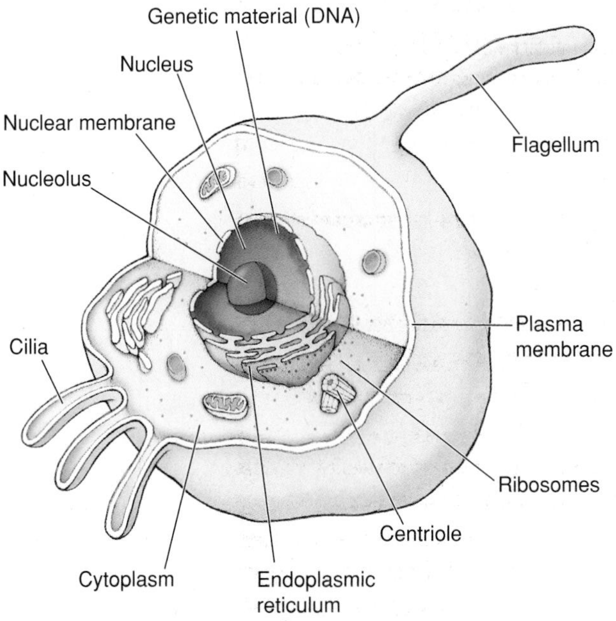

Figure 6-5 Basic animal cell with select structures.

- Centriole—rod-shaped material in the cytoplasm that begins cell division
- Cilia (singular *cilium*)—hairlike processes on the cell surface that move foreign particles along the cell surface
- Flagella (singular *flagellum*)—whiplike processes on the cell surface; accommodate cell movement

Cell Division

Cell division occurs when one cell splits into two identical cells. The process is as follows:

- Interphase—DNA duplicates and chromosomes double
- Mitosis—also referred to as cell division; comprises four phases:
  - Prophase—centrioles move to opposite ends of the cell, forming two poles; they stretch filaments between them, resembling longitudes on a globe
  - Metaphase—chromosomes line up along an equator-type line along centriole filaments
  - Anaphase—duplicated chromosomes separate, and one of each begins to move toward the opposite centriole or pole
  - Telophase—nucleus divides in the center, forming two distinct cells

Cellular Movement of Substances

The maintenance of homeostasis and fluid balance and the process of metabolism require constant movement of nutrients into the cell and the elimination of waste products from the cell. The movement occurs at the cell or plasma membrane. It is semipermeable, meaning it allows passage of some substances but not others. The types of movement are categorized either as not requiring or requiring cell energy.

- Movement without cellular energy
  - Diffusion—movement of molecules from area of higher to lower concentration
  - Osmosis—water diffusion (movement from area of higher to lower concentration) through a semipermeable membrane
  - Filtration—process of pushing water with dissolved materials through one side of a membrane; an example is kidney filtration
- Movement with cellular energy
  - Active transport—movement of molecules from area of lower to higher concentration
  - Phagocytosis—ingestion and digestion of bacteria and other substances by phagocytic cells

TISSUES

The body contains different types of **tissues** found in the diverse organs and systems. The study of tissue is called **histology**.

- Epithelial tissue—forms the outer surface of the body; lines body cavities and major tubes and passageways that open to the exterior
  - Cells—squamous (flat and irregular), cuboidal (square), or columnar (long and narrow)
  - Layers—simple (one layer) or stratified (more than one layer)
- Connective tissue—supports and connects other tissues and structures
  - Soft—areolar, adipose
  - Fibrous—tendons, ligaments, capsules, fascia
  - Hard—cartilage, bone
  - Liquid—blood, lymph
- Muscle tissue—produces movement
  - Skeletal muscle—moves muscle and bone (voluntary)
  - Cardiac muscle—forms the heart (involuntary)
  - Smooth muscle—forms visceral organs (involuntary)
- Nerve tissue—composed of neurons (nerve cells); provides networks to carry impulses

MEMBRANES

Membranes are thin sheets of tissue that line and protect body structures.

Epithelial Membranes

- Serous membranes—secrete watery fluid
  - Parietal membranes—line body cavities
  - Visceral membranes—cover internal organs (pleura and pericardium are examples)
- Mucous membranes—secrete mucus and line tubes or spaces open to the exterior
- Cutaneous membrane—the skin

Connective Tissue Membranes

- Synovial membranes—line joint cavities
- Meninges—surround the brain and spinal cord and are composed of three layers
- Fascia membranes—separate or bind muscles and permit movement of the skin
- Other connective tissue membranes:
  - Pericardium—surrounds heart
  - Periosteum—surrounds bone
  - Perichondrium—surrounds cartilage

BODY SYSTEMS

The chapter overview describes a *system* as a group of organs working together to perform a set of related functions. The human body comprises 12 interrelated systems and is described in detail in this section.

INTEGUMENTARY SYSTEM

Integumentary comes from the Greek word *integument*, meaning "cover." The **integumentary system** is the largest system in the body.

Functions of the Integumentary System

- Protects against infection and other "invaders" (e.g., radiation)
- Assists with prevention of dehydration
- Controls body temperature
- Receives sensory information
- Eliminates waste products
- Produces vitamin D

Components of the Integumentary System

- Skin—the largest organ; external covering of the body (Fig. 6-6)
  - Epidermis—the surface layer of the skin that contains strata (sublayers), melanin (pigment giving the skin its color), and keratin (protein that thickens skin and makes skin waterproof)
  - Dermis—the deeper layer of the skin that contains nerves, blood vessels, collagen, and other skin

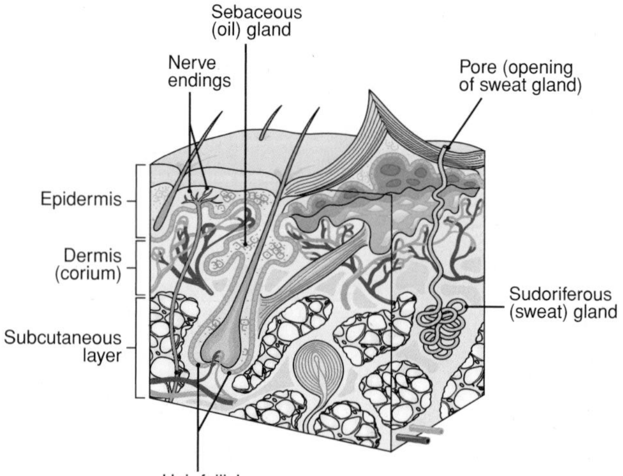

Figure 6-6 Cross section of skin. (Reprinted with permission from Cohen BJ, Wood DL. Memmler's The Human Body in Health and Disease. 9th Ed. Philadelphia: Lippincott Williams & Wilkins, 2000.)

structures or appendages. Collagen is a fibrous protein found in the dermis, connective tissues, tendons, and ligaments. It is sometimes referred to as the body's glue, providing strength and flexibility.

- Appendages—structures located in the dermis that perform special functions
  - Sweat glands—coiled tubes located in the dermis that produce and transport sweat to help regulate body temperature and remove waste
  - Ceruminous glands—structures located in the ear that secrete cerumen (earwax) for protection
  - Sebaceous glands—structures connected to hair follicles located in the dermis that secrete sebum to lubricate skin and hair
  - Hair—structures composed primarily of dead keratinized tissue that cover most of body
  - Nails—hard, keratinized structures located on tips of fingers and toes
  - Subcutaneous tissue—layer of tissue below the dermis composed of adipose and elastic fibers that connects the dermis to muscle surfaces

Common Diseases and Disorders of the Integumentary System

- Burns—tissue damage from exposure to heat, chemicals, or electricity
  - First degree (superficial)—involves the epidermis; has a red appearance with minimal or no edema
  - Second degree (partial thickness)—involves the epidermis and part of dermis; has a blistered red appearance with edema
  - Third degree (full thickness)—involves epidermis, entire dermis, and often the underlying tissues; has a pale white or charred appearance with broken skin and edema
- Carcinoma—skin cancer
  - Basal cell carcinoma—malignant disease of the basal cell layer of skin
  - Squamous cell carcinoma—malignant disease of the squamous cell layer of skin; more likely to metastasize than basal cell
  - Melanoma—highly malignant nevus (mole)

Other common diseases and disorders of the integumentary system appear in Box 6-2.

SKELETAL SYSTEM

The **skeletal system** is the framework of the body. The human skeleton is composed of **206 bones,** cartilage, and ligaments.

Box 6-2

Common Skin Diseases and Disorders

Abrasion—scrape
Acne—inflammation of sebaceous glands
Albinism—abnormal absence of pigment in skin, hair, and eyes
Alopecia—baldness
Avulsion—tearing away from body structure
Cyst—a sac containing a liquid
Decubitus—bedsore; ulceration resulting from pressure and poor circulation
Dermatitis—inflammation of the skin characterized by pruritus (itching), erythema (redness), and lesions
Eczema—form of dermatitis with a combination of vesicles and dry, leathery patches
Eschar—scab
Excoriation—abrasion (scrape) of the epidermis
Fissure—furrow, crack, groove, or crevice
Furuncle—boil
Herpes simplex—cold sore or fever blister
Herpes zoster (shingles)—painful vesicles along peripheral nerve tracts caused by the herpes zoster virus, which also causes varicella (chickenpox)
Impetigo—bacterial infection, usually around the mouth and nose, caused by staphylococci or streptococci; dry to crusty vesicles
Lesion—abnormal change in localized tissue caused by injury or disease
Macule—small spot or colored area (such as a freckle)
Nevus (mole)—raised congenital spot on skin surface
Papule—pimple
Pediculosis—infestation with lice
Psoriasis—chronic inflammatory skin disease characterized by scaly red patches on body surface
Pustule—pus- or lymph-filled vesicle
Scleroderma—disease causing thickened, rigid skin
Tinea corporis—ringworm; fungal infection
Tinea pedis—athlete's foot; fungal infection
Ulcer—open lesion on the skin or mucous membrane
Urticaria—hives
Verruca—wart
Vesicle—blisterlike sac on the skin
Vitiligo—skin disease with white milky patches surrounded by normal pigmentation
Wheal—round, elevated skin lesion with white center and red periphery

Functions of the Skeletal System

- Provides frame and strength to the body
- Produces body movement
- Provides protection for organs (e.g., the skull protects the brain)
- Serves as storehouse for calcium (Ca) salts
- Produces blood cells in the bone marrow

Components of the Skeletal System

- Bone—hard connective tissue impregnated with a calcium substance (206 bones in the adult skeleton)
- Cartilage—firm connective tissue found primarily in joints, thorax walls, larynx, airway passages, and ears
- Ligaments—bands of fibrous connective tissue that connect the articulating ends of bones to facilitate or limit movement; **do not confuse ligaments with tendons, which connect muscle to bone**
- Joints—areas where two or more bones come together or articulate, such as the knee, shoulder, and neck (see Box 6-3, which describes joint movements)

Box 6-3
Joint Movements

Abduction—moving away from the body midline (the opposite of adduction) (e.g., spreading the arms)
Adduction—moving toward the body midline (the opposite of abduction) (e.g., bringing the arms to the sides)
Circumduction—drawing an imaginary circle with a body structure (e.g., the arms)
Eversion—turning wrists or ankles outward, away from the body (the opposite of inversion), such as turning the foot away from the body
Extension—bringing the limbs or phalanges toward a straight position (the opposite of flexion), such as opening the fingers of a closed hand
Flexion—bending (the opposite of extension), such as closing the fingers of the hand
Hyperextension—extreme or abnormal extension, usually resulting in injury (e.g., dislocated finger)
Inversion—turning inside out (the opposite of eversion), such as turning the heels out so toes face each other
Plantar flexion—pointing toes downward, which flexes the arch of the foot (e.g., en pointe dancing in ballet)
Rotation—turning on an axis, such as turning the head to indicate "No"

Organization of the Skeletal System

The major bones are illustrated in Figure 6-7. These bones are divided into the axial segment and the appendicular segment.

Axial Skeleton

The **axial** segment of the skeleton consists of the bones of the skull, spine, and chest.

- Cranium—skull (Fig. 6-8)
  - Frontal—forehead
  - Parietal—sides and top
  - Temporal—lower sides
  - Mastoid process—lower portion of the temporal bone
  - Styloid process—projection inferior to the external ear
  - Zygomatic process—upper cheek
  - Occipital—base of the skull, contains the foramen magnum (the opening in the skull that connects the spinal cord to the brain)
  - Sphenoid—bat-shaped, lateral eye orbits
  - Ethmoid—bony area between the nasal cavity and the orbits
- Facial—14 bones form the face (major bones are listed in Fig. 6-8)
  - Nasal—two bones that form the bridge of the nose
  - Zygomatic—arch of the cheek
  - Mandible—lower jaw
  - Maxilla—upper jaw
- Vertebral column (spine)—26 vertebrae (bones) that cover the spinal cord (Fig. 6-9)
  - Cervical vertebrae (7 vertebrae)—neck bones; the first is called the *atlas* (supports the head); the second is called the *axis* (pivot for the head)
  - Thoracic vertebrae (12 vertebrae)—chest; attaches to the posterior portion of ribs
  - Lumbar vertebrae (5 vertebrae)—small of back; heavier and larger than other vertebrae
  - Sacrum (1 vertebra)—posterior of bony pelvis located between the two hip bones
  - Coccyx (1 vertebra)—tailbone
- Thorax—rib cage
  - Ribs—12 pair of bones that make up the thorax; the bars of the cage
  - Sternum—breast bone that, with the ribs, protects the heart
    - Manubrium—top of the breast bone that joins with the clavicle and first ribs
    - Xiphoid process—small tip at the lower end of the sternum

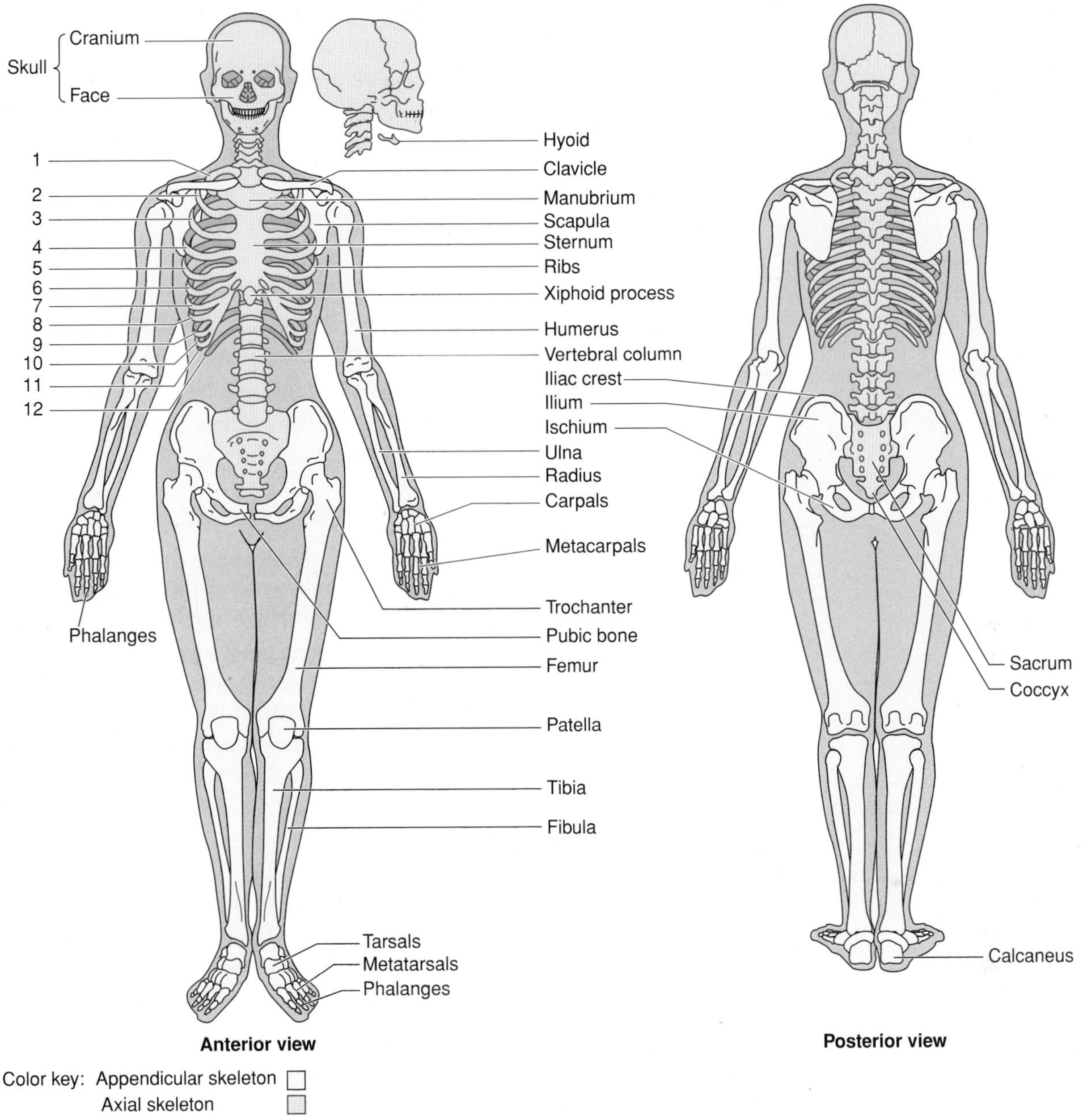

Figure 6-7 Human skeleton. (Reprinted with permission from Willis MC, CMA-AC. Medical Terminology: A Programmed Learning Approach to the Language of Health Care. Baltimore: Lippincott Williams & Wilkins, 2002.)

Appendicular Skeleton

The **appendicular skeleton** consists of the bones of the upper and lower extremities and the girdles attaching them to the axial skeleton portion.

- Shoulder girdle
  - Clavicle—collar bone, which joins the sternum at the anterior and the scapula laterally
  - Scapula—shoulder blade
- Upper extremities—arms, hands, fingers, and thumbs
  - Humerus—upper arm (largest arm bone)
  - Radius—lateral bone of forearm (in anatomic position, thumb side)
  - Ulna—medial bone of forearm (in anatomic position)
  - Carpals—the four bones that make up the wrist
  - Metacarpals—the five bones of the palm of the hand
  - Phalanges—fingers (three bones each) and thumbs (two bones each)
- Pelvic girdle—attaches lower extremities to axial skeleton
  - Ilium—superior wing-shaped portions of hip bones

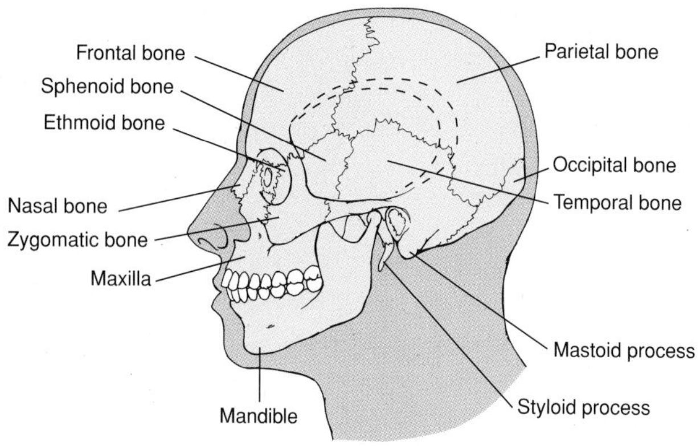

Figure 6-8 The adult skull. (Reprinted with permission from Oatis CA. Kinesiology: The Mechanics and Pathomechanics of Human Movement. Baltimore: Lippincott Williams & Wilkins, 2003.)

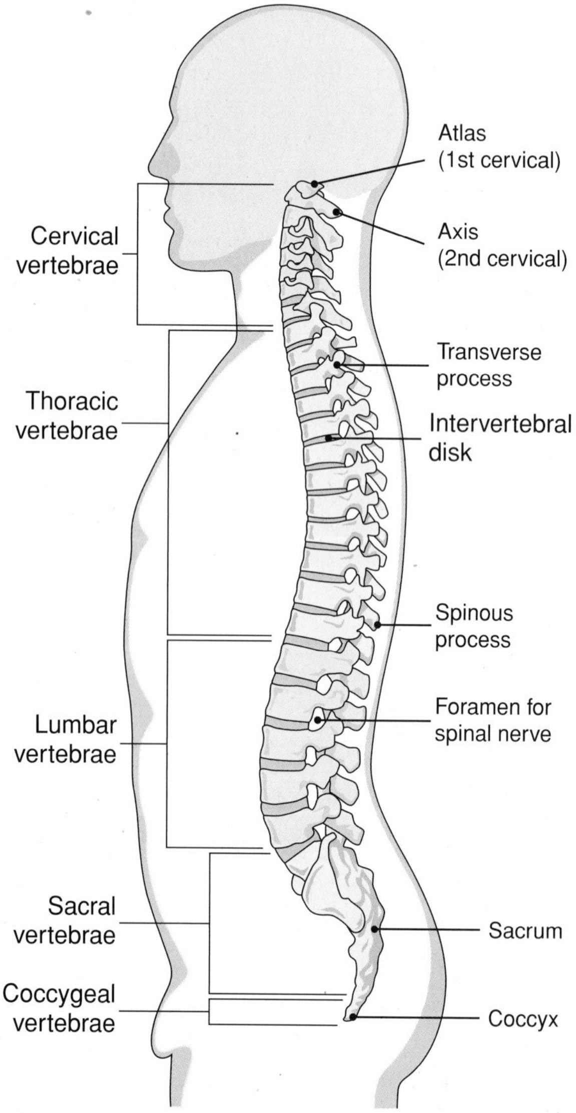

Figure 6-9 Adult vertebral column. (Reprinted with permission from Cohen BJ, Wood DL. Memmler's The Human Body in Health and Disease. 9th Ed. Philadelphia: Lippincott Williams & Wilkins, 2000.)

- Ischium—inferior portion of hip bones that supports weight when sitting
- Pubis—anterior union of the hip bones

■ Lower extremities—legs, feet, and toes

- Femur—thigh bone; **the body's largest, longest, and strongest bone**
- Patella—kneecap
- Tibia—shin bone
- Fibula—smaller leg bone, lateral to tibia
- Tarsals—the seven ankle and foot bones (largest is the calcaneus, or heel bone)
- Metatarsals—the five foot bones
- Phalanges—toe bones (three bones each), great toes (two bones each)

Common Diseases and Disorders of the Skeletal System

■ Congenital or developmental disorders—skeletal abnormalities resulting from birth defects or occurrences during the developmental stages

- Cleft palate—congenital deformity caused by a malunion of the maxilla, leaving an opening in the roof of the mouth (palate)
- Spina bifida—congenital deformity caused by malformation of vertebrae that exposes the spinal column
- Scoliosis—abnormal lateral curvature of the vertebral column
- Kyphosis (hunchback)—an excessive curvature in the thoracic portion of the vertebral column
- Lordosis (swayback)—excessive curvature in the lumbar portion of the vertebral column

Note: Know the differences between scoliosis, kyphosis, and lordosis.

- Rickets—structural deformities of the bone resulting from lack of vitamin D

■ Arthritis—inflammation of the joints

- Osteoarthritis—degenerative joint disease resulting in deformities and chronic pain; usually occurs as part of the aging process, but excessive joint use (such as long-distance running) and trauma are also contributory factors
- Rheumatoid arthritis—inflammation and overgrowth of synovial membranes and joint tissues characterized by swelling of joints, usually occurring in young adults
- Gout—inflammation and pain, usually of the great toes or thumbs, caused by accumulation of uric acid crystals; the highest incidence occurs in late-middle-aged men
- Septic arthritis—serious bloodstream bacterial infection attacking the joints; common pathogens are *Streptococcus*, *Staphylococcus*, and tuberculosis

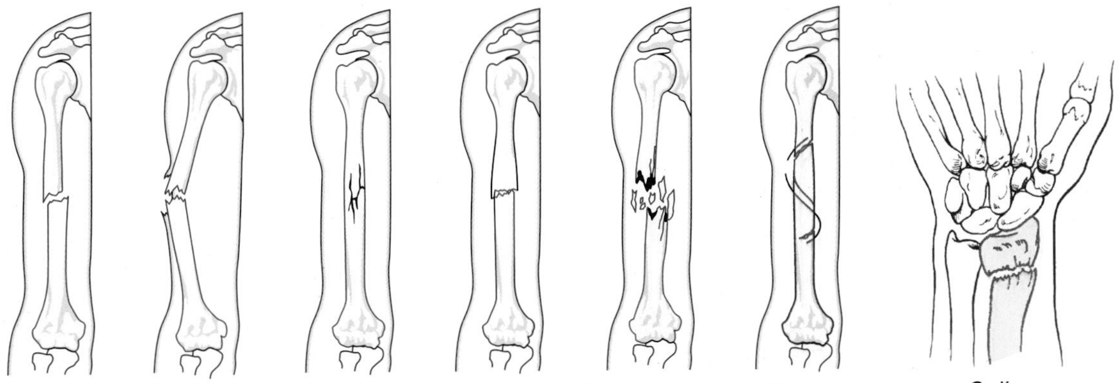

Figure 6-10 Types of fractures.

- Fractures—a break or rupture in the bone; Figure 6-10 illustrates the following types of fractures:
  - Simple—closed fracture with no open wound
  - Compound—open fracture with an external wound
  - Greenstick—incomplete break or a bending of the bone, usually in children
  - Impacted—broken ends of the bone are forced into each other
  - Comminuted—splintering or crushing of the bone with several fragments
  - Spiral—fracture caused by a twisting motion
  - Colles—displaced fracture of the distal radius, proximal to the wrist
- Neoplasms—tumors
  - Malignant—cancerous tumors (e.g., osteosarcoma, osteochondroma)
  - Nonmalignant—benign tumors such as cysts
  - Osteomyelitis—inflammation of the bone or marrow caused by pathogens
  - Osteoporosis—porous, brittle bones resulting from low levels of calcium salts; common in menopausal women

MUSCULAR SYSTEM

The **muscular system** contains approximately 650 muscles that make up the general form of the body.

Functions of the Muscular System

- Produces body movement through chemical reactions at cellular level
- Maintains body posture and alignment
- Protects bones and internal organs
- Generates heat

Muscle Traits

- Excitability—receive and respond to a stimulus
- Contractility—shorten
- Extensibility—stretch or lengthen
- Elasticity—return to original length after shortening or lengthening

Types of Muscle Tissues

- Smooth muscle—forms the walls of hollow organs, blood vessels, and respiratory passages; moves substances through the systems (involuntary); striated
- Skeletal muscle—attached to bones, moves muscle and bones (voluntary)
- Cardiac muscle—forms the wall of heart, creates pumping action of the heart (involuntary); striated

Components of the Muscular System

- Muscles—tissue made up of contractile fibers that effect movement of organs and body parts; Figure 6-11 illustrates anterior and posterior muscles
- Tendons—**connective tissue that attaches muscle directly to the periosteum (covering) of the bone**
- Aponeurosis—broad sheet that attaches muscle to muscle or muscle to select bones, such as the skull
- Synapses—neuromuscular junctions transmitting messages from the nerves that stimulate muscles to act

Body Mechanics

- Lever—bone acts as fixed bar moving around a pivot
- Fulcrum—joint acts as pivot to the bone
- Force—muscle contracts and pulls bone

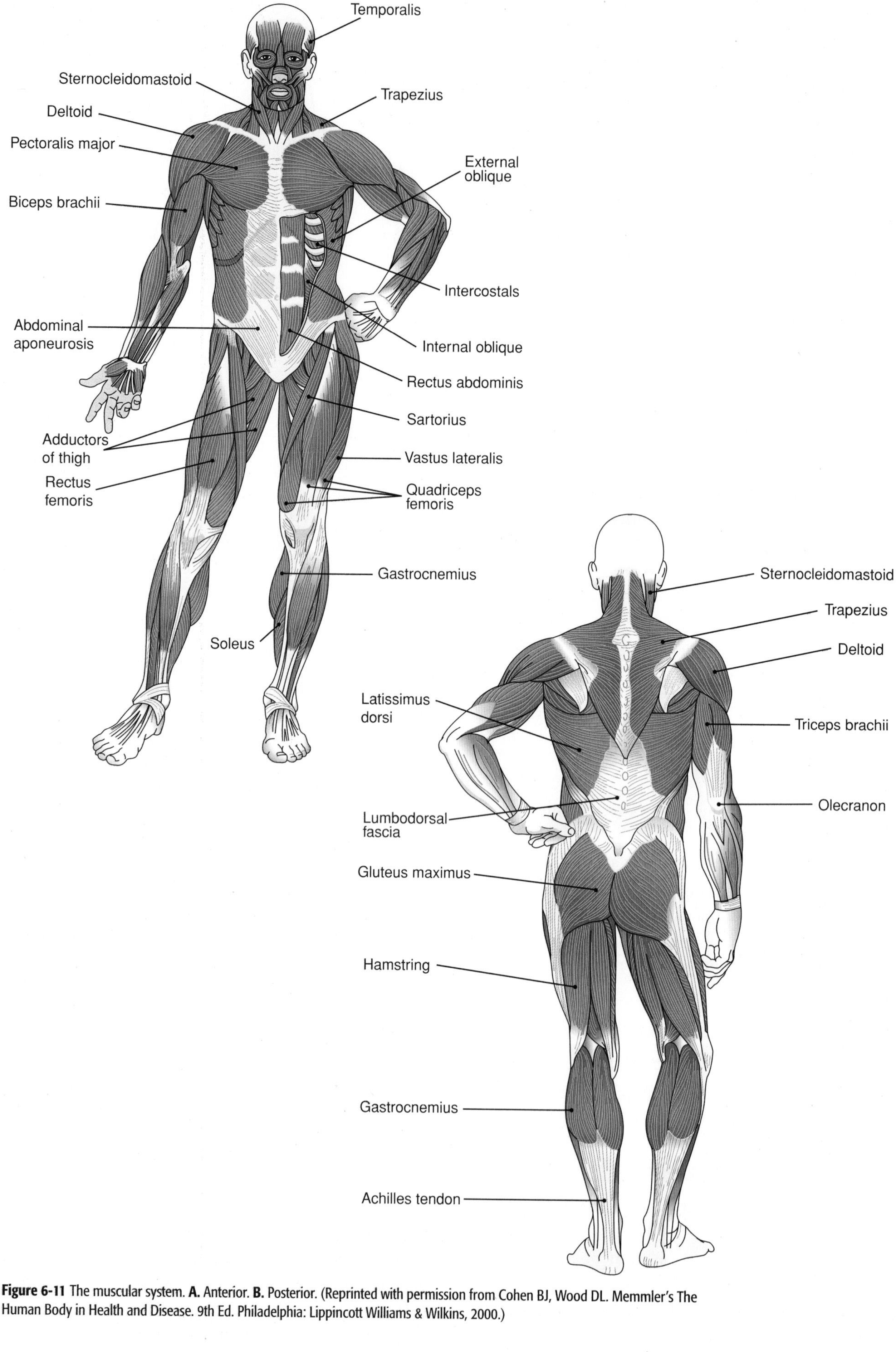

Figure 6-11 The muscular system. **A.** Anterior. **B.** Posterior. (Reprinted with permission from Cohen BJ, Wood DL. Memmler's The Human Body in Health and Disease. 9th Ed. Philadelphia: Lippincott Williams & Wilkins, 2000.)

Common Diseases and Disorders of the Muscular System

- Muscular dystrophy—progressive weakening of muscles that leads to paralysis; may be congenital
- Myasthenia gravis—progressive neuromuscular disease characterized by great muscle weakness and fatigue that results from poor adenosine triphosphate (ATP) production; may be an autoimmune disorder
- Tendonitis—inflammation of the tendon
- Sprain—overstretching of the ligament
- Strain—overstretching of the tendon
- Atrophy—wasting of muscle, often resulting from nonuse

NERVOUS SYSTEM

The **nervous system** is the coordinating agent of the body. Similar to a command post and communication center, it carries messages to and from points and decides on actions and responses.

Functions of the Nervous System

- Regulates body functions and processes
- Communicates stimuli and responses throughout the body
- Generates thoughts, sensations, emotions, and perceptions

Organization of the Nervous System

- Central nervous system (CNS)—brain and spinal cord; integrates sensory information and responses
- Peripheral nervous system (PNS)—nerves originating in the brain and spinal cord that extend outside the CNS and transmit sensory information and responses
    - Somatic nervous system—transmits sensory information to skeletal muscle; voluntary
    - Autonomic nervous system—transmits sensory information to smooth and cardiac muscles (visceral) and glands; involuntary
        - Sympathetic nervous system—prepares the body for stressful situations (i.e., "fight or flight")
        - Parasympathetic nervous system—returns the body to rest and replenishment of energy
    - Afferent (sensory) division of systems—transmits information to the brain
    - Efferent (motor) division of systems—transmits information from the brain to organs and other body structures

Components of the Nervous System

- Neurons—nerve cells, the structural and functional units of the nervous system
    - Dendrites—neuron fibers conducting impulses *to* the cell body
    - Axons—neuron fibers conducting impulses *away from* the cell body
    - Myelin sheath—fatty material that covers and protects neuron fibers; speeds conduction
- Nerves—bundles of neurons that conduct impulses and connect to the brain and spinal cord
- Neuroglia—nonconducting cells that support and protect nervous tissue
- Synapses—neuromuscular junctions (gaps) between neurons
- Neurotransmitters—chemicals released by the axons that stimulate the next cell to continue the transmission of the impulse; the three main neurotransmitters are acetylcholine, epinephrine, and norepinephrine
- Meninges—three layers of connective tissue covering and completely enclosing the brain and spinal cord
    - Dura mater—outer layer, thickest and toughest of the meninges; from the Latin *mater*, meaning "mother"
    - Arachnoid—middle layer, attached to deepest meninges by weblike fibers with space for movement of cerebral spinal fluid; from the Latin *arachnoid*, meaning "spider"
    - Pia mater—innermost layer, attached directly to nervous tissue of brain and spinal cord
- Cerebrospinal fluid (CSF)—clear fluid that flows through the brain and spinal cord and into the subarachnoid spaces of the meninges; cushions and supports nervous tissue and transports nutrients and waste products from the cells
- Brain—organ acting as the primary center for regulating and coordinating body functions and activities (Fig. 6-12); divided into right and left hemispheres
    - Lobes—five areas of the brain located in each hemisphere; each lobe has a corresponding bone that protects it
        - Frontal—controls speech and voluntary muscle movement
        - Parietal—contains the sensory area and interprets impulses from skin (e.g., pain, heat); also estimates distance, size, and shapes
        - Temporal—interprets sound (auditory sense) and smell (olfactory sense); also associated with personality, behavior, emotion, and memory
        - Occipital—interprets sight
        - Insula—believed to be associated with visceral functions
    - Cerebrum—**largest part of the brain,** divided into right and left hemispheres by the longitudinal fissure; contains auditory, visual, gustatory, and olfactory areas and areas of higher mental faculties

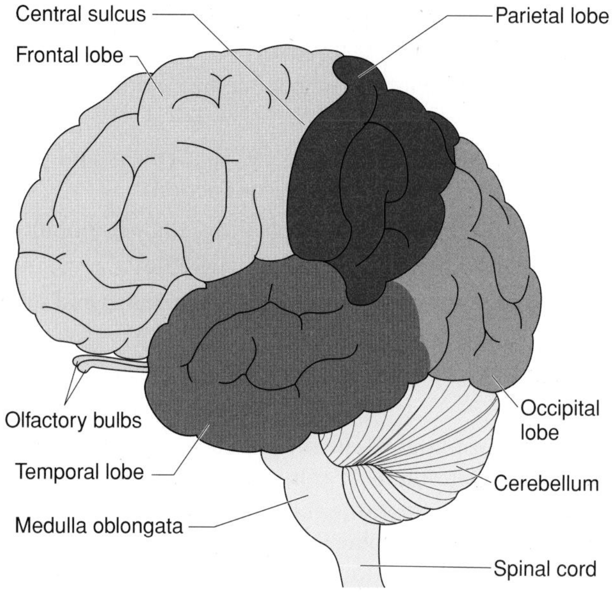

Figure 6-12 Surfaces of the brain. (Reprinted with permission from Willis MC, CMA-AC. Medical Terminology: A Programmed Learning Approach to the Language of Health Care. Baltimore: Lippincott Williams & Wilkins, 2002.)

- Cerebellum ("little brain")—involved in synergic control of skeletal muscles and coordination of voluntary muscular movements; connected to the cerebrum, brainstem, and spinal cord by the pons
- Pons—area where nerves cross, resulting in nerves located on one side of the brain controlling the opposite side of the body; connects the cerebellum with the nervous system
- Medulla oblongata—portion of the brain connecting with the spinal cord; contains centers for control of heart beat, respiratory rate, and blood pressure
- Midbrain—connects the pons and cerebellum with the cerebrum; functions as relay for certain eye and ear reflexes
- Diencephalon—located between the cerebral hemispheres and the brainstem; **contains the thalamus and hypothalamus**
  - Thalamus—located in diencephalon, serves as relay for sensory input
  - Hypothalamus—located in diencephalon, contains nerve cells that assist with maintenance of water balance, fat and sugar metabolism, secretion of endocrine glands, and regulation of body temperature
- Ventricles—cavities or spaces in the brain and spinal cord where CSF is formed, filtered, and circulated

■ Cranial nerves (see Box 6-4)—12 pairs of nerves located in the cranium that control sensory, special sensory, somatic motor, and visceral motor impulses; these nerves are identified by Roman numerals

Box 6-4
Cranial Nerves

I. Olfactory nerve—transmits smells from the nasal mucosa to the brain
II. Optic nerve—transmits vision from the eye to the brain
III. Oculomotor nerve—facilitates contraction of many of the eye muscles
IV. Trochlear nerve—innervates eyeball muscles
V. Trigeminal nerve—composed of three branches that innervate the face transmitting sensory (pain, temperature, touch), motor (muscles of mastication), and lingual (taste) impulses
VI. Abducens nerve— innervates the lateral rectus muscle; responsible for abduction of the eye (outward movement)
VII. Facial nerve—controls facial expressions; combines with the fibers of the trigeminal nerve providing the sense of taste to the anterior two-thirds of the tongue
VIII. Auditory nerve—also known as the vestibulocochlear or acoustic nerve; transmits impulses for hearing and equilibrium
IX. Glossopharyngeal nerve—contains sensory and motor fibers that supply the posterior tongue, pharynx, and parotid gland (largest salivary gland); controls swallowing
X. Vagus nerve—the longest cranial nerve supplying organs in the thoracic and abdominal cavities; innervates glands that produce digestive juices and other secretions
XI. Accessory nerve—divides into two branches, cranial and spinal; the cranial branch innervates the muscles of the larynx, and the spinal branch innervates two muscles of the neck, the sternocleidomastoid and the trapezius.
XII. Hypoglossal nerve—transmits impulses to control the muscles of the tongue

A pneumonic used to remember the 12 pairs of cranial nerves is:
On **O**ld **O**lympus **T**iny **T**ops **A** **F**in **A**nd **G**erman **V**iewed **A**mber **H**ops

■ Spinal cord—continuous tubelike structure located within the spinal vertebrae that extends from the occipital bone to the coccyx; contains ascending and descending nerve tracts that carry transmissions to and from the brain

■ Spinal nerves—31 pairs of nerves arising from the spinal cord, with extending branches to the body parts

- Ganglia (singular *ganglion*)—small, raised areas of gray matter, located outside the CNS, that contain cells of neurons

Common Diseases and Disorders of the Nervous System

Brain or Spinal Cord

- Trauma—injuries as a result of blunt or penetrating force (e.g., gunshot and knife wounds, motor vehicle accidents, diving accidents)
- Neoplasms—malignant and benign tumors
- Paralysis—loss of movement and sensation to a body part or area because of disease or trauma
  - Hemiplegia—paralysis of one side of body
  - Paraplegia—paralysis of the trunk or lower extremities
  - Quadriplegia—paralysis of all extremities and usually the trunk

Brain and Cranial Nerves

- Alzheimer disease—degenerative disorder of the brain beginning with dementia-like symptoms and progressing to a nonfunctioning of neuron fibers that prevents communication between cells for ordinary tasks (e.g., swallowing) and leads to death; etiology is unknown
- Bell palsy—unilateral facial muscle paralysis (drooping of eye and mouth) resulting from dysfunction of cranial nerve VII
- Cerebral palsy—loss of mental function or sensation and control of movement resulting from birth injury or defect
- Cerebrovascular accident (CVA)—stroke; occlusion or hemorrhage of vessel(s) in the brain that results in impairment of mental functions or paralysis
- Dementia—irrecoverable deterioration of mental functions that begins with memory loss and progresses to excitability, defective judgment, delusions, and loss of control of body functions; multiple causes (e.g., alcohol abuse, epilepsy, strokes, lesions)
- Encephalitis—inflammation of the brain
- Epilepsy—abnormal electrical activity of the brain that results in seizures; multiple causes, such as head trauma, high fevers, disease processes, poisoning, or overdose
- Hydrocephalus—accumulation of CSF in the brain caused by an obstruction that results in mounting pressure and destruction of brain tissue
- Narcolepsy—uncontrollable episodes of falling asleep, also known as sleep epilepsy
- Parkinson disease—chronic progressive neurologic disease characterized by fine tremors and muscle weakness and rigidity; etiology believed to be associated with low dopamine production
- Transient ischemic attack (TIA)—ministrokes; temporary episodes of impaired neurologic function resulting from decreased blood flow to the brain

Spinal Cord and Nerves

- Amyotrophic lateral sclerosis (ALS, Lou Gehrig disease)—progressive disease of the motor neurons that causes muscle atrophy and weakness
- Herpes zoster—shingles; an infection caused by the herpes zoster virus (the same virus that causes varicella), resulting in blisterlike lesions and pain along the nerve trunks
- Multiple sclerosis—progressive inflammation and hardening of the myelin sheath in the nervous system
- Neuritis—inflammation of the nerve
- Poliomyelitis—vaccine-preventable disease that attacks the gray matter of the spinal cord; paralysis or partial paralysis may occur
- Sciatica—neuritis and associated pain of the sciatic nerve and its branches

SENSORY SYSTEM

The sensory system is closely aligned with the nervous system and serves to protect the body by recognizing the environment and detecting changes. These functions allow the nervous system to transmit stimuli, determine responses, and send reactive messages.

General Senses

General or somatic sensors are located throughout the body.

- Pressure—receptors in skin and internal organs
- Temperature—receptors in skin and internal organs
- Touch—receptors in skin and internal organs
- Position/orientation—receptors in muscles, tendons, and joints
- Pain—receptors in skin, internal organs, muscles, tendons, and joints

Special Senses

The special senses are sight, hearing, smell, and taste. The components of these senses are located in special organs and structures.

Vision (Sight)

Figure 6-13 illustrates the following structures of the eye; Box 6-5 lists common diseases and disorders of the eye.

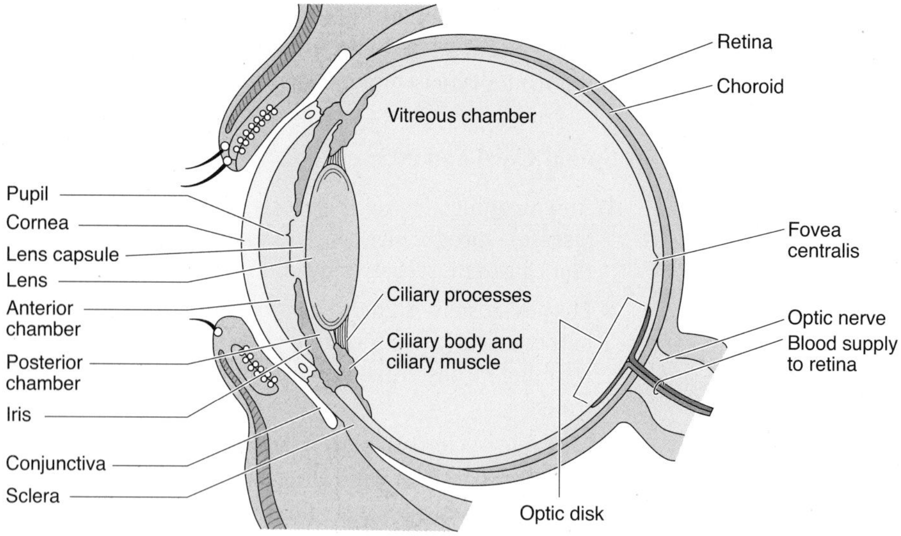

Figure 6-13 The eye. (Reprinted with permission from Willis MC, CMA-AC. Medical Terminology: A Programmed Learning Approach to the Language of Health Care. Baltimore: Lippincott Williams & Wilkins, 2002.)

Box 6-5

Common Diseases and Disorders of the Eye

Astigmatism—impaired vision from irregular curve of cornea; image focuses improperly on retina; may be mild to severe; usually corrected with glasses or contact lenses

Cataract—cloudy or opaque lens; usually corrected by surgery

Conjunctivitis—inflammation of the conjunctiva caused by infection or irritation

Diabetic retinopathy—damage to the retina in diabetic patients resulting from hemorrhage of vessels; usually progressive and related to the control of the person's diabetes

Exophthalmia—protrusion of the eyeballs, usually resulting from endocrine disorder

Glaucoma—disease causing damage to optic nerve from increased intraocular pressure; often results in blindness if uncontrolled

Hyperopia—farsightedness; a condition in which distant objects can be seen more clearly than closer objects

Macular degeneration—progressive, abnormal growth of blood vessels or other materials in retina; usually leads to blindness, although laser surgery may slow process

Myopia—condition of nearsightedness; can see objects close by but not far away

Presbyopia—most common eye condition associated with aging

Strabismus—inability of both eyes to simultaneously focus on a subject; known as "lazy eye" or as being "cross-eyed"

- Eye—organ containing receptors for sight
  - Sclera—white outer coat of eye
    - Cornea—anterior transparent cover of sclera; focuses light rays
  - Choroid—middle layer of the eye between sclera and retina
    - Iris—colored portion of eye; regulates amount of light entering eye
    - Pupil—hole in the middle of the iris
  - Retina—innermost layer of the eye; contains photoreceptors
    - Rods—function in dark, recognize shades of gray; located throughout the retina
    - Cones—function in light, recognize color; located throughout the retina
    - Optic disc—blind spot, area where the optic nerve exits the eye
  - Chambers
    - Anterior—between the lens and cornea; contains aqueous humor (clear, watery fluid that maintains the slight curve of the cornea)
    - Posterior—between the lens and the retina; contains vitreous humor (gelatin-like fluid that maintains shape of eyeball) and some aqueous humor
  - Lens—transparent refractory structure between the iris and vitreous humor
- Accessory structures
  - Eyebrows and lashes—help protect against foreign objects entering the eye
  - Eyelids—moisturize eyes, also protect against foreign objects

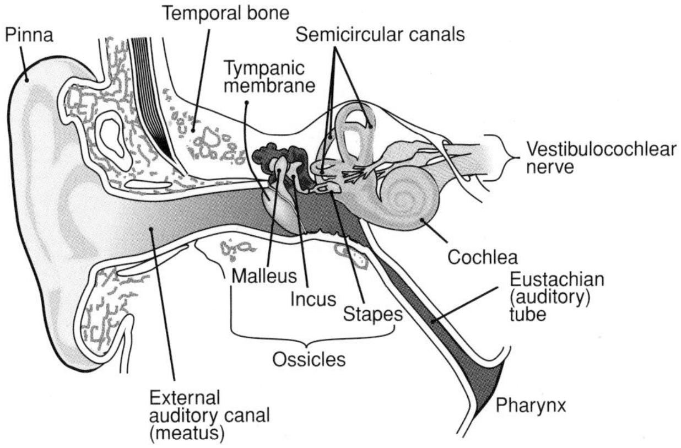

Figure 6-14 The ear. (Reprinted with permission from Cohen BJ, Wood DL. Memmler's The Human Body in Health and Disease. 9th Ed. Philadelphia: Lippincott Williams & Wilkins, 2000.)

- Lacrimal structures—glands and ducts that secrete and drain tears
- Conjunctiva—mucous membrane lining of the eyelid
- Optic nerve—second cranial nerve; carries visual impulses from the rods and cones to the brain

Hearing (Auditory Sense)

Figure 6-14 illustrates the following structures of the ear; Box 6-6 lists common diseases and disorders of the ear.

- Ear—sense organ for hearing and equilibrium
- Outer ear
  - Pinna (auricle)—external ear; directs waves to the canal

Box 6-6

Common Diseases and Disorders of the Ear

Deafness—partial or complete hearing loss; many causes, such as trauma, disease, nerve damage
Ménière's disease—chronic disturbance in labyrinth resulting in dizziness, loss of equilibrium, and deafness; unknown cause; treatment is palliative (attempting to provide relief for signs and symptoms)
Otitis media—infection of middle ear; most common in infants and toddlers; usually treated with antibiotics
Otosclerosis—partial deafness resulting from bone growth involving the ossicles; may be improved by surgery
Tinnitus—ringing in the ears
Vertigo—dizziness

  - External auditory canal—tubelike opening or meatus from the pinna to the tympanic membrane
    - Ceruminous glands—glands in beginning of the ear canal that produce cerumen (earwax) to protect the internal ear structures
    - Tympanic membrane (eardrum)—boundary between external and middle ear canals; vibrates to transmit sound waves to inner ear
- Middle ear—contains three auditory (hearing) ossicles (bones) that amplify sound from the tympanic membrane and transmit to fluid in inner ear
  - Malleus (hammer)—first ossicle
  - Incus (anvil)—second ossicle
  - Stapes (stirrup)—third ossicle
- Eustachian tube—connects the middle ear with the throat and pharynx; equalizes pressure on the tympanic membrane
- Inner ear (labyrinth)—contains vestibule, semicircular canal, and cochlea, with receptors for hearing and balance
  - Vestibule—middle section of the inner ear that involves balance
  - Semicircular canal—curved passageway in the inner ear that detects motion and regulates balance
  - Cochlea—snail-shaped tube that contains the receptor for hearing

Smell (Olfactory Sense)

- Nasal cavity
  - Olfactory epithelium—contains receptors for smell
  - Olfactory nerve—first cranial nerve leading from olfactory center in the temporal lobe of the brain to olfactory sensors in epithelium

Taste (Gustatory)

- Tongue
  - Glossal papillae—taste receptors, or taste buds, located on the tongue that sense bitter, sour, sweet, and salty tastes
  - Cranial nerves—facial and glossopharyngeal cranial nerves associated with taste

ENDOCRINE SYSTEM

The endocrine system contains glands producing regulatory chemicals or hormones (Fig. 6-15). This system, in conjunction with the nervous system, regulates and coordinates other body systems. The nervous system communicates to the endocrine system the need for hormone adjustments resulting from environmental changes. The hormones are secreted into the bloodstream and carried to

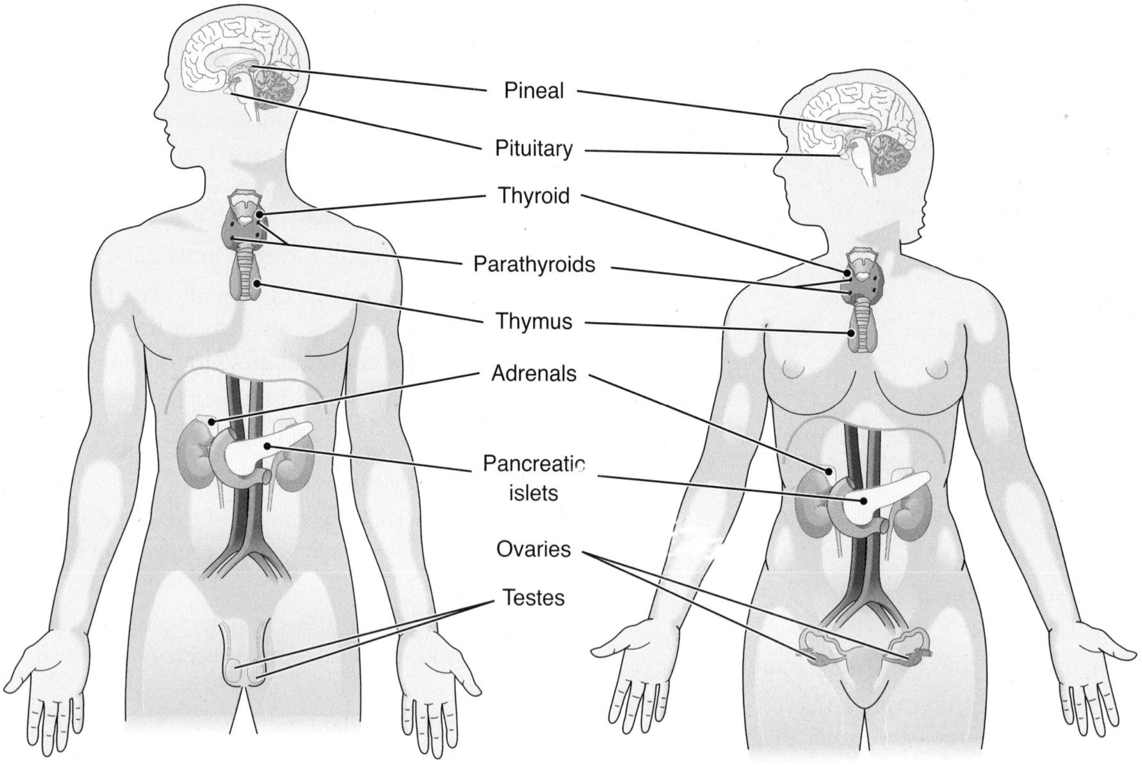

Figure 6-15 Endocrine glands. (Reprinted with permission from Cohen BJ. Medical Terminology. 4th Ed. Philadelphia: Lippincott Williams & Wilkins, 2003.)

target cells where the reactions occur. **The term *endocrine* comes from the Greek word *endon*, meaning "within" (because the secretions are within the gland).** Table 6-1 summarizes the endocrine glands and their hormones and functions. Other glands, called ***exocrine glands*, secrete externally or into ducts.** These glands and hormones will be discussed with the appropriate systems.

Functions of the Endocrine System

- Regulates growth, metabolism, reproduction, and behavior
- Coordinates and stimulates many body functions by secreting and sending hormones to specific cells

Common Diseases and Disorders of the Endocrine System

Pineal Gland

- Seasonal affective disorder (SAD)—overproduction of melatonin during long periods of darkness (winter), resulting in depression

Anterior Pituitary Gland

- Dwarfism—decreased production of growth hormone (GH) that results in abnormally small size
- Giantism—overproduction of GH that results in abnormally large size
- Acromegaly—overproduction of GH after puberty that results in wide, large face, hands, and feet

Thyroid Gland

- Goiter—enlarged thyroid
- Hypothyroidism—underactivity of the thyroid
  - Cretinism—hypothyroidism; decreased secretion of thyroxine in infants that results in impaired physical and mental development
  - Myxedema—atrophy of the thyroid in adults that results in decreased secretion of thyroxine, causing forms of physical and mental decline
- Hyperthyroidism—overactivity of the thyroid
  - Graves disease—hyperthyroidism; increased secretion of thyroxine characterized by goiter, exophthalmia (bulging eyes), weight loss, extreme nervousness, and rapid metabolism

Parathyroid Gland

- Tetany—spasms resulting from low blood calcium

Table 6-1 **Endocrine Glands, Hormones, and Select Functions**

Gland	Hormones and Select Functions
Pineal gland	**Melatonin**—regulates sexual development and sleep/wake cycles
Pituitary gland, "Master gland"	**Anterior pituitary (adenohypophysis)** **Growth hormone (GH)**—promotes growth of bone and soft tissue **Thyroid-stimulating hormone (TSH)**—stimulates thyroid to produce thyroid hormones **Adrenocorticotropic hormone (ACTH)**—stimulates adrenal cortex to produce hormones for stress and water/electrolyte balance **Follicle-stimulating hormone (FSH)**—stimulates secretion of estrogen and growth of testes; promotes development of sperm cells **Luteinizing hormone (LH)**—causes development of corpus luteum in females and stimulates secretion of testosterone in males **Prolactin**—stimulates female breast development and milk secretion **Posterior pituitary** **Vasopressin or antidiuretic hormone (ADH)**—increases reabsorption in kidney and stimulates blood vessels to contract **Oxytocin**—increases uterine contractions and causes breast milk secretion
Thyroid gland	**Thyroid hormone (thyroxine, T_4; T_3)**—increases metabolic rate; necessary for normal cell growth **Calcitonin**—reduces plasma calcium concentrations
Parathyroid gland	**Parathyroid hormone (PTH)**—increases calcium level in blood
Thymus gland	**Thymosin**—stimulates production of T cells, facilitating immunity
Adrenal glands	**Aldosterone**—regulates sodium and potassium levels
Adrenal cortex	**Cortisol (glucocorticoid)**—increases blood glucose and assists in stress
Adrenal medulla	**Androgens**—stimulate development of secondary sex characteristics **Epinephrine**—increases heart rate and blood pressure **Norepinephrine**—aids neurotransmission
Pancreas	**Insulin**—decreases sugar levels **Glucagon**—increases sugar levels
Gonads (sex glands) *Ovaries (female)*	**Estrogens**—stimulate growth of breasts, uterus, and secondary sex characteristics **Progesterone**—prepares and maintains the uterine lining for pregnancy
Testes (male)	**Testosterone**—stimulates development of sex characteristics and sperm

Adrenal Cortex Gland

- Addison disease—hyposecretion of cortisol by the adrenal cortex, resulting in muscle atrophy, tissue weakness, and skin pigmentation
- Cushing syndrome—overproduction of cortisol by the adrenal cortex, resulting in round face, excessive weight gain, thin skin, and high blood sugar

Pancreas

- Diabetes mellitus—most common endocrine disorder; low production of insulin, resulting in cells retaining sugar
  - Insulin-dependent diabetes mellitus (IDDM)—type 1 diabetes
  - Non–insulin-dependent diabetes (NIDDM)—type 2 diabetes

CARDIOVASCULAR SYSTEM

The **cardiovascular** (or circulatory) **system** pumps blood, carrying life-sustaining oxygen and other substances throughout the body. The primary components are blood, blood vessels, and the heart.

Functions of the Cardiovascular System

- Transports oxygen, nutrients, and other needed substances to body tissues
- Assists in removal of body wastes
- Regulates acidity (pH) of body fluids
- Assists in regulating body temperature

Components of the Cardiovascular System

Blood

Blood is the connective tissue containing cells and fluid in a viscous consistency that circulates in vessels throughout the body.

- Plasma—liquid portion of blood (55%)
  - Albumin—the most abundant plasma protein; maintains osmotic pressure
  - Fibrinogen—the smallest amount of plasma protein; assists in the coagulation (clotting) process
  - Globulin—plasma protein used for gamma globulin
  - Serum—clear, liquid portion of blood that remains after the blood clots
- Cellular components of blood (45%)
  - Erythrocytes—red blood cells (RBCs); contain hemoglobin to carry oxygen; mature cells do not have a nucleus
  - Leukocytes—white blood cells (WBCs); fight infection
  - Platelets (thrombocytes)—cell fragments; function in coagulation

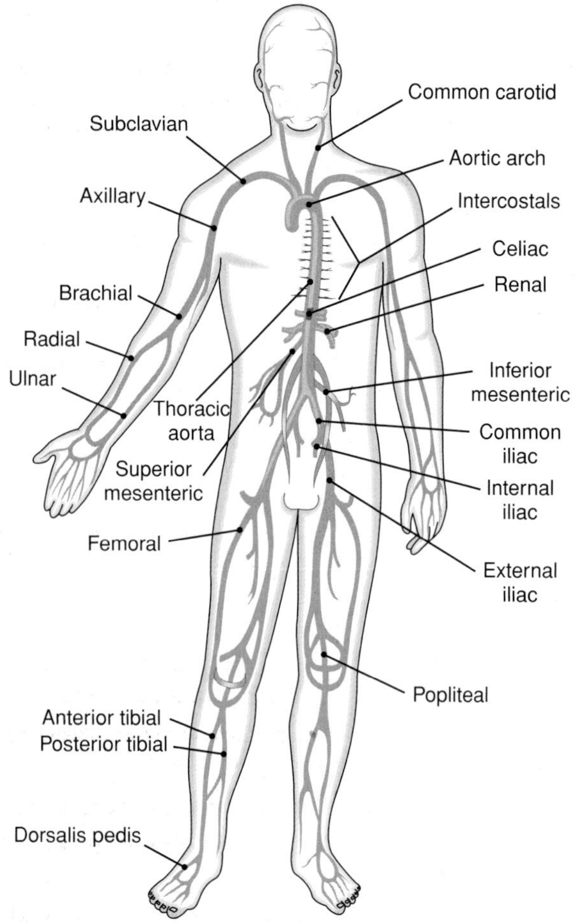

Figure 6-16 Major arteries. (Reprinted with permission from Cohen BJ, Wood DL. Memmler's The Human Body in Health and Disease. 9th Ed. Philadelphia: Lippincott Williams & Wilkins, 2000.)

Blood Vessels

Blood vessels are the arteries, veins, and capillaries that carry blood throughout the body.

- Arteries (Fig. 6-16)—blood vessels throughout the body that carry oxygenated blood away from the heart
- Veins (Fig. 6-17)—blood vessels throughout the body carrying deoxygenated blood toward the heart; contain valves
- Capillaries—small blood vessels connecting veins and arteries

Heart

The heart is the body's pump, a fist-sized muscular organ composed of three layers and an outer covering.

- Endocardium—inner layer
- Myocardium—middle layer
- Epicardium—outer layer
- Pericardium—outer fibrous sac that covers and protects the heart
- Chambers—four heart chambers: two superior and two inferior
  - Right atrium (plural *atria*)—superior chamber that receives deoxygenated blood from the systemic vessels
  - Left atrium—superior chamber that receives oxygenated blood from the pulmonary veins
  - Right ventricle—inferior chamber that pumps blood to the lungs
  - Left ventricle—inferior chamber that pumps blood to the body tissues
- Valves—flaplike structures that open and close, allowing blood to flow through the heart in one direction
  - Atrioventricular valves (AV)—located between the atria and ventricles; their closing prevents backflow of blood into the atria
    - Tricuspid valve (three flaps)—AV valve located between the right atrium and ventricle

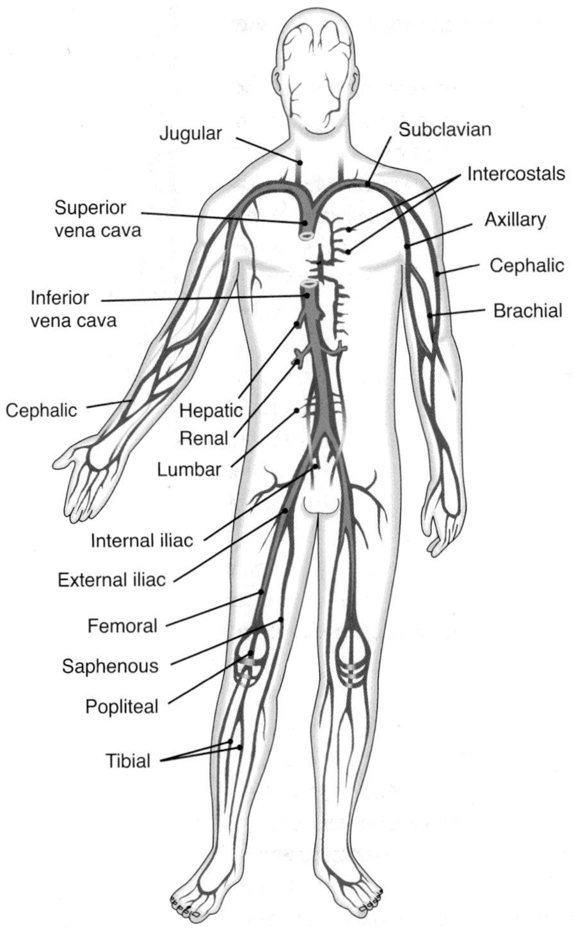

Figure 6-17 Major veins. (Reprinted with permission from Cohen BJ, Wood DL. Memmler's The Human Body in Health and Disease. 9th Ed. Philadelphia: Lippincott Williams & Wilkins, 2000.)

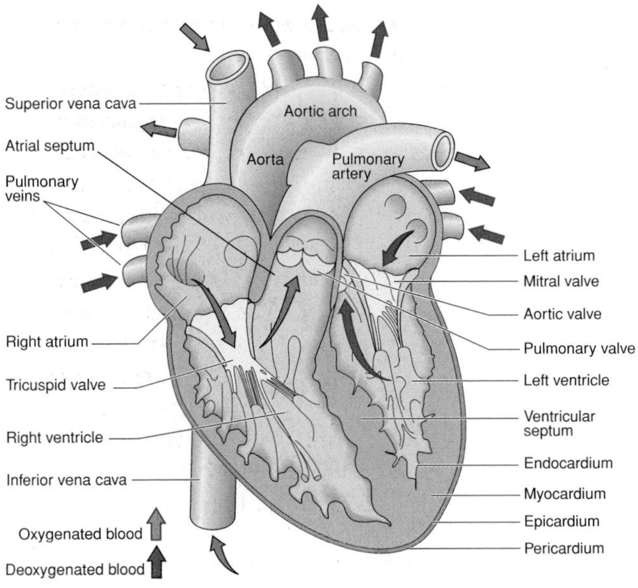

Figure 6-18 The heart and great vessels. (Reprinted with permission from Willis MC, CMA-AC. Medical Terminology: A Programmed Learning Approach to the Language of Health Care. Baltimore: Lippincott Williams & Wilkins, 2002.)

  - ❍ Mitral valve (bicuspid; two flaps)—AV valve located between the left atrium and ventricle
- • Semilunar valves (SL)—located between the ventricles and the pulmonary artery and aorta; their closing prevents backflow of blood into the ventricles
  - ❍ Aortic valve—located between the left ventricle and the aorta
  - ❍ Pulmonary valve—located between the right ventricle and the pulmonary artery

■ Great vessels of the heart—Figure 6-18 identifies structures and demonstrates how blood flows through the heart

- • Aorta—largest body artery; consists of three parts: ascending, aortic arch, and descending
- • Coronary arteries (right and left)—supply blood to the myocardium; significant blockage of these arteries results in myocardial infarction (MI; heart attack)
- • Pulmonary artery—only artery that carries deoxygenated blood; transports blood from the heart to the lungs to be oxygenated
- • Vena cava—**largest body vein**; has inferior and superior branches
  - ❍ Inferior vena cava—brings deoxygenated blood to the heart from the lower extremities, pelvis, and some abdominal organs
  - ❍ Superior vena cava—brings deoxygenated blood to the heart from the head, neck, upper limbs, thorax, and some abdominal organs

■ Pulmonary veins (four)—right and left superior and inferior veins bring oxygenated blood from the lungs to the left atrium of the heart for circulation throughout the body; **the only veins that carry oxygenated blood**

The Cardiac Cycle

The main function of the cardiovascular system is to circulate blood (Fig. 6-19). The major portion of this function is accomplished through the pumping of the heart in a rhythmic cycle of contraction and relaxation called the *cardiac cycle*.

■ Atrial systole **(contraction)**—the atria contract, forcing blood into ventricles through the tricuspid and mitral valves, which close at the end of the contraction

■ Ventricular diastole **(relaxation)**—the ventricles relax, filling with blood from the atria

■ Ventricular systole **(contraction)**—the ventricles contract, forcing blood through the SL valves to the aorta and pulmonary artery

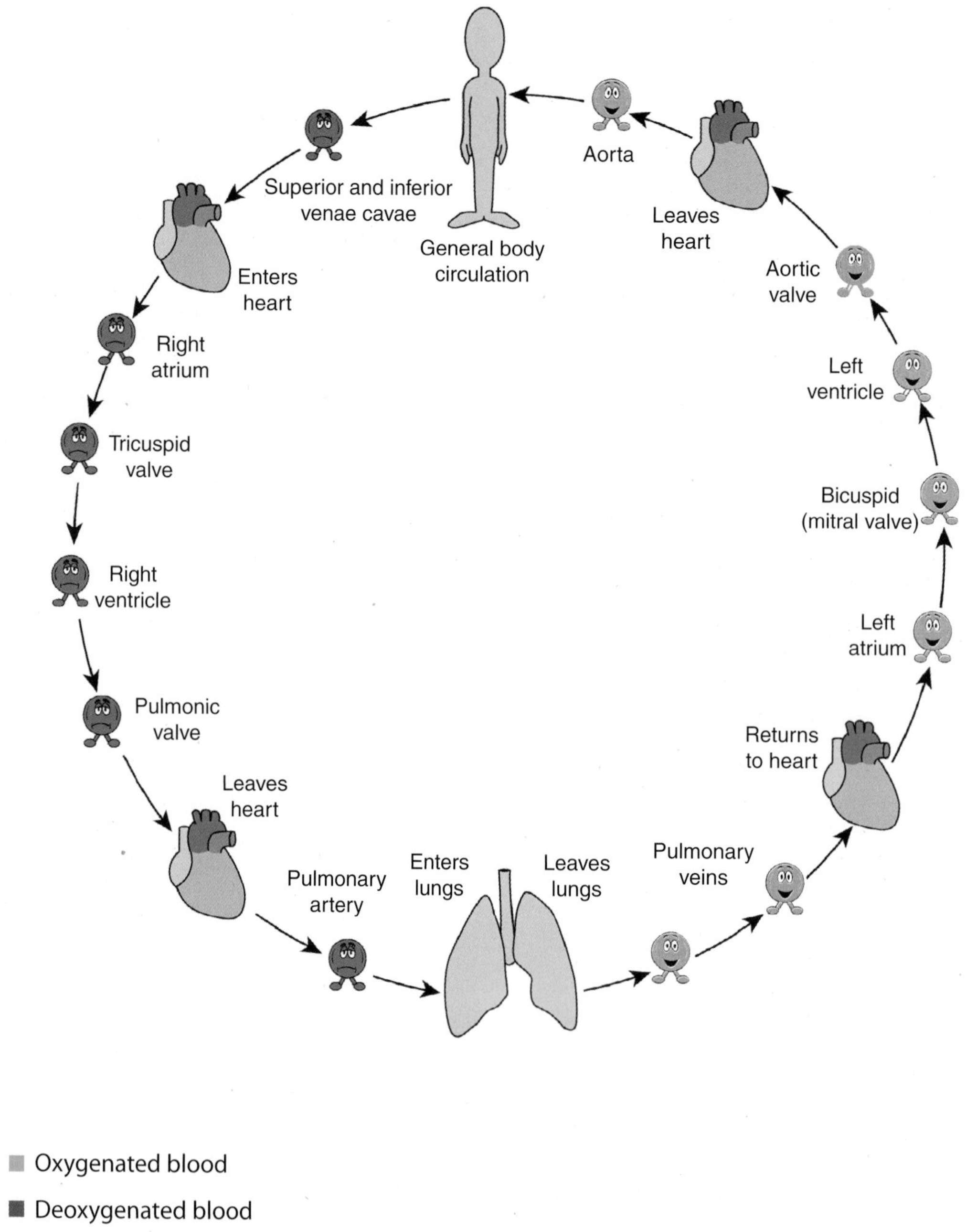

Figure 6-19 Blood circulation through the body.

- Atrial diastole **(relaxation)**—the atria relax, filling with blood from the vena cava and pulmonary veins
- Cycle repeats beginning with atrial systole

Cardiac Conduction

The heart is stimulated to contract through a series of electrical impulses or signals located throughout the heart itself. The impulses are carried or relayed through a group of structures that make up the conduction system (Fig. 6-20). These conduction paths, with the cardiac cycle, produce the electrocardiogram, which will be discussed in Chapter 20.

- Sinoatrial (SA) node—located in the upper wall of the right atrium, the **SA node is the pacemaker of the heart** and initiates a normal heart beat and rate of **60 to 80 beats per minute (sinus rhythm)**; it causes the atria to contract
- AV node—located in the atrial septum at the lower right, the AV node picks up the impulse or signal from the SA node that causes the atria to contract; if the SA node

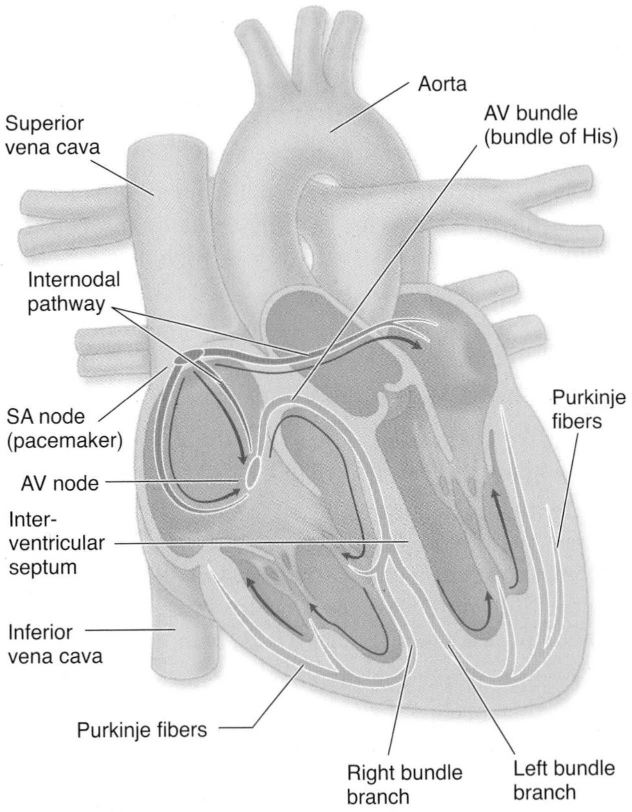

Figure 6-20 Cardiac conductive system. (Reprinted with permission from Cohen BJ, Wood DL. Memmler's The Human Body in Health and Disease. 9th Ed. Philadelphia: Lippincott Williams & Wilkins, 2000.)

fails, the AV node may initiate the impulse; the resulting heart rate is slower, at 40 to 60 beats per minute

- Bundle of His—specialized cells in the ventricular septum, carrying the impulse from the AV node; should the SA and AV nodes fail, the bundle of His may initiate the impulse; the resulting heart rate is 20 to 40 beats per minute
- Bundle branches—two branches extending from the bundle of His that carry the impulse down the ventricular septum
- Purkinje fibers—smaller fibers arising from the bundle branches that carry the impulse to the ventricular walls, causing them to contract

Common Diseases and Disorders of the Cardiovascular System

Diseases and Disorders of the Blood

- Anemia—abnormally low hemoglobin or RBCs, decreasing oxygen supply to the tissues; anemia has many causes and types; main symptoms are fatigue and weakness
  - Aplastic anemia—anemia that results from bone marrow damage decreasing the production of RBCs
  - Pernicious anemia—anemia that results from **vitamin B_{12}** deficiency
  - Sickle cell anemia—chronic inherited disease found in Africans and their descendants, causing the hemoglobin cell to mutate its shape
- Leukemia—type of malignancy; rapid and abnormal development of leukocytes (WBCs) in spleen, bone marrow, and lymph nodes
- Hemophilia—genetic bleeding disorder; deficiency of specific clotting factors that results in abnormal bleeding, especially into the joints, from minor trauma; the causative gene is transmitted from mother to sons

Diseases and Disorders of the Blood Vessels

- Aneurysm—genetic or traumatic weakness of a blood vessel wall demonstrated by a "bubble" or outpouching caused by pressure of blood; an abdominal aortic aneurysm is called an *AAA* or *triple A*
- Arteriosclerosis—hardening of the artery and loss of elasticity resulting from thickening of the vessel wall
  - Atherosclerosis—most common form of arteriosclerosis, with irregular fatty deposits on artery wall that result in narrowing and occlusion of vessel; may cause MIs, CVAs, gangrene, and other disorders associated with blood vessel blockage

Note: The difference between atherosclerosis and arteriosclerosis is a highly probable exam question.

  - Coronary artery disease (CAD)—arteriosclerosis or atherosclerosis-type process of the coronary arteries, usually leading to myocardial ischemia (damage to tissue resulting from lack of oxygen caused by an occlusion)
- Embolus (plural *emboli*)—a detached thrombus or other substance that occludes a vessel
- Thrombophlebitis—inflammation of a vein with clots
- Thrombus (plural *thrombi*)—an attached blood clot located within the cardiovascular system

Diseases and Disorders of the Heart

- Angina pectoris—severe constricting chest pain resulting from lack of blood supply to the heart; associated with CAD
- Arrhythmias—abnormal heart rhythms
  - Bradycardia—slow heart rate
  - Tachycardia—fast heart rate
  - Flutters—rapid, coordinated heart beats
  - Fibrillation—rapid, uncoordinated contractions of the heart (may be atrial or ventricular)
  - Heart blocks—interruption of the heart's electrical conduction

- Congenital heart disease—disorder present at birth
  - Patent ductus arteriosis—opening between the aorta and pulmonary artery in fetal circulation that does not close after birth
  - Ventricular septal defect—most common congenital heart problem; a hole in the septum between the two ventricles
  - Tetralogy of Fallot—presence of four specific congenital heart defects
- Congestive heart failure—venous and pulmonary congestion and general edema (swelling) resulting from decreased blood circulation
- Hypertension—high blood pressure (beginning at 140/90)
- Myocardial infarction—heart attack; necrosis (death) of an area in the myocardium resulting from cessation of blood supply, usually from coronary thrombosis
- Rheumatic heart disease—inflammation and hardening of the heart valve(s) resulting from a streptococcal infection associated with rheumatic fever
- Stenosis of the heart valves (aortic, mitral, tricuspid, or pulmonary)—narrowing of the valve that prevents normal blood flow

LYMPHATIC SYSTEM

The lymphatic system is sometimes considered part of the cardiovascular (circulatory) system. It is similar in that it has a fluid called *lymph*, which is circulated throughout the body in a network of vessels. The lymph and lymphatic tissues cleanse and filter, protecting against and combating disease.

Functions of the Lymphatic System

- Defends against disease
- Assists in developing immunities
- Returns excess interstitial fluid to the blood

Components of the Lymphatic System

- Lymph—clear fluid resembling blood plasma that contains some RBCs and WBCs and lymphocytes
- Lymphocytes—white cells that protect the body against infection and aid in establishing immunity
- Lymph vessels—similar to veins, they carry lymph and contain valves and lymph nodes
  - Lymph capillaries—microscopic vessels
  - Lymphatic ducts (two)—narrow tubular channels carrying lymph to the bloodstream
    - Thoracic duct—the larger lymph duct; it drains the entire body except the right side above the diaphragm
    - Right lymphatic duct—the smaller lymph duct; it drains the right side of the body above the diaphragm
- Lymph nodes—oval-shaped fibrous capsules that filter and cleanse the lymph as it enters the blood
- Tonsils—three pairs of masses of lymphoid tissue that filter foreign organisms entering the body through the mouth or nose and assist in the formation of white cells
  - Palatine tonsils—located on each side of the soft palate, these lymph masses are the ones commonly referred to as the "tonsils"
  - Pharyngeal tonsils—adenoids; located on upper pharynx
  - Lingual tonsils—located at back of tongue
- Spleen—organ located in the upper left hypochondriac region of the abdomen under the diaphragm dome; contains lymph tissue; cleanses blood, destroys old RBCs, produces RBCs before birth, and reserves blood in case of emergencies (e.g., hemorrhage)
- Thymus—gland, considered part of the endocrine system, that produces thymosin, which is necessary for growth and the function of lymphocytes

Common Diseases and Disorders of the Lymphatic System

- Splenomegaly—enlarged spleen, associated with certain infectious diseases
- Lymphoma—benign or malignant tumor of lymph tissue
  - Hodgkin's disease—chronic malignant lymphoma(s) with enlarged spleen; treated by chemotherapy and radiation; generally seen in young men
  - Non-Hodgkin's lymphoma—widespread malignant disease in lymph tissues; responds poorly to therapy; generally seen in older adults
- Acquired immunodeficiency syndrome (AIDS)—decreased immunity resulting from infection with the human immunodeficiency virus (HIV); leaves patient susceptible to opportunistic diseases
- Mononucleosis (mono)—acute infectious disease caused by Epstein-Barr virus, resulting in lymph tissue involvement, including enlarged spleen; generally seen in young adults

Overview of Immunity

Immunity is the individual's resistance to specific diseases or disorders, usually by acquiring the corresponding antibody to that disease or disorder. Immunity is a function of the lymphatic system. The national exams often contain questions concerning active and passive immunity, which are described in Box 6-7.

Box 6-7

Types of Immunity

Immunity: resistance or the condition of not being susceptible to a disease

Active Immunity

Long-term immunity—produced by the body's own production of antibodies

- **Natural active immunity**—acquired from exposure to disease-causing organisms
- **Artificial active immunity**—acquired from immunization with killed or attenuated organisms, toxins, or recombinant DNA

Passive Immunity

Short-term immunity: produced by introducing antibodies manufactured outside the body

- **Natural passive immunity**—acquired from maternal antibodies while in the uterus or breast-feeding
- **Artificial passive immunity**—acquired from immunization with antibodies or globulins of disease-causing organisms

Additional Terms Associated With Immunity

- Antigen—a substance (e.g., bacteria/viruses, bacterial/viral toxins, foreign blood cells) that causes the formation of antibodies
- Antibody—a substance produced in the body in response to the presence of an antigen; antibodies enhance activities of leukocytes and produce globulins protecting the body against further assault from the specific antigen
- Phagocytosis—ingestion of bacteria and particles by phagocytes (a form of leukocyte)
- Globulins—the fraction of the blood serum protein associated with antibodies; vaccination with globulins produces passive immunity
- Immunization (vaccination)—protection from communicable diseases by administration of living attenuated agents (e.g., measles), killed organisms (e.g., pertussis), inactivated toxins (e.g., tetanus), or recombinant DNA (e.g., hepatitis B); Box 6-8 identifies common vaccine-preventable diseases

Box 6-8

Common Vaccine-Preventable Diseases

Diphtheria
Haemophilus influenzae b
Hepatitis A
Hepatitis B
Human papilloma virus
Influenza (select strains)
Measles
Meningitis (select strains)
Mumps
Pertussis (whooping cough)
Pneumonia (select strains)
Polio
Rotavirus
Rubella (German measles)
Tetanus (lockjaw)
Varicella (chickenpox)

RESPIRATORY SYSTEM

The **respiratory system** is a group of body structures (Fig. 6-21) responsible for breathing or ventilation. The process involves taking in oxygen (O_2), which is needed to sustain human cells, and giving off carbon dioxide (CO_2), which is the waste product of respiration.

Functions of the Respiratory System

- Obtains O_2 and other gases from the external environment
- Delivers gases to the blood (diffusion)
- Removes CO_2, a waste product of respiration, from the cells
- Transports CO_2 to the external environment

Components of the Respiratory System

Respiratory Center

The respiratory center is the bundled nerve cells, located in the medulla oblongata and pons of the brain, controlling breathing and responding to changing levels of O_2 and CO_2 in the blood.

Upper Respiratory Tract

The upper respiratory tract is the passageway for gases. It is composed of the following:

- Nose—projection on the face that warms and moistens air as it enters the body; contains cilia and hair to prevent foreign particles from entering the respiratory system
- Pharynx (throat)—passageway from nose to larynx
- Larynx (voice box)—organ between the pharynx and trachea containing the vocal cords, which vibrate to produce speech

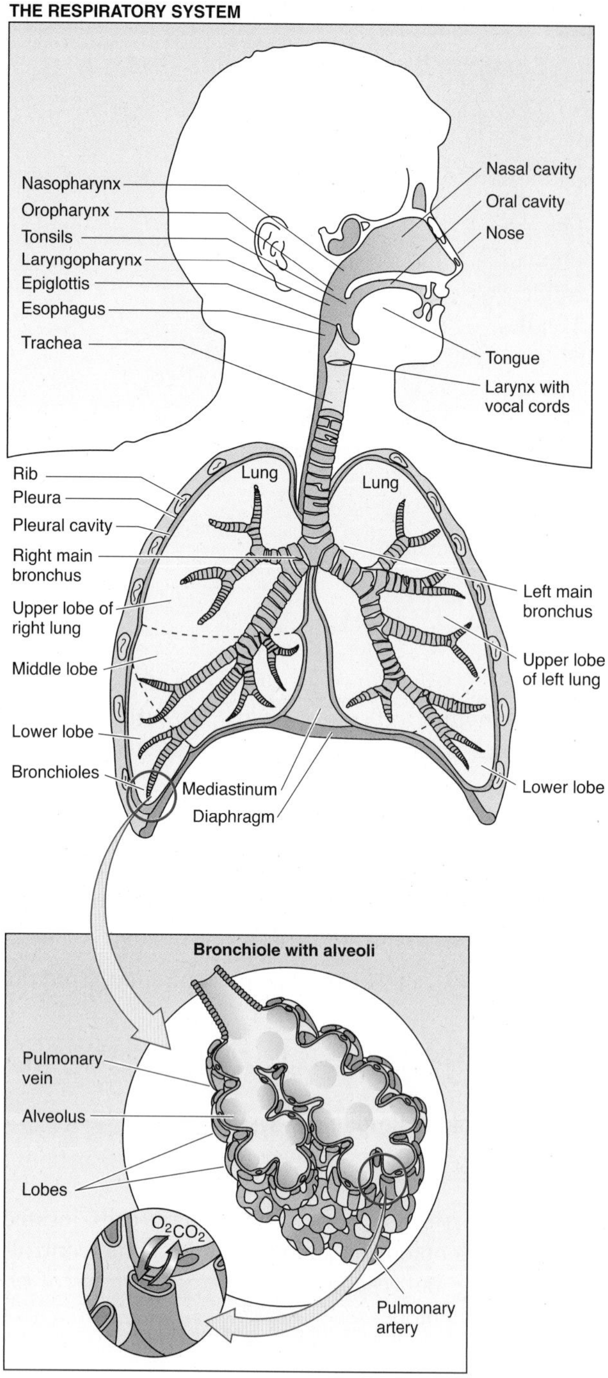

Figure 6-21 The respiratory system. (Reprinted with permission from Willis MC, CMA-AC. Medical Terminology: A Programmed Learning Approach to the Language of Health Care. Baltimore: Lippincott Williams & Wilkins, 2002.)

- Epiglottis—flaplike structure that covers the larynx during swallowing

Lower Respiratory Tract

The lower respiratory tract is composed of the following:

- Trachea—tube branching into two bronchi, which lead into the lungs
- Bronchi (singular *bronchus*)—tubes from the trachea entering the lungs that subdivide into two more branches in the lungs
  - Bronchioles—smaller branches of the bronchi
  - Alveoli (singular *alveolus*)—air sacs at the ends of the bronchioles where the exchange of gases occurs
- Lungs (two)—main organ of the respiratory system, located in the thoracic cavity; distributes and exchanges gases
  - Right lung—contains three lobes
  - Left lung—contains two lobes
  - Pleura—lung linings containing pleural fluid to protect lungs and reduce friction during respiration
- Thorax—cavity containing the lungs
- Diaphragm—muscle tissue separating thoracic and abdominal cavities that contracts and expands during respiration, allowing lungs to fill and empty air

Additional Respiratory System Terms

- Cheyne-Stokes respiration—irregular breathing pattern of slow and shallow, then rapid and deep respirations, with pauses for 20 to 30 seconds; frequently occurs before death
- Inspiration (inhalation)—bringing air into lungs; the diaphragm contracts, increasing the size of the thoracic cavity and allowing air to enter the lungs
- Expiration (exhalation)—releasing air from the lungs; the diaphragm relaxes, decreasing the size of the thoracic cavity and pushing air out
- External respiration—exchange of O_2 and CO_2 in the lungs and capillaries
- Internal respiration—exchange of O_2 and CO_2 between the capillaries and the tissue cells
- Pulmonary—referring to the lungs
- Rales—sometimes referred to as rhonchi; a crackling breath sound resulting from increased secretions in the bronchi
- Stridor—high-pitched breath sounds resembling wind, caused by partial obstruction of air passages
- Wheeze—squeaking or whistling breath sound, usually caused by narrowed tracheobronchial airways, as in asthma

Common Diseases and Disorders of the Respiratory System

- Asthma—episodic chronic respiratory disorder resulting from constricted bronchi, associated with allergens, infection, pollutants, cold air, exercise, or stress; characterized by wheezing and low oxygen levels

- Atelectasis—decreased or absence of air in part or in all of the lung and alveoli resulting from collapse of these structures
- Bronchitis—chronic or acute inflammation of the bronchi
- Carcinoma (cancer)—malignant tumor of lung or other areas of respiratory system
- Chronic obstructive pulmonary disease (COPD)—usually progressive respiratory system disorder with irreversible obstruction of air exchange in the bronchi, alveoli, and lungs; emphysema is a form of COPD
- Croup—acute viral infection, usually in infants, characterized by barking cough
- Cystic fibrosis—a genetic disorder that produces abnormally thick mucous secretions blocking and impairing the bronchi, pancreatic and bile ducts, and intestines
- Emphysema—a form of COPD characterized by irreversible loss of elasticity in alveoli that impedes respiration
- Legionnaires' disease—a type of pneumonia caused by the *Legionella pneumophila* bacteria
- Pertussis (whooping cough)—a vaccine-preventable bacterial infection (*Bordetella pertussis*) producing a "whoop" coughing sound; may be fatal in infants
- Pharyngitis—sore throat, inflammation of the pharynx
- Pleurisy—inflammation of the pleura
- Pneumonia—viral or bacterial infection causing inflammation of the lungs
- Pneumothorax—partial or complete collapse of the lung(s) resulting from air in the pleural cavity
- Pulmonary edema—fluid accumulation in the lungs, often associated with congestive heart failure
- Tuberculosis—an infectious bacterial disease characterized by tubercles in the tissue; the lung is the most common disease site

DIGESTIVE SYSTEM

The **digestive system** consists of the digestive tract, or alimentary canal, and its accessory organs, including the liver, pancreas, and gallbladder (Fig. 6-22). These organs take food and process it into usable energy for the body's growth, maintenance, and survival. The nutrients are absorbed and circulated, and the solid waste is eliminated.

Functions of the Digestive System

- Digestion—physical and chemical processes changing food into simple nutrients to be used by the cells for energy and building materials

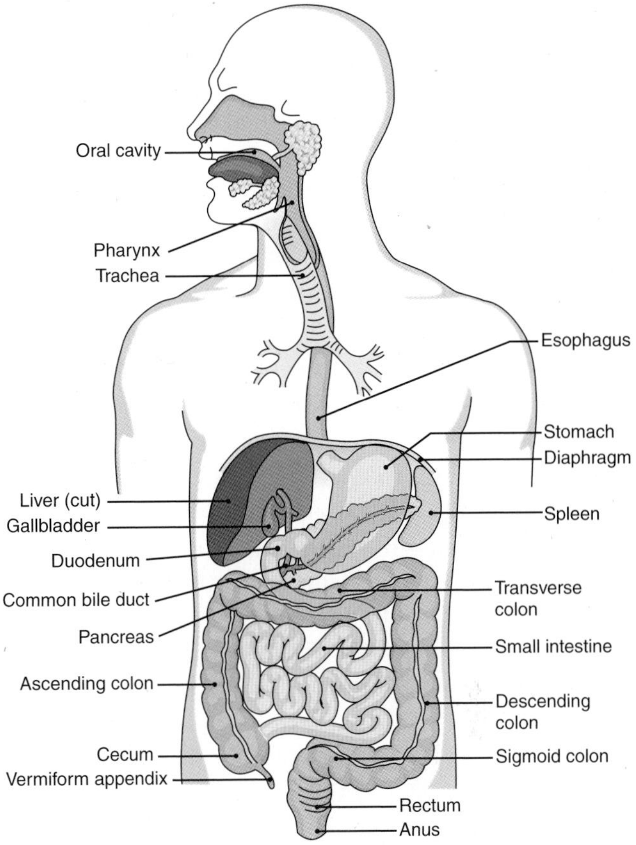

Figure 6-22 The digestive system. (Reprinted with permission from Cohen BJ, Wood DL. Memmler's The Human Body in Health and Disease. 9th Ed. Philadelphia: Lippincott Williams & Wilkins, 2000.)

- Absorption—the transfer of the products of digestion into the blood and lymph for circulation
- Elimination—excretion of the solid waste products of digestion in the form of feces

Components of the Digestive System

Digestive Tract

The digestive tract, or alimentary canal, is the system of tubelike organs in which digestion occurs; it begins at the mouth and ends at the anus.

- Mouth (oral cavity)—orifice in the lower face where food enters the body; chewing (mastication) and mixing with saliva occurs, forming a bolus
  - Salivary glands—three pair of glands located in the mouth that secrete saliva to moisten food and to begin the chemical breakdown of carbohydrates
  - Teeth—hard dentine structures located in the upper and lower jaws used for chewing (mastication); adults have 32 teeth
- Pharynx (throat)—this organ is part of the respiratory system and also allows masticated food to pass from the mouth to the esophagus

- Esophagus—tube from the pharynx to the stomach
- Stomach—J-shaped organ between the esophagus and the duodenum that produces a churning action, mixing food with gastric acids and enzymes as part of digestion; also stores food
- Small intestine—longest portion of digestive tract; it digests fats, proteins, and carbohydrates and absorbs the nutrient products into the blood
  - Duodenum—upper portion of the small intestine, separated from the stomach by the pyloric sphincter
  - Jejunum—middle portion of the small intestine
  - Ileum—lower portion of the small intestine, opening into the cecum
  - Villi (singular *villus*)—tiny projections in the small intestine lining where absorption of nutrients occurs
- Large intestine—the final organ of the digestive tract, it connects to the small intestine by the ileum and ends at the anus; manufactures vitamins K and B; absorbs fluids and electrolytes; forms, stores, and excretes feces
  - Cecum—upper portion of the large intestine; contains the appendix
  - Colon—largest portion of large intestine; divided into four parts
    - Ascending colon—portion of colon vertically positioned along right side of abdominal cavity
    - Transverse colon—portion of colon positioned horizontally and bridging the ascending and descending colons
    - Descending colon—portion of colon vertically positioned along the left side of the abdominal cavity
    - Sigmoid—lower S-shaped portion of colon connected to the descending colon and the rectum
  - Rectum—the lower portion of the large intestine, connecting the sigmoid to the anus and containing the reflexes for defecation
  - Anus—the final portion of the digestive tract, where feces are excreted
    - Internal sphincter—involuntary-control sphincter located in the anus
    - External sphincter—voluntary-control sphincter located in the anus

Note: The exams generally contain questions requiring knowledge of the different portions of the large and small intestines.

Accessory Digestive Organs

The organs outside the digestive tract that are involved in the digestive system functions are:

- Liver—largest gland in the body, located in the upper right portion of the abdominal cavity; produces bile, detoxifies blood, removes bilirubin, manufactures plasma protein involved in the production of prothrombin and fibrinogen, and aids metabolism
- Pancreas—an endocrine gland located behind the stomach producing pancreatic juice, which is transported to the duodenum to aid in digestion, and insulin and glucagon, which regulate carbohydrate metabolism
- Gallbladder—pear-shaped sac located on the inferior surface of the liver; stores bile to aid in digestion and fat absorption; bile is carried from the gallbladder to the duodenum via the common bile duct

Additional Digestive System Terms

- Enzymes—proteins that act as catalysts increasing the speed of digestion; each enzyme is specific to a certain type of food and reaction
- Hepatic—referring to the liver
- Jaundice—yellowing of skin, white of eyes, and mucous membranes resulting from increased bilirubin in blood; most common causes are obstruction of bile flow, liver dysfunction, or excess destruction of RBCs
- Peristalsis—rhythmic contractions that move food throughout the digestive tract
- Rugae—folds in the lining of the stomach and certain other organs

Common Diseases and Disorders of the Digestive System

- Anorexia—diminished appetite and aversion to food
- Botulism—serious food poisoning, usually found in contaminated canned foods, caused by *Clostridium botulinum* bacteria
- Cancer—malignant disease that may occur in any organ of the digestive system
- Cholelithiasis—gallstones
- Cirrhosis—end-stage liver disease interfering with blood flow, resulting in jaundice, portal hypertension, and function failure
- Crohn disease—inflammatory bowel disease; chronic inflammatory disease of ileum or colon resulting in diarrhea, pain, weight loss, and sometimes rectal bleeding; generally affects young female adults
- Diverticula (singular *diverticulum*)—abnormal pouches in the walls of an organ, usually found in the colon
- Diverticulosis—diverticula of the colon
- Gastroesophageal reflux disease (GERD)—backflow of stomach acids into the esophagus due to an incompetent esophageal sphincter, resulting in burning and discomfort; can lead to ulcers
- Giardiasis—infectious diarrhea caused by *Giardia lamblia*, which is found in contaminated water

- Hemorrhoids—inflammation and dilation of veins in rectum and anus
- Hepatitis—acute or chronic inflammation of the liver; there are at least eight types of identified hepatitis (A, B, C, D, E, F, G, H), with different causes and prognoses
- Hernia—protrusion of an organ or part of an organ through the wall normally containing it; the intestine is the most common organ to herniate
  - Hiatal hernia—protrusion of the stomach into the diaphragm
  - Incarcerated hernia—protrusion of the intestine that becomes swollen and obstructed
  - Inguinal hernia—protrusion of the intestine through the inguinal opening
  - Strangulated hernia—constriction of the herniated organ; may result in gangrene
  - Umbilical hernia—protrusion of the intestine through the abdominal wall around the umbilicus
- Intussusception—one part of the intestine slipping into another, leading to bowel obstruction and gangrene if not quickly treated; most common in male infants
- Thrush—yeast infection of the mouth caused by *Candida albicans*
- Ulcerative colitis—inflammation and ulceration of the mucosa of the colon and rectum
- Ulcers—lesions of the mucosa of any organ; most common in the stomach and intestine

URINARY SYSTEM

Reviewing the muscular, nervous, endocrine, cardiovascular, respiratory, and other systems demonstrates their interdependence on each other. The urinary system is no different. The main role of the **urinary system** is to remove liquid waste products from the blood and excrete them (Fig. 6-23). The urinary system works closely with the other systems to carry out these functions; other functions are listed in the next section with the male reproductive system.

Functions of the Urinary System

- Excretes nitrogen waste products and excess water and salts from the blood in the form of urine
- Assists the liver in detoxification
- Assists in maintaining pH balance
- Assists in maintaining blood volume

Components of the Urinary System

Kidneys

The kidneys are two muscular, bean-shaped organs located in the back of the abdominal cavity that filtrate, reabsorb selected substances, and excrete urine; Figure 6-24 illustrates the anatomy of the kidney and an enlarged nephron.

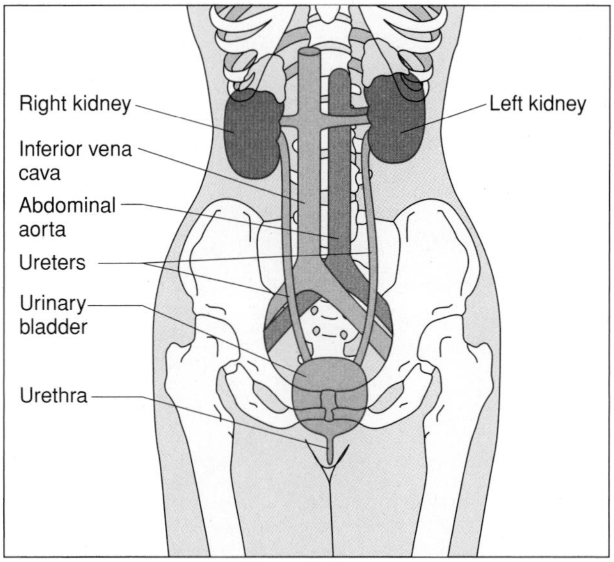

Figure 6-23 The urinary system. (Reprinted with permission from Willis MC, CMA-AC. Medical Terminology: A Programmed Learning Approach to the Language of Health Care. Baltimore: Lippincott Williams & Wilkins, 2002.)

- Cortex—outer layer
- Medulla—inner layer
  - Renal pyramids—triangular wedges in the medulla containing nephrons
    - Nephrons—group of microscopic coiled tubules (more than 1 million in each kidney) located in the renal pyramids that filter blood and form urine; the main structures are collecting tubules and glomeruli (enclosed in Bowman's capsule) and arterioles; the bottom of the paperclip-shaped segment of the nephron is called the loop of Henle
    - Calices (singular *calix*)—group of renal pyramid points forming the renal pelvis, where urine collects; also spelled *calyces* (singular *calyx*)

Ureters

The **ureters** are two slim tubes that carry urine from the kidneys to the urinary bladder.

Urinary Bladder

The **urinary bladder** is a saclike organ behind the symphysis pubis that temporarily stores urine.

Urethra

The **urethra** is the tube that takes urine from the bladder out of the body.

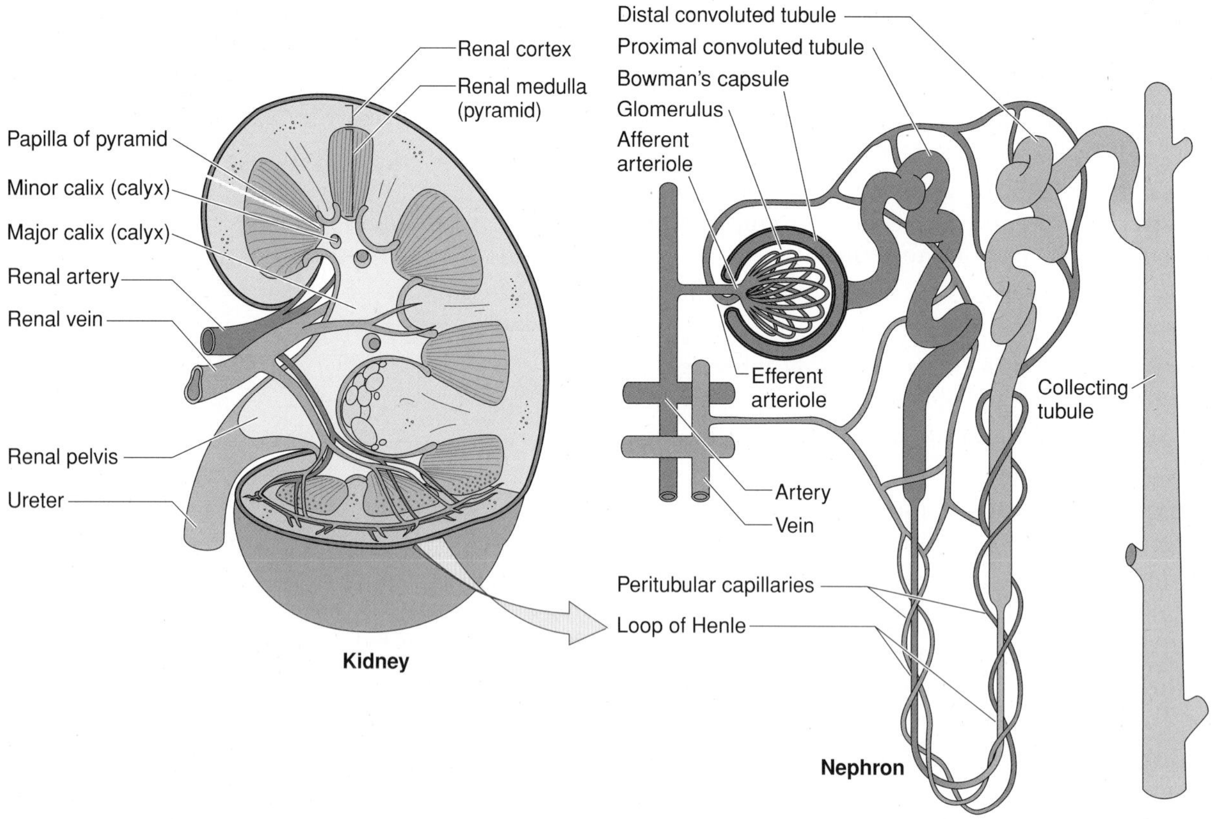

Figure 6-24 Longitudinal section of the kidney and enlarged nephron. (Reprinted with permission from Willis MC, CMA-AC. Medical Terminology: A Programmed Learning Approach to the Language of Health Care. Baltimore: Lippincott Williams & Wilkins, 2002.)

Additional Urinary System Terms

- Dehydration—water deficit
- Dialysis—a form of osmosis removing certain impurities from the blood (two types: **peritoneal dialysis** and **hemodialysis**)
- Edema—local or generalized excess retention of tissue fluid
- Glomerular filtration—the movement of fluid and materials under pressure from the blood through the glomerular membrane; the beginning of urine formation
- Tubular reabsorption—the process that follows glomerular filtration; the filtered water and other needed materials leave the tubule by diffusion and active transport to enter tissue fluids
- Urination—voiding or micturition; discharge of urine from the bladder through the urethra
- Urine—fluid waste from the blood secreted by the kidneys; stored in the urinary bladder and excreted from the urethra

Common Diseases and Disorders of the Urinary System

- Enuresis—involuntary discharge of urine
- Glomerulonephritis—acute or chronic inflammation of the kidney glomeruli; symptoms include edema, blood and protein in the urine, and possible uremia
- Hydronephrosis—distention of the renal pelvis resulting from obstructed flow of urine
- Hypospadias—congenital disorder in which the male urethra opens on the under side of the penis
- Incontinence—inability to retain urine, semen, or feces
- Nephrolithiasis (renal calculi)—kidney stones
- Polycystic kidney disease—familial disorder producing cysts in the kidney tubules and leading to kidney failure
- Pyelonephritis—inflammation and pyogenic infection of the renal pelvis
- Renal failure—acute or chronic loss of kidney function resulting in buildup of nitrogen waste in the body
- Uremia—high levels of nitrogen waste in the body

REPRODUCTIVE SYSTEMS

The male and female each has a different **reproductive system**. The male sperm uniting with the female ovum results in the formation of a new and distinct human.

The function of reproductive systems is to perpetuate the human species.

Male Reproductive System

The male of the human species is characterized by having an X and a Y chromosome.

Functions of the Male Reproductive System

- Produces sperm
- Deposits sperm into the female reproductive canal
- Produces hormones for male sex characteristics

Components of the Male Reproductive System

Figure 6-25 illustrates the components of the male reproductive system.

- Scrotum—external pouch suspended from the male perineum that contains the testes and epididymis
- Testes (testicles)—two glandular organs in the male scrotum that produce sperm, some semen (seminal fluid), and testosterone
- Epididymis—two coiled tubules on the posterior of the testes that store and carry sperm from the testes to the vas deferens
- Vas deferens (vas)—tubule that carries sperm from epididymis to seminal vesicles
- Seminal vesicles—a pair of accessory glands in the male, posterior to the urinary bladder, that secrete nutrient fluid for sperm

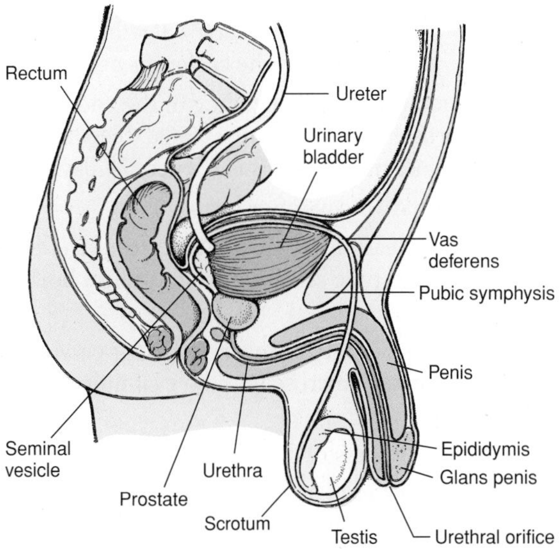

Figure 6-25 The male reproductive system. (Reprinted with permission from Stedman's Medical Dictionary. 27th Ed. Baltimore: Lippincott Williams & Wilkins, 2000.)

- Ejaculatory duct—passage formed by the seminal vesicles and vas deferens that allows semen to enter the urethra
- Prostate gland—donut-shaped gland around the male urethra at the bladder neck that secretes alkaline fluid to protect sperm
- Cowper gland—two small glands located at the base of the penis that secrete lubricant during intercourse
- Penis—external male sex organ that contains the urethra; during sexual arousal, it becomes engorged with blood and firm and erect, allowing entry to the female vagina where the sperm is ejected (ejaculated)
  - Glans penis—acorn-shaped head of penis
  - Prepuce—foreskin; a fold of skin covering the glans penis

Additional Male Reproductive System Terms

- Circumcision—surgical removal of foreskin
- Gamete—male (sperm) or female (ovum) reproductive cell
- Genitalia—external sex organs
- Spermatozoa—sperm
- Vasectomy—male sterilization procedure; tying off or removing part or all of vas deferens

Common Diseases and Disorders of the Male Reproductive System

- Benign prostatic hyperplasia (BPH)—nonmalignant enlargement of the prostate
- Cancers of the male reproductive system—malignancies, usually in the testes or prostate
- Cryptorchidism—failure of testes to descend into the scrotum
- Hypospadias—congenital anomaly; the male urethra opens on the posterior of the penis
- Impotence—inability of the male to achieve erection or ejaculation
- Orchiditis (also spelled orchitis)—inflammation of the testes
- Phimosis—inability to retract the foreskin over the glans penis because of tightness of the skin
- Priapism—abnormal, painful, prolonged penile erection, usually resulting from spinal cord injury or disease

Female Reproductive System

The female of the human species is characterized by two X chromosomes.

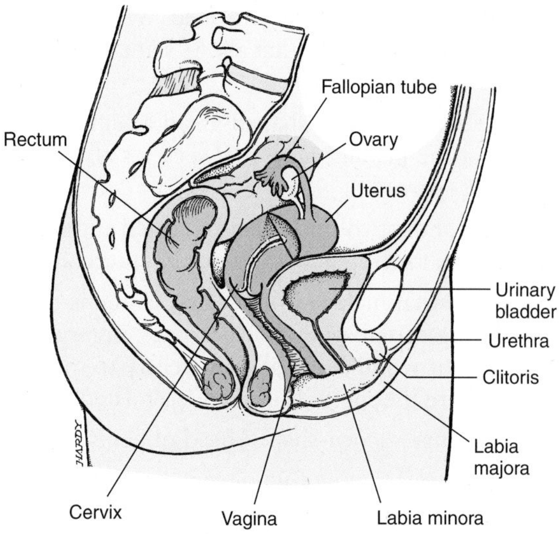

Figure 6-26 The female reproductive system. (Reprinted with permission from Stedman's Medical Dictionary. 27th Ed. Baltimore: Lippincott Williams & Wilkins, 2000.)

Functions of the Female Reproductive System

- Produces ova (eggs) for fertilization
- Carries and nurtures developing fetus
- Gives birth
- Provides food source for newborn
- Produces hormones for female sex characteristics, reproduction, and lactation

Components of the Female Reproductive System

Figure 6-26 depicts the components of the female reproductive system.

- Ovaries—two female sex glands located in the pelvis that form ova (the female egg or germ cell) and secrete estrogen
- Uterus—female organ located in pelvic cavity between the oviducts and the vagina; it houses and nourishes the growing fetus and placenta
  - Fundus—upper region of the uterus
  - Body—large central area of the uterus
  - Cervix—lower uterine region opening to the vagina
  - Endometrium—lining of the uterus that sloughs off during menstruation; provides nourishment and protection during pregnancy
- Fallopian tubes (oviducts)—canals that pick up ova released by the ovaries and carry them to the uterus
- Vagina—part of the birth canal; muscular tube connecting the cervix of the uterus to the external female genitalia
- Vulva—external female genitalia
  - Mons pubis—soft pad over the symphysis pubis
  - Labia majora—two large folds covering the vaginal opening, extending from the mons pubis to the perineum
  - Labia minora—two small folds of skin inside the labia majora
  - Clitoris—small nodule of erectile tissue located in the superior junction of the labia majora; contributes to sexual arousal
  - Bartholin glands—glands at the vaginal opening that provide lubrication during sexual intercourse
  - Perineum—area between the vaginal opening and rectum
- Breasts—two mammary glands and fatty tissue situated over the pectoral muscles that produce milk

Additional Female Reproductive System Terms

- Antepartum—time before delivery
- Fertilization—impregnation of the female's ovum (egg) with the male's sperm
- Fetus—term given to developing baby in the uterus after the first trimester
- Gestation—period of pregnancy
- Menarche—first female menses; usually occurs between 9 and 15 years of age
- Menopause—cessation of menses and female reproduction as a result of aging or surgical removal of the ovaries or uterus
- Menstrual cycle—an approximately 28-day phase beginning with menstruation, followed by the thickening of the endometrium; midcycle, ovulation occurs, followed by secretion of progesterone by the corpus luteum to prepare the uterus for a fertilized ovum; if pregnancy does not occur, the cycle repeats
- Menstruation (menses)—shedding of the endometrium of the uterus in the form of vaginal bleeding when pregnancy does not occur, usually every 28 days
- Neonatal—first 30 days after birth
- Ovulation—release of an ovum (egg) from the follicle into the ovarian tube resulting from cyclical hormonal function
- Papanicolaou smear (Pap smear)—test for cervical cancer that involves microscopically examining cervical scrapings
- Parturition—process of delivery; giving birth
- Placenta—oval vascular structure in the uterus during pregnancy that supplies nutrients to the fetus
- Pregnancy—gestation; period of fetal development in the uterus from fertilization to birth, usually lasting 40 weeks

Common Diseases and Disorders of the Female Reproductive System

- Abortion—termination of pregnancy before fetal viability; may be spontaneous (naturally occurring) or medically/surgically induced
- Abruptio placentae—premature separation of the placenta
- Amenorrhea—absence of menstrual flow
- Carcinomas—malignancies of the female reproductive system that most commonly occur in the breasts, ovaries, uterus, and cervix
- Eclampsia—toxemia of pregnancy with high blood pressure, albuminuria, oliguria, seizures, and sometimes coma and death
- Ectopic pregnancy (extrauterine)—implantation of fertilized ovum outside the uterus, most commonly in the fallopian tubes
- Endometriosis—condition caused by abnormal location of endometrium tissue outside the uterus; causes pain and, sometimes, cyst formation
- Fibroids—nonmalignant tumors of the uterus
- Menorrhagia—painful menses
- Miscarriage—spontaneous abortion; natural interruption of a pregnancy before the seventh month
- Pelvic inflammatory disease (PID)—inflammation of the pelvic cavity organs resulting from widespread infection
- Placenta previa—implantation of the placenta in the lower uterus
- Premenstrual syndrome (PMS)—irritability, bloating, and depression preceding menses

Sexually Transmitted Diseases

Sexually transmitted diseases (STDs) or infections (STIs) affect both males and females. The act of intercourse results in passing and intermingling of body secretions between the sexual partners. These secretions may contain pathogens that are then sexually transmitted from one person to another. The more sexual partners a person has, the higher the risk of becoming infected.

- AIDS—decreased immunity resulting from infection with HIV; leaves victim susceptible to opportunistic diseases
- Chlamydia—caused by *Chlamydia trachomatis*; the most prevalent STD; symptoms are frequently undetected and result in female PID; babies born to mothers with chlamydia are at risk for chlamydial pneumonia
- Genital herpes—viral infection of the male and female genital tracts' mucous membranes with painful lesions; incurable and may lead to cervical cancer in women; newborns become infected through the female birth canal
- Genital warts—infection caused by human papilloma viruses; a potential cause of cervical cancer
- Gonorrhea—contagious inflammation of the genital mucous membrane of either sex, caused by *Neisseria gonorrhoeae*
- HIV—the virus causing AIDS
- Syphilis—chronic STD resulting in lesions (chancres) that may spread to the bone and other body systems; disease may be congenital

TERMS

Anatomy and Physiology Review

The following list reviews the terms discussed in this chapter, **as well as other important terms that you may see on the exam.**

abduction moving away from the body midline (the opposite of adduction) (e.g., spreading the arms)

abortion termination of pregnancy before viability; may be spontaneous (naturally occurring) or medically/surgically induced

abruptio placentae premature separation of the placenta

absorption the transfer of the products of digestion into the blood and lymph for circulation

acquired immunodeficiency syndrome (AIDS) decreased immunity resulting from infection with the human immunodeficiency virus (HIV), leaving victim susceptible to opportunistic diseases

acromegaly overproduction of the growth hormone after puberty, resulting in wide, large face, hands, and feet

active transport movement of molecules from area of lower to area of higher concentration

Addison disease hyposecretion of cortisol by the adrenal cortex, resulting in muscle atrophy, tissue weakness, and skin pigmentation

adduction moving toward the body midline (the opposite of abduction) (e.g., bringing the arms to the sides)

adrenal glands endocrine glands located on top of each kidney; refer to Table 6-1 for functions

alveoli (singular *alveolus*) air sacs at the ends of the bronchioles where the exchange of gases occurs

Alzheimer disease degenerative disorder of the brain beginning with dementia-like symptoms and progressing to a nonfunctioning of neuron fibers that prevents communication between cells for ordinary tasks (such as swallowing), which results in death; etiology is unknown

amenorrhea absence of menstrual flow

amyotrophic lateral sclerosis (ALS) progressive disease of the motor neurons, causing muscle atrophy and weakness; also known as *Lou Gehrig disease*

anabolism phase of metabolism in which cells are built or repaired

anaphase third phase of mitosis; duplicated chromosomes separate, and one of each begins to move toward opposite centrioles or poles

anatomy the study of body structure

anemia abnormally low hemoglobin or red blood cells, decreasing oxygen supply to the tissues; many causes and types; the main symptoms are fatigue and weakness

aneurysm congenital or traumatic weakness of the vessel wall demonstrated by a "bubble" or outpouching caused by pressure of blood; an abdominal aortic aneurysm is called *AAA* or *triple A*

angina pectoris severe constricting chest pain from lack of blood supply to the heart; associated with coronary artery disease

anorexia diminished appetite and aversion to food

antepartum time before delivery

anterior in front (ventral)

antibody a substance produced in the body in response to the presence of an antigen; antibodies enhance activities of leukocytes and produce globulins protecting the body against further assault from the specific antigen

antigen a substance (e.g., bacteria/viruses, bacterial/viral toxins, foreign blood cells) that causes the formation of antibodies

anus the final portion of the digestive tract, where feces are excreted

aorta the largest body artery; consists of three parts: ascending, aortic arch, and descending

aponeurosis broad sheet of muscle fibers attaching muscle to muscle or muscle to select bones, such as the skull

appendicular skeleton consists of the bones of the upper and lower extremities and the girdle attaching them to the axial skeleton.

arrhythmias abnormal heart rhythms

arteriosclerosis hardening of the arteries and loss of elasticity resulting from thickening of the vessel wall

arthritis inflammation of the joints

asthma an episodic chronic respiratory disorder resulting from constricted bronchi; associated with allergens, infection, pollutants, cold air, exercise, or stress; characterized by wheezing and low oxygen levels

astigmatism impaired vision resulting from irregular curve of cornea; the image focuses improperly on the retina; may be mild to severe; usually corrected with glasses or contact lenses

atelectasis a decrease or absence of air in part or all of the lung and alveoli, resulting in a collapse of these structures

atherosclerosis the most common form of arteriosclerosis; irregular fatty deposits on arterial wall result in narrowing and occlusion of vessel; may cause myocardial infarctions, cerebrovascular accidents, gangrene, and other disorders associated with blood vessel blockage

atrioventricular (AV) node located at the lower right of the atrial septum, it picks up the impulse or signal from the sinoatrial (SA) node that causes atrial contraction; if the SA node fails, the AV node may initiate the impulse; the resulting heart rate is slower, at 40 to 60 beats per minute

axial skeleton consists of the bones of the skull, spine, and chest

Bell palsy unilateral facial muscle paralysis (drooping of eye and mouth) resulting from dysfunction of the seventh cranial nerve

benign prostatic hyperplasia (BPH) nonmalignant enlargement of the prostate

bile a substance produced by the liver and stored in the gallbladder that aids in digestion and fat absorption

body organism; a group of systems working together to maintain life

body cavities spaces within the body that house internal organs

botulism serious food poisoning, usually found in contaminated canned foods, caused by *Clostridium botulinum* bacteria

brain an organ acting as the primary center for regulating and coordinating body functions and activities; divided into right and left hemispheres

bronchi (singular *bronchus*) tubes from trachea entering the lungs that subdivide into two more branches in the lungs

bronchioles smaller branches of the bronchi

bronchitis chronic or acute inflammation of the bronchi

bundle branches two branches extending from the bundle of His in the heart that carry the electrical impulse down the ventricular septum

bundle of His specialized cells in the cardiac ventricular septum that carry the electrical impulse from the atrioventricular (AV) node; should the sinoatrial and AV nodes fail, the bundle of His may initiate the impulse; the resulting heart rate is 20 to 40 beats per minute

cardiovascular system the body system containing the heart and blood vessels to circulate blood, transport nutrients, and remove waste from tissues

carpals four wrist bones

cartilage firm connective tissue found primarily in joints, thorax walls, larynx, and airway passages and ears

catabolism the phase of metabolism in which cells are broken down

cataract a cloudy or opaque lens that impairs sight; usually corrected by surgery

caudal the location near the sacral region of the spinal column

cecum the upper portion of the large intestine; contains the appendix

cells the structural and functional units of life

central nervous system (CNS) made up of the brain and spinal cord; integrates sensory information and responses

centriole rod-shaped material in the cytoplasm that begins cell division

cerebellum "little brain"; portion of the brain involved in synergic control of skeletal muscles and coordination of voluntary muscular movements; connected to the cerebrum, brainstem, and spinal cord by the pons

cerebral palsy loss of mental function, sensation, or control of movement resulting from birth injury or defect

cerebrospinal fluid (CSF) clear fluid that flows through the brain and spinal cord and into the subarachnoid spaces of the meninges; it cushions and supports nervous tissue and transports nutrients and waste products from the cells

cerebrovascular accident (CVA) stroke; occlusion or hemorrhage of vessel(s) in the brain, resulting in impairment of mental functions or paralysis or both

cerebrum the largest part of the brain, divided into right and left hemispheres by the longitudinal fissure; it contains auditory, visual, gustatory, and olfactory areas as well as areas of higher mental faculties, and regulates balance

Cheyne-Stokes respiration an irregular breathing pattern of slow and shallow, then rapid and deep respirations with pauses for 20 to 30 seconds; frequently occurs before death

chlamydia the most prevalent sexually transmitted disease, caused by *Chlamydia trachomatis*; symptoms are frequently undetected, resulting in female pelvic inflammatory disease

cholelithiasis gallstones

chronic obstructive pulmonary disease (COPD) a usually progressive respiratory system disorder with irreversible obstruction of air exchange in the bronchi, alveoli, and lungs; emphysema is a form of COPD

cilia hairlike processes that trap and move foreign particles

circumcision surgical removal of foreskin

circumduction drawing an imaginary circle with a body structure (e.g., the arms)

cirrhosis end-stage liver disease with interference with blood flow, resulting in jaundice, portal hypertension, and liver failure

clavicle collar bone joining the sternum at the anterior and the scapula laterally

cochlea snail-shaped tube in ear containing receptor for hearing

collagen a fibrous protein found in the dermis, connective tissues, tendons, and ligaments; it is sometimes referred to as the body's glue, providing strength and flexibility

Colles fracture displaced fracture of the distal radius, proximal to the wrist

colon largest portion of large intestine; divides into four parts: ascending colon, transverse colon, descending colon, and sigmoid

congestive heart failure (CHF) venous and pulmonary congestion and general edema (swelling) resulting from decreased blood circulation

conjunctivitis inflammation of the conjunctiva caused by infection or irritation

coronary artery disease (CAD) arteriosclerosis or atherosclerosis of the coronary arteries, usually leading to myocardial ischemia (damage to tissue)

Cowper glands two small glands located at the base of the penis that secrete lubricant during intercourse

cranial location associated with the head

cretinism hypothyroidism; decreased secretion of thyroxine in infants resulting in failure of physical and mental development

Crohn disease inflammatory bowel disease; chronic inflammatory disease of ileum or colon resulting in diarrhea, pain, weight loss, and sometimes rectal bleeding; generally affects young female adults

croup acute viral infection, usually in infants, characterized by barking cough

cryptorchidism failure of testes to descend into the scrotum

Cushing syndrome overproduction of cortisol by the adrenal cortex, resulting in round face, overweight, thin skin, and high blood sugar

cystic fibrosis a genetic disorder producing abnormally thick mucous secretions that block and impair the bronchi, pancreatic and bile ducts, and intestines

cytoplasm colloidal substance (protoplasm) found in the cell; holds other structures in place

dendrites neuron fibers conducting impulses to the cell body

dermis deeper layer of skin containing nerves, blood vessels, and other skin structures or appendages

diabetes mellitus most common endocrine disorder; low production of insulin, resulting in cells retaining sugar; two types: insulin-dependent diabetes mellitus (type 1 diabetes) and non–insulin-dependent diabetes mellitus (type 2 diabetes)

diabetic retinopathy damage to the retina in diabetic patients from hemorrhage of vessels; usually progressive and related to the control of the diabetes

dialysis a form of osmosis that removes certain impurities from the blood (two types: peritoneal and hemodialysis)

diaphragm muscle tissue separating thoracic and abdominal cavities that contracts and expands during respiration, allowing lungs to fill and empty air

diastole relaxation portion of the cardiac cycle

diffusion movement of molecules from area of higher to lower concentration
digestion physical and chemical processes changing food into simple nutrients to be utilized by the cells for energy and building materials and into solid waste to be eliminated from the body
digestive system body system containing mouth, esophagus, stomach, intestines, rectum, liver, gallbladder, and pancreas; the system ingests and processes food and eliminates solid waste products
distal away from the origin of a structure
diverticula (singular *diverticulum*) abnormal pouches in the walls of an organ, usually the colon
diverticulosis diverticula of the colon
dorsal posterior; in back
duodenum upper portion of small intestine, separated from the stomach by the pyloric sphincter
dwarfism decreased growth hormone, resulting in abnormally small size
eclampsia toxemia of pregnancy, with high blood pressure, albuminuria, oliguria, seizures, and sometimes coma
ectopic pregnancy extrauterine pregnancy; implantation of fertilized ovum outside the uterus, most commonly in the ovarian tubes
ejaculatory duct passage formed by the seminal vesicles and vas deferens allowing semen to enter the urethra
elimination excretion of the solid waste products of digestion in the form of feces
embolus (plural *emboli*) a detached thrombus or other substance occluding a vessel
emphysema a form of chronic obstructive pulmonary disease that impedes respiration; characterized by irreversible loss of elasticity in alveoli
endocardium inner layer of the heart
endocrine system body system containing glands and related structures that produce and secrete hormones
endometriosis condition caused by endometrium tissue located outside the uterus that causes pain and, sometimes, cyst formation
enucleation removal of the eyeball
enuresis involuntary discharge of urine
enzymes proteins that act as catalysts to increase the speed of digestion; each enzyme is specific to a certain type of food and reaction
epicardium outer layer of the heart
epidermis surface layer of skin containing strata and melanin
epididymis two coiled tubules on the posterior of the testes that store and carry sperm from the testes to the vas deferens
epiglottis flaplike structure covering larynx during swallowing
epilepsy abnormal electrical activity of the brain resulting in seizure; there are multiple causes, such as head trauma, high fevers, disease processes, poisoning, or overdose
erythrocytes red blood cells (RBCs); contain hemoglobin to carry oxygen; mature cells do not have a nucleus
esophagus tube from the pharynx to the stomach
eustachian tube connects middle ear with throat and pharynx; equalizes pressure on tympanic membrane
eversion turning wrists or ankles outward, away from the body (the opposite of inversion), such as turning the foot away from the body
exophthalmia protrusion of the eyeballs, usually resulting from an endocrine disorder
expiration exhalation; letting air out of the lungs; the diaphragm relaxes, decreasing the size of the thoracic cavity and pushing air out
extension bringing the limbs or phalanges toward a straight position (the opposite of flexion), such as opening the fingers of a closed hand
extracellular fluid body fluid outside the cell
fallopian tubes oviducts; canals leading from the ovaries to the uterus
femur thigh bone; the body's largest, longest, and strongest bone
fertilization impregnation of the female ovum (egg) with the male sperm
fetus term given after the first trimester to a developing baby in the uterus
fibroids nonmalignant tumors of the uterus
fibula smaller lower leg bone, lateral to tibia
filtration process of moving fluid containing dissolved particles through a membrane; an example is kidney filtration
flagella whiplike processes on the cell surface; accommodate cell movement
flexion bending (the opposite of extension), such as closing the fingers of the hand
fluid balance the regulation of the amount and composition of the body's fluids
frontal plane imaginary line or cut of the body made in line with the ears and then down the middle of the body, resulting in a front and a back portion; also called *coronal plane*
gallbladder pear-shaped sac located on the inferior surface of the liver; stores bile to aid in digestion and fat absorption
gamete male (sperm) or female (ovum) reproductive cell
ganglion marked swelling of gray matter, located outside the central nervous system, containing cells of neurons
gastroesophageal reflux disease (GERD) backflow of stomach acids into the esophagus due to an incompetent esophageal sphincter, resulting in burning and discomfort; can lead to ulcers
genital herpes painful and incurable viral infection of the male or female genital tract's mucous membrane; may

lead to cervical cancer in women; newborns become infected through contact with the mother's birth canal

genitalia external sex organs

genital warts infection caused by the human papillomavirus; believed to be a precursor of female cervical cancer

gestation period of pregnancy

giantism overproduction of the growth hormone, resulting in abnormally large size

giardiasis infectious diarrhea caused by *Giardia lamblia* in contaminated water

glans penis acorn-shaped head of penis

glaucoma a disease of the eye characterized by increased intraocular pressure; causes damage to optic nerve; often results in blindness

globulins the fraction of the blood serum protein associated with antibodies; vaccination with globulins produces passive immunity

glomerular filtration the movement of fluid and materials under pressure from the blood through the kidney's glomerular membrane; the beginning of urine formation

glomerulonephritis acute or chronic inflammation of the kidney glomeruli; symptoms include edema, blood and protein in the urine, and possible uremia

goiter enlarged thyroid

gonorrhea contagious inflammation of the genital mucous membrane of either sex, caused by *Neisseria gonorrhoeae*

gout inflammation and pain, usually of the great toes or thumbs, caused by accumulation of uric acid crystals; usually occurs in late-middle-aged men

Graves disease hyperthyroidism; increased secretion of thyroxine; characterized by goiter, exophthalmia (bulging eyes), weight loss, extreme nervousness, and rapid metabolism

hemodialysis a form of dialysis that removes blood via a catheter placed directly into a vein; the blood then circulates through a dialysis machine to remove impurities

hemophilia genetic bleeding disorder involving a deficiency of specific clotting factors and resulting in excessive bleeding, especially into the joints

hemorrhoids inflammation and dilation of veins in rectum and anus

hepatic referring to the liver

hepatitis acute or chronic inflammation of the liver; there are at least eight types of identified hepatitis (A, B, C, D, E, F, G, H), with different causes and prognoses

hernia protrusion of an organ or part of an organ through the wall normally containing it; intestine is the most common organ to herniate

herpes zoster shingles; infection caused by the herpes zoster virus forming blister-type lesions and producing pain along the nerve trunks

histology study of tissues

homeostasis equilibrium or health of the body as measured by established norms for blood pressure, heart rate, temperature, respiration rate, and other indicators

human immunodeficiency virus (HIV) the virus causing acquired immunodeficiency syndrome

human papilloma virus (HPV) the virus associated with genital warts and cervical cancer

humerus upper arm bone

hydrocephalus accumulation of cerebrospinal fluid in the brain caused by an obstruction and resulting in mounting pressure and destruction of brain tissue

hydronephrosis distention of the renal pelvis resulting from obstructed flow of urine

hyperextension extreme or abnormal extension, usually resulting in injury (e.g., dislocated finger)

hyperopia farsightedness; a condition in which distant objects can be seen more clearly than closer objects

hypertension high blood pressure (beginning at 140/90)

hyperthyroidism overactivity of the thyroid

hypertonic solution fluid more concentrated than intracellular fluid; it draws fluid away from the cell and causes the cell to shrink

hypospadias congenital disorder; the male urethra opens on the under side of the penis

hypothalamus located in the diencephalon, the hypothalamus contains nerve cells assisting in maintenance of water balance, fat and sugar metabolism, secretion of endocrine glands, and regulation of body temperature

hypothyroidism underactivity of the thyroid

hypotonic solution fluid less concentrated than intracellular fluid; it results in excess fluid entering the cell and may cause the cell to rupture

ileum lower portion of the small intestine, opening into the cecum

ilium superior wing-shaped portion of hip bones

immunity the individual's ability to resist specific diseases or disorders, usually by acquiring the corresponding antibody

immunization vaccination; protection from communicable diseases by administration of living attenuated agents (e.g., measles), killed organisms (e.g., pertussis), inactivated toxins (e.g., tetanus), or recombinant DNA (e.g., hepatitis B)

impotence inability of the male to achieve erection or ejaculation

incontinence inability to retain urine, semen, or feces

incus anvil; second ossicle (bone) of the middle ear

inferior below

inspiration inhalation; bringing air into lungs; diaphragm contracts, increasing the size of the thoracic cavity and allowing air to enter the lungs

integumentary system the largest system of the body, it contains skin, glands, hair, nails, blood vessels, and nerves to protect against infection and other "invaders"; assists with prevention of dehydration; controls body temperature; receives sensory information; eliminates waste products; and produces vitamin D
intracellular fluid body fluid inside the cell
intussusception one part of the intestine slipping into another, leading to bowel obstruction and gangrene if not quickly treated; most common in male infants
inversion turning inside out (the opposite of eversion), such as turning the heels out so toes face each other
ischium inferior portion of hip bones supporting the body weight when sitting
isotonic solution with the same concentration as intracellular fluid, moves in and out of the cell at the same rate
jaundice yellow color of skin, white of eyes, and mucous membranes resulting from increased bilirubin in blood; most common causes are obstruction of bile flow, liver dysfunction, and excess destruction of red blood cells
joints areas where two or more bones come together or articulate
keratin a protein in the epidermis that thickens and waterproofs the skin
kidneys two muscular, bean-shaped organs located in the back of the abdominal cavity that filtrate, reabsorb selected substances, and excrete urine
kyphosis hunchback; an excessive curvature in the thoracic portion of the vertebral column
labyrinth inner ear; contains vestibule, semicircular canal, and cochlea with receptors for hearing and balance
large intestine the final organ of the digestive tract; connects to the small intestine at the ileum; sections include cecum, colon, rectum; ends at the anus; manufactures vitamins K and B; absorbs fluids and electrolytes; forms, stores, and excretes feces
larynx voice box; organ between the pharynx and trachea containing vocal cords, which vibrate to produce speech
lateral away from midline, toward the side
Legionnaires' disease a type of pneumonia caused by the *Legionella pneumophila* bacteria
leukemia type of malignancy characterized by rapid and abnormal development of leukocytes (white blood cells) in spleen, bone marrow, and lymph nodes
leukocytes white blood cells (WBCs); fight infection
ligaments bands of fibrous connective tissue connecting the articulating ends of bones to facilitate or limit movement
liver largest gland in the body, located in the upper right portion of the abdominal cavity; it produces bile, detoxifies blood, and aids metabolism
lordosis swayback; excessive curvature in the lumbar portion of the vertebral column
lungs two main organs of the respiratory system that are located in the thoracic cavity; they distribute and exchange gases
lymphatic system body system containing lymph, lymph nodes, and related organs to protect against and fight disease
macular degeneration progressive abnormal growth of blood vessels or other structures in the retina, usually leading to blindness
malleus hammer; first ossicle (bone) of the middle ear
mandible lower jaw bone
maxilla upper jaw bone
medial toward the middle or center
mediastinum small cavity within the thoracic cavity that lies between the lungs and contains the heart and large blood vessels
medulla oblongata portion of the brain connecting with spinal cord; contains centers for control of heart beat, respirations, and blood pressure
melanin pigment giving the skin its color
membranes thin sheets of tissue that line and protect body structures
menarche first female menses; usually occurs between 9 and 15 years of age
meninges (singular *meninx*) three layers of connective tissue covering that completely enclose the brain and spinal cord
menopause cessation of menses and female reproduction from aging or surgical removal of the ovaries
menorrhagia painful menses
menstrual cycle a phase lasting approximately 28 days, beginning with menstruation, followed by the thickening of the endometrium; midcycle, ovulation occurs, followed by secretion of progesterone by the corpus luteum to prepare the uterus for a fertilized ovum; if pregnancy does not occur, the cycle repeats
menstruation menses; the shedding of the endometrium of the uterus in the form of vaginal bleeding when pregnancy does not occur, usually in a 28-day cycle
metabolism energy transformation in living cells
metacarpals five bones that form the palm of the hand
metaphase second phase of mitosis; chromosomes line up along an equator-type line along centriole filaments
metatarsals the five foot bones
midbrain connects the pons and cerebellum with the cerebrum; functions as relay for certain eye and ear reflexes
miscarriage spontaneous abortion; a natural interruption of a pregnancy before the seventh month
mitosis cell division; comprises four phases: prophase, metaphase, anaphase, and telophase

mouth oral cavity; orifice in the lower face where food enters the body; chewing (mastication) and mixing with saliva occurs, forming a bolus
multiple sclerosis progressive inflammation and hardening of the myelin sheath in the nervous system
muscular system body system that contains muscles and related structures that accommodate movement
myocardial infarction (MI) heart attack; necrosis (death) of an area in the myocardium resulting from cessation of blood supply, usually from coronary thrombosis
myocardium middle layer of the heart
myopia condition of nearsightedness; can see objects close by but not far away
myxedema atrophy of thyroid in adults, resulting in decreased secretion of thyroxine, causing forms of physical and mental decline
narcolepsy uncontrollable episodes of falling asleep; also known as sleep epilepsy
neonatal first 30 days after birth
nephrolithiasis (renal calculi) kidney stones
nephrons group of microscopic coiled tubules (more than 1 million in each kidney), located in the renal pyramids, that filter blood and form urine; main structures are collecting tubules, glomeruli, and arterioles; the bottom of the paperclip-shaped segment of the nephron is called the loop of Henle
nervous system body system containing nerves and related structures that receive stimuli and initiate responses
neurotransmitter chemical released by the axons that stimulates the next cell to continue the transmission of an impulse
nucleolus small structure in the cell nucleus that holds ribonucleic acid (RNA) and ribosomes essential for protein formation
nucleus located in the center of the cell; controls cell activity and contains genetic material (DNA)
orchiditis (also spelled *orchitis*) inflammation of the testes
organ group of tissues working together to perform a function, such as the kidney
osmosis water diffusion (movement from area of higher to lower concentration) through a semipermeable membrane
osmotic pressure the tendency of a higher-concentration solution to draw in water from a lower-concentration solution
osteoarthritis degenerative joint disease that results in deformities and chronic pain; usually occurs as part of the aging process, but excessive use (e.g., in marathon runners) and trauma are also contributory factors
osteochondroma malignancy of the bone and cartilage
osteomyelitis inflammation of the bone or marrow caused by pathogens
osteoporosis porous, brittle bones resulting from low levels of calcium salts; common in menopausal women
osteosarcoma malignant tumor of the bone
otitis media infection of middle ear; most common in infants and toddlers; usually treated with antibiotics
ovaries two female endocrine sex glands (gonads) that secrete estrogen to stimulate growth of breasts, uterus, and secondary sex characteristics and form ova (the female gametes) and progesterone to prepare and maintain uterus in pregnancy; located in the pelvis
ovulation release of an ovum (egg) from the follicle into the ovarian tube resulting from cyclical hormone function
pancreas an endocrine gland located behind the stomach that produces pancreatic juice, which is transported to the duodenum to aid in digestion, and insulin and glucagon, which regulate carbohydrate metabolism
Papanicolaou smear (Pap smear) test for cervical cancer that involves microscopically examining cervical scrapings
parasympathetic nervous system portion of the nervous system that returns the body to rest and replenishes energy
parathyroid gland one of four pea-sized glands located on or embedded in the thyroid that secrete parathyroid hormone, increasing blood levels of calcium
Parkinson disease chronic progressive neurologic disease characterized by fine tremors and muscle weakness and rigidity; etiology believed to be associated with low dopamine production
parturition process of delivery; giving birth
patella kneecap
patent ductus arteriosus (PDA) opening between the aorta and pulmonary artery in fetal circulation that does not close as it should after birth
pathology the study of abnormal changes in body structure or function, usually caused by disease
pelvic inflammatory disease (PID) inflammation of the pelvic cavity organs resulting from widespread infection
penis external male sex organ containing the urethra; during sexual arousal, the penis becomes engorged with blood and firm and erect, allowing entry to the female vagina where the sperm is ejected (ejaculated)
peripheral nervous system (PNS) nerves outside the central nervous system originating from the brain and spinal cord; it transmits sensory information and responses
peristalsis rhythmic contractions that move food throughout the digestive tract
peritoneal dialysis a form of dialysis using the peritoneal membrane to filter wastes
pertussis whooping cough; a vaccine-preventable bacterial infection caused by *Bordetella pertussis*,

producing a "whoop" coughing sound; serious, sometimes fatal in infants

phagocytosis ingestion and digestion of bacteria and other substances by phagocytic cells

phalanges fingers (three bones each) and thumb (two bones each); toes (three bones each) and great toes (two bones each)

pharyngitis sore throat; inflammation of the pharynx

pharynx throat; passageway from nose to larynx

phimosis inability to retract the foreskin over the glans penis because of tightness of the skin

physiology the study of body function

pineal gland endocrine gland located in the brain behind the hypothalamus that secretes melatonin, which regulates the body's sleep/wake cycles

pinna auricle; external ear; directs sound waves to the canal

pituitary endocrine gland located at the base of the brain, called "master gland" because of the number of hormones it secretes and functions it serves; Table 6-1 lists its functions

placenta oval vascular structure present in the uterus during pregnancy that supplies nutrients to the fetus

placenta previa abnormal implantation of the placenta in the lower uterus

plantar flexion pointing toes downward, which flexes the arch of the foot (e.g., en pointe dancing in ballet)

plasma liquid portion of blood (55%)

platelets (thrombocytes) cell fragments; function in coagulation

pleura lung linings containing pleural fluid to protect lungs and reduce friction during respiration

pleurisy inflammation of the pleura

pneumonia viral or bacterial infection causing inflammation of the lungs

pneumothorax partial or complete collapse of the lung(s) resulting from air in the pleural cavity

polycystic kidney disease familial disorder producing cysts in the kidney tubules leading to kidney failure

pons area where nerves cross, resulting in nerves located on one side of the brain controlling the opposite side of the body; connects the cerebellum with the nervous system

pregnancy gestation; period of fetal development in the uterus from fertilization to birth, usually 40 weeks

premenstrual syndrome (PMS) irritability, bloating, and depression preceding menses

prepuce foreskin; a fold of skin on the penis covering the glans

presbyopia most common eye condition associated with aging

priapism abnormal, painful, prolonged penile erection, usually resulting from spinal cord injury or disease

prophase first stage of mitosis; centrioles move to opposite ends of the cell, forming two poles; they stretch filaments between them, resembling longitudes on a globe

prostate gland donut-shaped gland around the male urethra at the bladder neck that secretes alkaline fluid to protect sperm

proximal toward the origin of a structure

pubis anterior union of the hip bones

pulmonary edema fluid accumulation in the lungs, often associated with congestive heart failure

Purkinje fibers smaller fibers arising from the bundle branches located in the heart's conductive system that carry the electrical impulse to the ventricular walls, causing them to contract

pyelonephritis inflammation and pyogenic infection of the renal pelvis

radius lateral bone of forearm (in anatomic position)

rales crackling breath sound resulting from increased secretions in the bronchi; sometimes referred to as *rhonchi*

rectum the lower portion of the large intestine that contains the reflexes for defecation

renal failure acute or chronic loss of kidney function that results in buildup of nitrogen waste in the body

reproductive system body system containing gonads (ovaries or testes) and related sex-specific organs and structures to reproduce the species

respiratory system body system containing nose, pharynx, larynx, trachea, lungs, and related structures that transport oxygen and remove carbon dioxide

rheumatoid arthritis inflammation and overgrowth of synovial membranes and joint tissues characterized by swelling of joints, usually occurring in young adults

rotation turning on an axis, such as turning the head to indicate "no"

rugae folds in the lining of the stomach and some other organs

sagittal plane an imaginary line or cut through the body, bilaterally separating it into right and left halves

salivary glands three pairs of glands located in the mouth, secreting saliva that moistens food and begins the chemical breakdown of carbohydrates

scapula shoulder blade

scoliosis abnormal lateral curvature of the vertebral column

scrotum external pouch suspended from the male perineum containing the testes and epididymis

seminal vesicles a pair of accessory glands in the male, posterior to the urinary bladder, that secrete nutrient fluid for sperm

serum clear, liquid portion of blood that remains after the blood clots

sigmoid lower S-shaped portion of colon connected to the descending colon and the rectum

sinoatrial (SA) node located in the upper wall of the right atrium, it is the pacemaker of the heart and

initiates a normal heartbeat and rate of 60 to 80 beats per minute (sinus rhythm); causes atria to contract
skeletal system body system containing bones and related structures to provide structural support
small intestine longest portion of digestive tract; digests fats, proteins, and carbohydrates and absorbs the nutrient products into the blood; contains three sections: duodenum, jejunum, and ileum
spermatozoa sperm
spina bifida congenital deformity exposing the spinal column, resulting from malformation of vertebrae
spinal cord continuous tubelike structure located within the spinal vertebrae extending from the occipital bone to the coccyx; it contains cerebrospinal fluid and ascending and descending nerve tracts that carry transmissions to and from the brain
stapes stirrup; third ossicle (bone) of the middle ear
stomach J-shaped organ between the esophagus and the duodenum that produces a churning action that mixes food with gastric acids and enzymes as part of digestion; also stores food
strabismus inability of both eyes to simultaneously focus on a subject; commonly known as lazy eye or being cross-eyed
strata sublayers
stridor high-pitched breath sounds resembling wind; caused by a partial obstruction of air passages
superior above
sympathetic nervous system portion of the nervous system preparing the body for stressful situations ("fight or flight")
synapse neuromuscular junction between neurons
syphilis sexually transmitted disease resulting in lesions (chancre) that may spread to bone and other systems; if untreated, it may be terminal
systole contraction portion of the cardiac cycle
tarsals the seven ankle and foot bones; the largest is the calcaneus, or heel bone
telophase final phase of mitosis; the nucleus divides in the center, forming two distinct cells
tendons connective tissue attaching muscle directly to the periosteum (covering) of the bone
testes male endocrine sex glands (gonads) that secrete testosterone and stimulate the development of male sex characteristics and sperm
tetany spasms caused by low blood calcium
thalamus located in the diencephalon, serves as relay for sensory input
thorax cavity containing lungs
thrombophlebitis inflammation of a vein with clots
thrombus (plural *thrombi*) a blood clot attached to a vessel wall
thrush yeast infection of the mouth caused by *Candida albicans*
tibia shin bone
tinnitus ringing in the ears
tissues group of cells with similar structures and functions (e.g., renal)
trachea tube branching into two bronchi leading into the lungs
transient ischemic attack (TIA) ministroke; temporary episode of impaired neurologic function resulting from decreased blood flow to the brain
transverse plane an imaginary line or cut through the body horizontally dividing it into superior and inferior sections
tuberculosis an infectious bacterial disease characterized by tubercles in the tissue; the lung is the most common disease site
tubular reabsorption the process that follows glomerular filtration; the filtered water and other needed materials leave the tubule by diffusion and active transport and enter tissue fluids
tympanic membrane eardrum; boundary between external and middle ear canals; vibrates, transmitting sound waves to inner ear
ulcerative colitis inflammation and ulceration of the mucosa of the colon and rectum
ulcers lesions of the mucosa of any organ; most common in the stomach and intestine
ulna medial bone of forearm (in anatomic position)
uremia high levels of nitrogen waste in the body
ureters two slim tubes that carry urine from the kidneys to the urinary bladder
urethra tube from the bladder that allows urine to leave the body
urinary bladder saclike organ behind the symphysis pubis that temporarily stores urine
urinary system body system containing kidneys, ureters, bladder, and urethra that removes nitrogen-type waste and regulates water balance
urination voiding or micturition; discharge of urine from the bladder
uterus female organ located in pelvic cavity from the oviducts to the vagina; houses and nourishes the growing fetus and placenta
vas deferens tubule carrying sperm from epididymis to seminal vesicles
vasectomy male sterilization procedure; tying off or removing part or all of vas deferens
vena cava largest body vein, with inferior and superior branches
vertebral column spine; 26 vertebrae (bones that cover the spinal cord)
vertigo dizziness
vestibule middle section of inner ear involving balance
villi (singular *villus*) tiny projections in the small intestine lining where absorption of nutrients occurs
wheeze squeaking or whistling breath sound, usually caused by narrowed tracheobronchial airways, as in asthma
xiphoid process small tip at the lower end of sternum

REVIEW QUESTIONS

All questions are relevant for the CMA (AAMA), RMA (AMT), and CMAS (AMT) exams.

1. The thoracic and abdominal cavities of the body are separated by the:
   A. ribs.
   B. stomach.
   C. diaphragm.
   D. peritoneum.

Answer: **C**

Why: The diaphragm is a dome-shaped muscle under the lungs that flattens during inhalation. This structure separates the thoracic cavity, which contain the lungs, from the abdomen.

Review: Yes ❑ No ❑

---

2. The main tissue of the outer layer of the skin is:
   A. connective.
   B. adipose.
   C. mucosal.
   D. endothelial.
   E. epithelial.

Answer: **E**

Why: Epithelial tissue covers surfaces, such as skin. It also lines cavities and forms glands. Connective tissue supports and forms the framework of body parts. Adipose tissue contains cells that are able to store large amounts of fat. Mucosal tissue lines the tubes and other spaces that open to the outside of the body, for example, the lining of the nose.

Review: Yes ❑ No ❑

---

3. The glands that are saclike in structure and produce oily secretions that lubricate the skin are:
   A. sebaceous.
   B. ceruminous.
   C. ciliary.
   D. mammary.

Answer: **A**

Why: Ceruminous glands are found in the ear canal and secrete cerumen, or earwax. Mammary glands are found in the breast and secrete breast milk. Ciliary glands are sweat glands found around the margin of the eyelids.

Review: Yes ❑ No ❑

---

4. The portion of skeletal bone that manufactures blood cells is the:
   A. periosteum.
   B. red bone marrow.
   C. diaphysis.
   D. cartilage.
   E. epiphysis.

Answer: **B**

Why: Periosteum is the membrane covering the outside of bones. The diaphysis of a bone is the long, narrow shaft of the bone. The epiphysis is the end portion of a bone where the growth of the bone takes place. Cartilage is a tough, elastic, translucent material that covers the ends of the long bones. The red bone marrow is found in the center of bones and manufactures blood cells.

Review: Yes ❑ No ❑

---

5. The structures that attach muscles to bones are:
   A. fascia.
   B. ligaments.
   C. tendons.
   D. cartilage.

Answer: **C**

Why: Fascia consists of fibrous bands or sheets that support organs and hold them in place. Ligaments are structures that connect bone to bone. Cartilage is a tough, elastic, translucent material that covers the ends of the long bones.

Review: Yes ❑ No ❑

6. Nerve fibers are insulated and protected by a fatty material called:
   A. myelin.
   B. dendrites.
   C. neurons.
   D. axons.
   E. synapses.

Answer: **A**

Why: Neurons are the functional cells of the nervous system, and the axons and dendrites are the neuron fibers that conduct impulses away from and to cell bodies. A synapse is the contact point from one nerve cell to another nerve cell.

Review: Yes ❑ No ❑

---

7. The function of the lacrimal apparatus is to:
   A. refract light rays through the eye.
   B. assist in maintaining the shape of the cornea.
   C. produce tears to lubricate the eye.
   D. differentiate black-and-white vision.

Answer: **C**

Why: The lens of the eye is important in light refraction. Aqueous humor is a watery fluid that fills the eyeball in front of the lens and helps maintain the curve of the cornea. Rods and cones in the retinal layer are responsible for differentiating between black, white, and color.

Review: Yes ❑ No ❑

---

8. A bone that is part of the pelvic girdle is the:
   A. sphenoid.
   B. ethmoid.
   C. ischium.
   D. zygomatic.
   E. sternum.

Answer: **C**

Why: The sphenoid, ethmoid, and zygomatic are all bones of the skull. The sphenoid and ethmoid bones are part of the cranium, and the zygomatic is the cheekbone. The sternum is the chest bone.

Review: Yes ❑ No ❑

---

9. The cellular components of blood include:
   A. erythrocytes, leukocytes, and platelets.
   B. anticoagulants, antibodies, and electrolytes.
   C. plasma, serum, and hemoglobin.
   D. lipids, amino acids, and albumin.

Answer: **A**

Why: Cellular components include cells and cell fragments, including erythrocytes, leukocytes, and platelets. Lipids are fatty acids; anticoagulants found in the blood are clotting factors; electrolytes and amino acids are chemicals; and albumin is a form of protein. None of these substances are formed elements like cells.

Review: Yes ❑ No ❑

---

10. The chambers of the heart are the:
   A. septum and valves.
   B. endocardium and epicardium.
   C. apex and septum.
   D. ventricles and atria.
   E. AV node and SA node.

Answer: **D**

Why: The septum of the heart is a partition dividing the heart into two sides. The heart valves direct blood flow through the heart. Endocardium and epicardium are layers of heart. The apex of the heart refers to the region at the bottom tip of the heart. The SA and AV nodes are areas involved in the conduction cycle of the heart.

Review: Yes ❑ No ❑

---

11. An organ located in the left upper quadrant is the:
   A. thymus.
   B. spleen.
   C. appendix.
   D. liver.

Answer: **B**

Why: The thymus is located behind the sternum. The liver is in the right upper quadrant, and the appendix is in the right lower quadrant.

Review: Yes ❑ No ❑

12. An example of active immunity is:
    A. maternal antibodies passed through the uterus to the baby.
    B. immunization with antibodies.
    C. maternal antibodies acquired by the baby from breast milk.
    D. producing antibodies as a result of having a disease.
    E. injection of globulins of disease-causing organisms.

Answer: **D**

Why: Active immunity is obtained when the individual actually develops antibodies by having the disease or by injection of a killed or attenuated organism, forcing the body to produce antibodies. Passive immunity means that the antibodies are made outside of the body and are "passed" on to the person. The mother passing antibodies through her placenta or breast milk is an example of this type of immunity.

Review: Yes ❑ No ❑

---

13. The structure in the body also known as the voice box is the:
    A. pharynx.
    B. larynx.
    C. epiglottis.
    D. trachea.

Answer: **B**

Why: The pharynx is referred to as the throat. The epiglottis covers the larynx during swallowing to keep food and liquids out of the respiratory tract. The trachea is commonly called the windpipe.

Review: Yes ❑ No ❑

---

14. The wavelike movement that propels food through the digestive tract is called:
    A. osmosis.
    B. diffusion.
    C. metabolism.
    D. resorption.
    E. peristalsis.

Answer: **E**

Why: Diffusion is a process of movement of molecules from a higher concentration to a lower concentration. Metabolism is the combination of chemical processes resulting in growth and bodily functions within a living organism. Resorption is the loss of substance or bone. Osmosis is the movement of materials through a semipermeable membrane.

Review: Yes ❑ No ❑

---

15. The process that does not require oxygen for the breakdown of glucose is referred to as being:
    A. aerobic.
    B. anaerobic.
    C. catabolic.
    D. pyrogenic.

Answer: **B**

Why: Aerobic refers to a process that requires the presence of air or oxygen. The prefix *an-* at the beginning of a word means without air or oxygen. Pyrogenic means heat producing, and catabolic refers to the process in which substances are metabolized into smaller substances (i.e., digestion of food).

Review: Yes ❑ No ❑

---

16. The term that means the body is in a state of equilibrium or balance is:
    A. anabolism.
    B. catabolism.
    C. homeostasis.
    D. metabolism.
    E. osmosis.

Answer: **C**

Why: Homeostasis is a state of equilibrium or health in the body. Metabolism is the body process of transforming energy in living cells. Anabolism is the building phase and catabolism is the breaking down phase of transforming energy. Osmosis is the process of water diffusing through a semipermeable membrane.

Review: Yes ❑ No ❑

17. The funnel-shaped basin that forms the upper end of the ureter is the:
    A. glomerulus.
    B. renal cortex.
    C. renal pelvis.
    D. Bowman's capsule.

Answer: **C**

Why: The glomerulus and Bowman's capsule are part of the nephron, the basic unit of the kidney. There are about 1 million nephrons in each kidney. The renal cortex is the outer portion of the kidney.

Review: Yes ❑ No ❑

---

18. In both males and females, the entire pelvic floor is called the:
    A. vestibule.
    B. peritoneum.
    C. fundus.
    D. pons.
    E. perineum.

Answer: **E**

Why: The vestibule refers to the area near the vaginal opening, and the fundus is the region in the top of the uterus, above the fallopian tube openings. The peritoneum is a membrane that lines the abdominal cavity. The pons is an area in the brain.

Review: Yes ❑ No ❑

---

19. A pregnancy that develops in a location outside the uterine cavity is referred to as:
    A. previa.
    B. miscarriage.
    C. abruptio.
    D. ectopic.

Answer: **D**

Why: The placenta is usually attached to the upper part of the uterus. Previa refers to the attachment of the placenta near the internal opening of the cervix. Abruptio refers to the premature separation of the placenta from the wall of the uterus. Miscarriage refers to a termination of pregnancy before the twentieth week of gestation, usually because of a problem with the conception or the womb environment.

Review: Yes ❑ No ❑

---

20. Which of the following body systems includes the thyroid and pituitary glands?
    A. Excretory
    B. Integumentary
    C. Endocrine
    D. Circulatory
    E. Nervous

Answer: **C**

Why: The excretory system refers to the kidneys and urinary tract. The integumentary system includes the skin, hair, nails, and sweat and sebaceous glands. The circulatory system refers to the veins and arteries. The nervous system includes the brain and nerves.

Review: Yes ❑ No ❑

---

21. The term **inguinal** pertains to what area or structure of the body?
    A. Intestines
    B. Bladder
    C. Groin
    D. Umbilicus

Answer: **C**

Why: The umbilicus is also known as the belly button or navel. The bladder is the internal organ that serves as a reservoir for urine. The intestines are in the abdomen. The groin or inguinal area is the region where the abdomen and thighs meet.

Review: Yes ❑ No ❑

22. The measure of acidity or alkalinity of a solution is called:
    A. acid.
    B. base.
    C. pH.
    D. buffer.
    E. neutral.

Answer: **C**

Why: An acid is a substance that can donate a hydrogen ion to another substance, and base refers to a substance that can receive a hydrogen ion. A buffer is a substance that tends to control the hydrogen ion concentration in a solution by adding or releasing hydrogen ions.

Review: Yes ❑ No ❑

---

23. A term that describes a solution that has the same concentration as cell fluids is:
    A. hypotonic.
    B. osmosis.
    C. isotonic.
    D. intercellular.

Answer: **C**

Why: Osmosis refers to the movement of a pure solvent, such as water, through a semipermeable membrane to equalize the solution's concentration. Hypotonic refers to a solution that is less concentrated than the fluids within a cell. Intercellular means between cells. The prefix *iso*-means equal or the same.

Review: Yes ❑ No ❑

---

24. The fibrous bands that support organs to hold them in place are:
    A. meninges.
    B. periosteum.
    C. fascia.
    D. synovia.
    E. tendons.

Answer: **C**

Why: Synovia is transparent, thick fluid found in joints. Meninges are the coverings of the brain and spinal cord. Periosteum is the covering of bones. Tendons are structures that attach muscle to bone.

Review: Yes ❑ No ❑

---

25. The membrane that surrounds the heart is the:
    A. endocardium.
    B. epicardium.
    C. mesocardium.
    D. pericardium.

Answer: **D**

Why: The prefix *peri-* means to surround, and the pericardium is the membrane or sac that surrounds the heart. The other choices refer to layers of heart muscle.

Review: Yes ❑ No ❑

---

26. The small tip of cartilage at the lower end of the sternum is the:
    A. zygomatic process.
    B. manubrium.
    C. styloid process.
    D. xiphoid process.
    E. ethmoid.

Answer: **D**

Why: The manubrium is the top part of the sternum. The zygomatic process is a bone in the upper cheek, and the ethmoid is a bone between the nasal cavity and orbits of the eye. The styloid process is the bony projection behind the ear.

Review: Yes ❑ No ❑

---

27. A major muscle in the body that assists in raising the arm away from the body is the:
    A. extensor carpi.
    B. biceps femoris.
    C. sartorius.
    D. deltoid.

Answer: **D**

Why: The extensor carpi muscles are located near the wrist in the forearm and assist in flexing and extending fingers. The biceps femoris muscle is one of the hamstring muscles and is found in the posterior thigh. The sartorius muscle is located in the leg.

Review: Yes ❑ No ❑

28. Cells that carry or transmit impulses toward the central nervous system are called:
    A. afferent neurons.
    B. efferent neurons.
    C. motor neurons.
    D. receptors.
    E. meninges.

Answer: **A**

Why: Motor neurons are also known as efferent neurons and carry impulses away from the central nervous system. Receptors are sensory nerve endings that respond to various kinds of stimulation. The meninges are the coverings of the brain and spinal cord.

Review: Yes ❑ No ❑

---

29. The space(s) in the brain where cerebrospinal fluid is formed is/are the:
    A. arachnoid.
    B. meninges.
    C. ventricles.
    D. lobes.

Answer: **C**

Why: The meninges are three layers surrounding the brain and spinal cord. The arachnoid is one of the meningeal layers. The lobes are divisions of the brain.

Review: Yes ❑ No ❑

---

30. Impulses from the receptors for smell are carried to the brain by the:
    A. proprioceptors.
    B. glossopharyngeal nerve.
    C. vestibulocochlear nerve.
    D. olfactory nerve.
    E. myelin sheath.

Answer: **D**

Why: Proprioceptors are receptors located in muscles, tendons, and joints that relay impulses that aid in judging position and changes in the locations of body parts in relation to each other. The glossopharyngeal nerve contains sensory fibers for taste and secretion of saliva. The vestibulocochlear nerve carries impulses for hearing and equilibrium. The myelin sheath is the fatty material that covers and protects neuron fibers.

Review: Yes ❑ No ❑

---

31. The hormone that is essential for growth is produced in the:
    A. parathyroid glands.
    B. adrenal glands.
    C. pituitary gland.
    D. thymus gland.

Answer: **C**

Why: The parathyroid glands secrete a hormone that regulates exchange of calcium between blood and bones. The adrenal glands secrete hormones whose primary functions are to increase blood pressure and heart rate and aid metabolism of carbohydrates, proteins, and fats. The thymus gland hormone promotes immunity.

Review: Yes ❑ No ❑

---

32. Which of the following represent layers of the heart?
    A. Atria and ventricles
    B. Ventricles and myocardium
    C. Epicardium and myocardium
    D. Endocardium and septum
    E. Septum and atria

Answer: **C**

Why: The atria and ventricles are chambers of the heart. The septum is the dividing wall of the right and left sides of the heart.

Review: Yes ❑ No ❑

---

33. The blood vessel that brings blood from the head, chest, and arms back to the heart is the:
    A. aorta.
    B. pulmonary vein.
    C. carotid artery.
    D. superior vena cava.

Answer: **D**

Why: The aorta, pulmonary vein, and carotid artery all carry blood away from the heart. The superior vena cava is a vein that carries blood back to the heart from the upper body.

Review: Yes ❑ No ❑

34. Which of the following is the proper sequence for the flow of blood in the body?
A. Artery → vein → arteriole
B. Venule → arteriole → capillary
C. Vein → venule → capillary
D. Capillary → arteriole → venule
E. Artery → arteriole → capillary

Answer: **E**

Why: The sequence of blood flow through the body is from artery to arteriole to capillary, then to venule and vein. The artery and vein are larger vessels than arterioles and venules, and the capillaries are the smallest.

Review: Yes ❑ No ❑

---

35. The condition of inflammation of the lymphatic vessels is called:
A. lymphoma.
B. splenomegaly.
C. lymphangitis.
D. lymphocytopenia.

Answer: **C**

Why: Lymphoma refers to a tumor in the lymph tissue. Splenomegaly means enlargement of the spleen. Lymphocytopenia refers to a decrease in the number of lymphocytes in the blood.

Review: Yes ❑ No ❑

---

36. The lymphatic system includes the following organs and tissue EXCEPT:
A. hypothalamus.
B. thymus.
C. spleen.
D. tonsils.
E. adenoids.

Answer: **A**

Why: The hypothalamus is not a part of the lymphatic system, but is in the brain. It activates and controls the autonomic nervous system and aids in regulating body temperature, sleep, and appetite.

Review: Yes ❑ No ❑

---

37. The process in which white blood cells take in and destroy waste and foreign material is called:
A. immunity.
B. phagocytosis.
C. hemolysis.
D. leukocytosis.

Answer: **B**

Why: Hemolysis refers to destruction of red blood cells. Leukocytosis is an abnormal increase in the number of white blood cells. Immunity refers to a condition of being unaffected by a particular disease.

Review: Yes ❑ No ❑

---

38. The structure common to the respiratory and digestive systems is the:
A. trachea.
B. larynx.
C. esophagus.
D. pharynx.
E. ileum.

Answer: **D**

Why: The larynx is known as the voice box, and the trachea is known as the windpipe. Both allow airflow in and out of the lungs. The esophagus transports food from the pharynx to the stomach. The pharynx transports both food to the digestive system and air to the respiratory system. The ileum is the lower part of the small intestine.

Review: Yes ❑ No ❑

---

39. An accumulation of air in the pleural space that may lead to collapse of the lung is called:
A. hemothorax.
B. thoracentesis.
C. pleurisy.
D. pneumothorax.

Answer: **D**

Why: Hemothorax refers to blood in the pleural space, and pneumothorax is an accumulation of air in the pleural space. Thoracentesis is a procedure in which a needle is inserted into the pleural space below the lung to remove fluid. Pleurisy refers to inflammation of the pleura, the covering or sac around each lung.

Review: Yes ❑ No ❑

40. The leaf-shaped cartilage that covers the opening of the larynx is the:
A. epiglottis.
B. soft palate.
C. uvula.
D. pharynx.
E. villus.

Answer: **A**

Why: The pharynx is also known as the throat. The soft palate is the tissue that forms the back of the roof of the mouth; the uvula is the soft projection that hangs down from this area and is used in speech production. The epiglottis is the cartilage that guards the entrance of the trachea during swallowing so food will move into the esophagus, not the larynx and trachea. A villus is one of many tiny projections in the small intestine lining.

Review: Yes ❑ No ❑

---

41. Most of the digestive process occurs in the:
A. stomach.
B. large intestine.
C. small intestine.
D. esophagus.

Answer: **C**

Why: The esophagus is a muscular tube that transports food from the pharynx to the stomach. No digestion occurs in the esophagus. In the stomach, food is churned and mixes with digestive juices that begin to liquefy and break down food. The large intestine reabsorbs water and eliminates undigested waste. The small intestine secretes enzymes that digest proteins and carbohydrates. Digested food is absorbed through the walls of the small intestine.

Review: Yes ❑ No ❑

---

42. The lining of the stomach has many folds called:
A. diverticula.
B. rugae.
C. villi.
D. mesentery.
E. ulcers.

Answer: **B**

Why: Diverticula are the saclike bulges in the intestinal wall. Villi are the tiny fingerlike projections in the small intestine. Mesentery is a fold of peritoneum connecting the jejunum and the ileum with the dorsal wall of the abdomen. Ulcers are lesions of the mucosa of any organ.

Review: Yes ❑ No ❑

---

43. The first portion of the small intestine is the:
A. jejunum.
B. ileum.
C. duodenum.
D. pylorus.

Answer: **C**

Why: The pylorus is in the distal region of the stomach leading into the small intestine. The small intestine has three portions. The first is the duodenum, the second is the jejunum, and the third is the ileum.

Review: Yes ❑ No ❑

---

44. An accumulation of excessive fluid in the intercellular spaces is called:
A. acidosis.
B. alkalosis.
C. edema.
D. effusion.
E. osmosis.

Answer: **C**

Why: The condition that results from a decrease in the pH of body fluids is called acidosis; an increase in the pH of body fluids is alkalosis. Effusion refers to the fluid that escapes into a cavity or space.

Review: Yes ❑ No ❑

45. The kidneys are located in the:
A. retroperitoneal space.
B. renal pelvis.
C. dorsal cavity.
D. hypogastric region.

Answer: **A**

Why: Both the kidneys and ureters lie behind the peritoneum in the retroperitoneal space. The renal pelvis is the funnel-shaped basin that forms the upper end of the ureter. The dorsal cavity houses the brain and spinal cord, and the hypogastric region is the lowest area in the mid-abdomen.

Review: Yes ❑ No ❑

---

46. The term **hydronephrosis** means:
A. inability to retain urine.
B. involuntary discharge of urine.
C. inflammation and infection of the renal pelvis.
D. distention of the renal pelvis resulting from obstructed flow of urine.
E. excessive urine.

Answer: **D**

Why: Pyelonephritis is the term for inflammation and infection of the renal pelvis. Enuresis is the involuntary discharge of urine. Incontinence is the inability to retain urine. Polyuria is excessive urine.

Review: Yes ❑ No ❑

---

47. The sex glands of the male and female reproductive system are the:
A. sperm and ova.
B. prostate and uterus.
C. testes and ovaries.
D. penis and vagina.

Answer: **C**

Why: The sperm and ova are actually the sex cells of reproduction. The prostate is a gland that secretes a substance that enhances the motility of the sperm through the reproductive tract. The uterus is the structure in which the developing fetus grows to maturity. The penis and vagina are the structures that provide a transport system for sperm from the male to the female for fertilization of an ovum. The vagina is also the birth canal.

Review: Yes ❑ No ❑

---

48. The bone that lies between the hip and the knee is the:
A. patella.
B. femur.
C. pelvis.
D. ilium.
E. tibia.

Answer: **B**

Why: The femur is the largest bone in the body and is also known as the thigh bone. It connects the hip to the knee. The patella is the kneecap. The pelvis is the bony structure at the lower end of the trunk. The bones of the pelvis include the ilium, ischium and pubic bone, sacrum, and coccyx. The tibia is the larger bone of the lower leg below the knee.

Review: Yes ❑ No ❑

---

49. The largest artery in the body is the:
A. superior vena cava.
B. inferior vena cava.
C. carotid artery.
D. abdominal aorta.

Answer: **D**

Why: The superior and inferior vena cava are both veins. The carotid artery is in the neck and is smaller than the aorta.

Review: Yes ❑ No ❑

50. The term that refers to absence of menstrual flow in a woman of reproductive age is:
A. menses.
B. uremia.
C. dysmenorrhea.
D. menopause.
E. amenorrhea.

Answer: E

Why: Menses refers to the normal menstrual period or flow. Dysmenorrhea is painful menstruation, and menopause is the term that means the total cessation of menstruation. Uremia is a condition of high levels of nitrogen waste in the body.

Review: Yes ❑ No ❑

---

51. The hormone produced by the embryonic cells of the fetus is:
A. human chorionic gonadotropin hormone.
B. adrenocorticotropic hormone.
C. oxytocin.
D. follicle-stimulating hormone.

Answer: A

Why: Adrenocorticotropic hormone, known as ACTH, and follicle-stimulating hormone, known as FSH, are hormones produced by the anterior pituitary gland. Oxytocin is produced by the posterior pituitary.

Review: Yes ❑ No ❑

---

52. A substance necessary for proper formation of a blood clot is:
A. macrophage.
B. lipid.
C. hemoglobin.
D. thrombin.
E. albumin.

Answer: D

Why: Macrophages are a type of phagocyte that assist in disposing of foreign material in the blood. Lipids are fats and cholesterol. Hemoglobin is a protein that contains iron and allows oxygen to bond to red blood cells for transport through the bloodstream. Albumin is a protein found in the blood.

Review: Yes ❑ No ❑

---

53. The left atrioventricular (AV) valve in the heart is also known as the:
A. pulmonary valve.
B. aortic valve.
C. mitral valve.
D. tricuspid valve.

Answer: C

Why: The pulmonary and aortic valves are semilunar valves that are exit valves. AV valves are entrance valves and include the mitral and tricuspid valve. The tricuspid valve is on the right, and the mitral valve is on the left.

Review: Yes ❑ No ❑

---

54. The only artery in the body that carries deoxygenated blood is the:
A. superior vena cava.
B. aorta.
C. pulmonary artery.
D. coronary artery.
E. interior vena cava.

Answer: C

Why: The aorta and coronary arteries both carry oxygenated blood to supply the heart and body. The superior vena cava and inferior vena cava are veins, not arteries.

Review: Yes ❑ No ❑

---

55. A localized dilation resulting from weakness of a blood vessel wall is a(n):
A. embolus.
B. thrombus.
C. septal defect.
D. aneurysm.

Answer: D

Why: An embolus is a foreign object, air, gas, or a piece of blood clot circulating in the blood that may become lodged in a blood vessel. A thrombus is a blood clot. A septal defect is an abnormality, usually congenital, in the wall that divides the heart chambers.

Review: Yes ❑ No ❑

56. An example of a chronic obstructive pulmonary disease is:
    A. asthma.
    B. emphysema.
    C. croup.
    D. pleurisy.
    E. pertussis.

Answer: **B**

Why: Asthma is characterized by recurring episodes of wheezing and coughing. Croup is caused by a viral infection, usually in infants. Pleurisy is inflammation of the pleura. Pertussis is known as whooping cough.

Review: Yes ❑ No ❑

---

57. A portion of the large intestine is the:
    A. pylorus.
    B. jejunum.
    C. ileum.
    D. sigmoid.

Answer: **D**

Why: The pylorus is the section of the stomach at the lowest end that connects to the duodenum. The jejunum and ileum are parts of the small intestine.

Review: Yes ❑ No ❑

---

58. A chronic degenerative disease of the liver is:
    A. Crohn disease.
    B. jaundice.
    C. colitis.
    D. cholecystitis.
    E. cirrhosis.

Answer: **E**

Why: Crohn disease is a chronic inflammation of the intestine, usually the ileum. Colitis is inflammation of the colon, and jaundice is a condition of yellowing of the skin resulting from excess bilirubin in the blood caused by liver disorders. Cholecystitis is inflammation of the gallbladder.

Review: Yes ❑ No ❑

---

59. The tube that permits urine to pass from the bladder to the outside of the body is the:
    A. urethra.
    B. ureter.
    C. renal pelvis.
    D. urinary meatus.

Answer: **A**

Why: The ureter is the tube that extends from the kidney to the urinary bladder. The renal pelvis is the funnel-shaped portion of the kidney where urine collects in the kidney. The urinary meatus is not a tube, but rather is the external opening of the urethra to the outside of the body.

Review: Yes ❑ No ❑

---

60. The innermost layer of the uterus is the:
    A. perineum.
    B. myometrium.
    C. endometrium.
    D. epimetrium.
    E. cervix.

Answer: **C**

Why: The perineum refers to the region between the vagina and rectum. The myometrium is the middle muscular layer of the uterus, and the epimetrium is the outer layer. The cervix is the lower end of the uterus.

Review: Yes ❑ No ❑

---

61. The frontal or coronal plane of the body divides the body into:
    A. right and left halves.
    B. equal top and bottom halves.
    C. unequal right and left sides.
    D. front and rear.

Answer: **D**

Why: The transverse or horizontal plane divides the body into top and bottom halves. The sagittal plane divides the body into right and left sides but not necessarily equal halves. If divided into equal halves, it is called the midsagittal plane.

Review: Yes ❑ No ❑

62. The membrane attached to internal organs is the:
   A. mucous membrane.
   B. cutaneous membrane.
   C. visceral layer.
   D. parietal layer.
   E. epithelial layer.

Answer: **C**

Why: The internal organs are the viscera, and the membrane surrounding them is the visceral layer. The mucous membranes line tubes and spaces open to the outside of the body. The cutaneous membrane is commonly known as the skin. The parietal layer is a serous membrane that is attached to the wall of a cavity or sac. The epithelial layer is the outer layer of the skin.

Review: Yes ❑ No ❑

---

63. The term that describes a disorder that breaks down tissues in a body system is:
   A. degenerative.
   B. infection.
   C. metabolic.
   D. neoplastic.

Answer: **A**

Why: Infection is an invasion of the body by pathogenic microorganisms. A metabolic disorder refers to a condition caused by disruption of the reactions involved in cellular metabolism in the body. Neoplastic refers to cancer or new growth.

Review: Yes ❑ No ❑

---

64. The study of the cause of any disease or of all factors that may be involved in the development of a disease is:
   A. physiology.
   B. anatomy.
   C. histology.
   D. incidence.
   E. etiology.

Answer: **E**

Why: Physiology is the study of body function; anatomy is the study of body structure. Histology is the study of tissue. Incidence refers to the range of occurrence of a disease and its tendency to affect certain groups of individuals more than other groups.

Review: Yes ❑ No ❑

---

65. The chronic skin condition characterized by a red, flat area covered with silvery scales is:
   A. decubitus ulcer.
   B. urticaria.
   C. psoriasis.
   D. shingles.

Answer: **C**

Why: A decubitus ulcer, also known as a bedsore, is due to constant pressure on a part of the body, which impairs blood supply to the area of skin that is pressed between bone and the patient's bed. Urticaria, known as hives, appears as elevated red patches or wheals. Hives are usually a result of an allergic reaction. Shingles, caused by the herpes zoster virus, produces vesicle (blister)-type lesions.

Review: Yes ❑ No ❑

---

66. Which of the following is not one of the cranial bones?
   A. Frontal
   B. Parietal
   C. Ethmoid
   D. Temporal
   E. Maxilla

Answer: **E**

Why: The maxilla, the upper jaw bone, is part of the skull but is one of the facial bones.

Review: Yes ❑ No ❑

67. The bone that is part of the shoulder girdle and is between the sternum and the scapula is the:
    A. clavicle.
    B. humerus.
    C. ulna.
    D. manubrium.

Answer: **A**

Why: The humerus is the upper arm bone, and the ulna is the smaller medial bone of the forearm. The manubrium is the top portion of the sternum.

Review: Yes ❑ No ❑

---

68. The type of muscle responsible for producing peristalsis is:
    A. cardiac.
    B. skeletal.
    C. smooth.
    D. voluntary.
    E. diaphragmatic.

Answer: **C**

Why: Cardiac muscle is only found in the heart wall. Skeletal muscle is voluntary muscle attached to bones allowing movement of joints. Smooth muscle is involuntary and is found in the walls of internal organs and passageways such as the intestines, where peristalsis takes place. The term **diaphragmatic** refers to the diaphragm.

Review: Yes ❑ No ❑

---

69. The type of joint motion that allows movement away from the midline of the body, such as moving the arms straight out to the sides, is:
    A. circumduction.
    B. flexion.
    C. extension.
    D. abduction.

Answer: **D**

Why: Circumduction is movement in a circular pattern. Flexion is a bending motion decreasing the angle between bones, and extension is a straightening motion increasing the angle between bones.

Review: Yes ❑ No ❑

---

70. The sympathetic system of the autonomic nervous system is responsible for:
    A. constriction of the pupil of the eye.
    B. decrease in rate of heart beat.
    C. dilation of bronchi of the lungs.
    D. constriction of blood vessels to skeletal muscles.
    E. slowing the pulse.

Answer: **C**

Why: The sympathetic system is responsible for stimulating the body's fight-or-flight response (stress). This response includes dilation of the bronchi. The parasympathetic system returns the body to normal activity by constricting the pupil and the blood vessels and by decreasing the heart rate or slowing the pulse.

Review: Yes ❑ No ❑

---

71. The portion of the brain that aids in the coordination of voluntary muscle action is the:
    A. cerebellum.
    B. thalamus.
    C. medulla oblongata.
    D. midbrain.

Answer: **A**

Why: The thalamus is responsible for relaying sensory impulses to the cerebral cortex of the brain. The medulla oblongata contains the respiratory center, which controls the muscles of respiration; the cardiac center, which helps regulate the rate and force of the heartbeat; and the vasomotor center, which regulates the contraction of smooth muscle in the blood vessel walls. The midbrain contains a relay center for certain eye and ear reflexes.

Review: Yes ❑ No ❑

72. Strabismus is a condition of the eye causing:
   A. nearsightedness.
   B. farsightedness.
   C. drooping eyelids.
   D. cross-eyed appearance.
   E. redness of the sclera.

Answer: **D**

Why: Myopia is nearsightedness, and hyperopia is farsightedness. The term for drooping eyelids is blepharoptosis (blephar/o = eyelid, optosis = drooping, falling). The sclera is the visible white portion of the eye that can become red from inflammation and irritation.

Review: Yes ❑ No ❑

---

73. A structure found in the inner ear is the:
   A. pinna.
   B. tympanic membrane.
   C. malleus.
   D. cochlea.

Answer: **D**

Why: The earlobe is the pinna. The tympanic membrane, or eardrum, separates the external and middle ear. The malleus is one of the three small bones of the middle ear. The other bones are the stapes and incus.

Review: Yes ❑ No ❑

---

74. The clusters of cells called the islets of Langerhans are located in the:
   A. adrenal glands.
   B. anterior pituitary gland.
   C. pancreas.
   D. pituitary gland.
   E. parathyroid glands.

Answer: **C**

Why: The islets of Langerhans, located in the pancreas, secrete insulin, which aids in the transport of glucose into cells, decreasing the blood sugar level.

Review: Yes ❑ No ❑

---

75. A goiter is associated with abnormal function of the:
   A. thyroid gland.
   B. parathyroid glands.
   C. spleen.
   D. pituitary gland.

Answer: **A**

Why: A goiter is a swelling in the neck region surrounding the thyroid gland. It is caused by hypertrophy, or chronic enlargement, of the thyroid gland.

Review: Yes ❑ No ❑

---

76. The Rh factor in blood is:
   A. an antigen that affects a person's blood type.
   B. responsible for protecting against infection.
   C. used to transport oxygen.
   D. one of the clotting factors.
   E. an enzyme that breaks down cholesterol.

Answer: **A**

Why: Rh is a red cell antigen (protein) that contributes to a person's blood type. A person is Rh-positive if the antigen is present in the blood and Rh-negative if it is absent from the blood. This antigen can cause incompatibility problems in pregnancies and blood transfusions.

Review: Yes ❑ No ❑

---

77. The area of the heart that initiates a heartbeat is the:
   A. atrioventricular node.
   B. sinoatrial node.
   C. right bundle branches.
   D. Purkinje fibers.

Answer: **B**

Why: The SA node (sinoatrial node) initiates the heart contractions. Impulses travel next to the AV node (atrioventricular node), then to the bundle of His, to the right and left bundle branches, and, last, to the Purkinje fibers.

Review: Yes ❑ No ❑

78. A heart disease that is present at birth is:
   A. atherosclerosis.
   B. rheumatic heart disease.
   C. congenital heart disease.
   D. angina pectoris.
   E. maternal.

Answer: C

Why: The term **congenital** means "born with" or "at birth." Atherosclerosis is a degeneration of the inside of the blood vessels that causes a narrowing of the opening as the walls become thicker. Angina pectoris is caused by inadequate blood flow to the heart muscle and results in chest pain. Rheumatic heart disease is caused by an attack of rheumatic fever, usually in childhood. **Maternal** is a term meaning "to the mother" or "from the mother."

Review: Yes ❑ No ❑

---

79. Which of the following blood vessels is proximal to the heart?
   A. Iliac artery
   B. Carotid artery
   C. Ascending aorta
   D. Renal artery

Answer: C

Why: The term **proximal** means closest to a body part. The ascending aorta is an extension of the aorta and is the largest vessel in the body. It is the first blood vessel to exit the heart with oxygenated blood. The iliac artery is located in the hip area. The carotid arteries, right and left, are found in the neck, and the renal artery supplies blood to the kidneys.

Review: Yes ❑ No ❑

---

80. Acquired, natural, active immunity is achieved by:
   A. injection of immune serum.
   B. nursing babies with mother's milk.
   C. contracting the disease.
   D. injection of a vaccine.
   E. immunizing with antibodies of a disease.

Answer: C

Why: Injection of any serum or vaccine is an artificial means of acquiring immunity. Nursing a baby is a method of passing on antibodies from the mother to the baby, which is passive. If someone comes in contact with a disease and naturally manufactures antibodies, this is an active method of acquiring immunity.

Review: Yes ❑ No ❑

---

81. The human immunodeficiency virus is the cause of which disease?
   A. Hodgkin's disease
   B. Leukemia
   C. Acquired immunodeficiency syndrome
   D. Sarcoma

Answer: C

Why: Acquired immunodeficiency syndrome (AIDS) is caused by the human immunodeficiency virus (HIV). Hodgkin's disease, leukemia, and sarcoma are all forms of malignancy (cancer).

Review: Yes ❑ No ❑

---

82. Which of the following statements is accurate about the lungs?
   A. The bronchioles branch to form smaller structures called bronchi.
   B. The right and left lungs both have three lobes.
   C. The sac covering the lungs is the pleural sac.
   D. The least amount of gas exchange takes place in the alveoli.
   E. External respiration is the exchange of oxygen and carbon dioxide in the lungs.

Answer: C

Why: The bronchi are larger structures than the bronchioles. The right lung has three lobes, and the left has only two lobes. The most gas exchange takes place in the millions of tiny alveolar sacs. External respiration is the exchange of oxygen and carbon dioxide in the lungs. Internal respiration is the exchange of these gases in the capillaries and tissue cells.

Review: Yes ❑ No ❑

83. A communicable, infectious disease of the lungs is:
    A. emphysema.
    B. chronic obstructive pulmonary disease.
    C. asthma.
    D. tuberculosis.

Answer: **D**

Why: Emphysema, chronic obstructive pulmonary disease (COPD), and asthma are not infectious or communicable. COPD is a condition in which there is an obstruction of normal airflow. Air is trapped in the lung spaces, and there is no proper exchange of oxygen and carbon dioxide. Emphysema is one type of lung disorder classified as a COPD. Asthma is a condition that creates spasms of the involuntary muscles of the bronchial tube walls and causes labored breathing. Asthma may be caused by allergens such as dust, pollen, or foods.

Review: Yes ❑ No ❑

---

84. An example of inflammatory bowel disease is:
    A. gastritis.
    B. pyloric stenosis.
    C. Crohn disease.
    D. Vincent's disease.
    E. Hodgkin's disease.

Answer: **C**

Why: Gastritis is inflammation of the stomach. Pyloric stenosis is a constriction of the pyloric sphincter, the ring of muscle between the stomach and small intestine. Vincent's disease is a form of gum disease of the mouth. Hodgkin's disease is a chronic malignant disease characterized by enlargement of the lymph nodes and spleen.

Review: Yes ❑ No ❑

---

85. A function of the liver is to:
    A. detoxify harmful substances, such as alcohol and certain drugs.
    B. produce insulin to metabolize glucose.
    C. absorb nutrients into the bloodstream.
    D. assist in digestion by producing hydrochloric acid.

Answer: **A**

Why: Insulin is a product of the pancreas. The small intestine is where most nutrients are absorbed into the bloodstream. Hydrochloric acid is produced in the stomach and is used to start the digestive process.

Review: Yes ❑ No ❑

---

86. The fluid contained within the body cells is called:
    A. lymph.
    B. plasma.
    C. interstitial fluid.
    D. isotonic.
    E. intracellular fluid.

Answer: **E**

Why: Lymph is the fluid that drains from the tissues into the lymphatic system. Plasma is the liquid part of blood, and interstitial fluid is tissue fluid found in the spaces between cells. Isotonic means the same concentration of fluid inside and outside a cell.

Review: Yes ❑ No ❑

---

87. Two important electrolytes found in the body are:
    A. zinc and magnesium.
    B. sodium and potassium.
    C. protein and carbohydrates.
    D. nitrogen and carbon dioxide.

Answer: **B**

Why: Zinc and magnesium are minerals, protein and carbohydrates are nutrients, and nitrogen and carbon dioxide are gases.

Review: Yes ❑ No ❑

88. A condition resulting from renal failure and causing high levels of blood urea nitrogen is:
A. uremia.
B. anemia.
C. edema.
D. hematuria.
E. dehydration.

Answer: **A**

Why: Dehydration is an excessive loss of body fluid. Anemia is a condition of decreased amount of hemoglobin, or red blood cells, in the blood. Edema is an accumulation of fluid in tissue spaces. Hematuria is a condition of blood in the urine.

Review: Yes ❑ No ❑

---

89. The period of pregnancy is called:
A. gestation.
B. menarche.
C. fertilization.
D. ovulation.

Answer: **A**

Why: The term **menarche** refers to the first time a female has a menstrual cycle, usually occurring between ages 9 and 15. Fertilization is the impregnation of the female egg with the male sperm; the release of an egg from the ovary is ovulation.

Review: Yes ❑ No ❑

---

90. The hormone that causes contraction of uterine muscle during labor is:
A. oxytocin.
B. progesterone.
C. follicle-stimulating hormone.
D. testosterone.
E. estrogen.

Answer: **A**

Why: Estrogen and progesterone are produced by the ovaries. Estrogen is important in the growth and development of sexual organs, and progesterone helps in development of mammary glands and preparation of the uterus lining for implantation of a fertilized ovum. Follicle-stimulating hormone is produced by the anterior pituitary and stimulates the growth of ovarian follicles. In the male, it promotes the development of sperm cells and growth of the testes. Testosterone is male hormone.

Review: Yes ❑ No ❑

---

91. The region located directly below the umbilical region is the:
A. right iliac region.
B. hypogastric region.
C. hypochondriac region.
D. epigastric region.

Answer: **B**

Why: The hypogastric region is the region below the umbilicus (navel), in the middle of the lower abdomen. The hypochondriac regions are on the right and left at the base of the ribs. The epigastric region is above the umbilicus and is located over the stomach area.

Review: Yes ❑ No ❑

---

92. An example of exocrine glands are:
A. sebaceous glands.
B. parathyroid glands.
C. adrenal glands.
D. ovaries.
E. testes.

Answer: **A**

Why: The parathyroid, adrenal glands, ovaries, and testes are examples of endocrine glands that secrete their hormones directly into the bloodstream and do not require ducts or tubes to transport the hormones.

Review: Yes ❑ No ❑

93. The order of the vertebral column from top to bottom is:
A. cervical, thoracic, sacral, lumbar, coccyx.
B. thoracic, lumbar, sacral, coccyx, cervical.
C. coccyx, sacral, lumbar, thoracic, cervical.
D. cervical, thoracic, lumbar, sacral, coccyx.

Answer: **D**

Why: The spine starts at the top with the cervical area in the neck region and ends with the coccyx, or the tailbone.

Review: Yes ❑ No ❑

---

94. The muscle located on the anterior thigh and that functions to extend the leg is the:
A. tibialis anterior.
B. quadriceps femoris.
C. sternocleidomastoid.
D. sacrospinalis.
E. gluteus maximus.

Answer: **B**

Why: Muscles frequently are named for the bone or area located in proximity to the muscle. The tibialis anterior lies in front, or anterior to, the tibia, the lower leg bone. The sternocleidomastoid connects the sternum, the mastoid process, and the clavicle. The sacrospinalis is located in the region of the sacrum, ilium (hip), and lumbar vertebrae of the spine. The gluteus maximus is the largest muscle in the posterior hip area.

Review: Yes ❑ No ❑

---

95. The artery located in the upper arm is the:
A. brachial artery.
B. carotid artery.
C. radial artery.
D. subclavian artery.

Answer: **A**

Why: The brachial artery is located in the upper arm and subdivides near the elbow to form the radial and ulnar arteries, which lie over the radius and ulna bones of the forearm. The carotid arteries are located in the neck. The subclavian arteries are located in the armpit (axillary) area.

Review: Yes ❑ No ❑

---

96. Any foreign substance that enters the body and induces an immune response is a(n):
A. antibody.
B. antigen.
C. enzyme.
D. immunoglobulin.
E. globulin.

Answer: **B**

Why: An immunoglobulin, also known as an antibody, is a substance produced in response to an antigen. An enzyme is a protein produced in the body that causes a breakdown of food. A globulin is a protein in the blood associated with antibodies.

Review: Yes ❑ No ❑

---

97. The smaller leg bone, lateral to the tibia, is the:
A. femur.
B. tarsal.
C. patella.
D. fibula.

Answer: **D**

Why: The femur, the largest bone in the body, is the thigh bone. The patella is the kneecap. Tarsal refers to any one of the seven ankle bones.

Review: Yes ❑ No ❑

98. The small pouch that is the first part of the large intestine is the:
    A. pylorus.
    B. duodenum.
    C. cecum.
    D. ileum.
    E. jejunum.

Answer: **C**

Why: The jejunum, duodenum, and ileum are parts of the small intestine; the pylorus is the region between the stomach and small intestine.

Review: Yes ❑ No ❑

---

99. The hormone that regulates the amount of water that is eliminated with urine is:
    A. ADH.
    B. ACTH.
    C. FSH.
    D. TSH.

Answer: **A**

Why: ADH, antidiuretic hormone, aids in regulating water retention or expulsion from the body. ACTH, adrenocorticotropic hormone, stimulates the adrenal cortex to produce cortical hormones that aid in protecting the body in stress and injury. FSH, follicle-stimulating hormone, stimulates the growth and activity of the ovarian follicle. TSH, thyroid-stimulating hormone, stimulates the thyroid gland to produce thyroid hormones.

Review: Yes ❑ No ❑

---

100. An excessive curvature in the thoracic portion of the spinal column, also known as hunchback, is:
    A. kyphosis.
    B. arthritis.
    C. lordosis.
    D. spina bifida.
    E. spondylitis.

Answer: **A**

Why: Arthritis is inflammation of the joints. Lordosis is an excessive curvature of the lumbar spine, also known as swayback. Spina bifida is a congenital deformity exposing the spinal column. Spondylitis is inflammation of the joints of the spine.

Review: Yes ❑ No ❑

---

101. Diabetic retinopathy is a result of damage to the:
    A. heart.
    B. lungs.
    C. eyes.
    D. brain.

Answer: **C**

Why: Diabetic retinopathy causes damage to the retina of the eye from hemorrhage of vessels; it is usually progressive and related to the control of the diabetes.

Review: Yes ❑ No ❑

---

102. Which of the following statements is TRUE?
    A. Diabetes mellitus is an uncommon endocrine disorder.
    B. Insulin-dependent diabetes mellitus is known as type 2 diabetes.
    C. Diabetes mellitus results from an overproduction of insulin.
    D. Type 2 diabetes is non–insulin-dependent diabetes.
    E. Insulin assists glucose into the cells.

Answer: **D**

Why: Diabetes mellitus results from a low production of insulin. Diabetic persons who are diagnosed with type 1 diabetes require insulin as part of their treatment of this disease. Persons with type 2 diabetes do not require insulin. Insulin does not assist glucose into the cells but promotes the synthesis of carbohydrates.

Review: Yes ❑ No ❑

---

103. Which of the following is a protein found in the epidermis that makes the skin waterproof?
    A. Melanin
    B. Keratin
    C. Collagen
    D. Cilia

Answer: **B**

Why: Melanin is a substance that provides pigment for the skin. Collagen is a protein found in the dermis that provides strength and flexibility. Cilia are hairlike processes that trap and move foreign particles.

Review: Yes ❑ No ❑

104. What is the most common condition of the eye associated with aging?
   A. Astigmatism
   B. Strabismus
   C. Macular degeneration
   D. Hyperopia
   E. Presbyopia

Answer: **E**

Why: Astigmatism is a condition causing impaired vision from an irregular curve of the cornea. Strabismus is an inability of both eyes to simultaneously focus on a subject. Macular degeneration is a progressive, abnormal growth of blood vessels or other materials in the retina. Hyperopia is a condition of farsightedness in which distant objects can be seen more clearly than closer objects.

Review: Yes ❑ No ❑

---

105. What structure is at the neck of the bladder and surrounds the urethra?
   A. Prostate
   B. Epididymis
   C. Prepuce
   D. Vas deferens

Answer: **A**

Why: The epididymis consists of two coiled tubules on the posterior of the testes that store and carry sperm. The prepuce is known as the foreskin. The vas deferens is a tubule that carries sperm from the epididymis to the seminal vesicles.

Review: Yes ❑ No ❑

---

106. The epigastric anatomical region of the abdomen is located:
   A. posterior to the kidneys.
   B. inferior to the colon.
   C. anterior to the pelvis.
   D. distal to the sternum.

Answer: **D**

Why: The epigastric anatomical region of the abdomen is located below the sternum and above the umbilical region.

Review: Yes ❑ No ❑

---

107. Collagen, a substance found in the dermis, is a/an:
   A. neurotransmitter.
   B. fibrous protein.
   C. catecholamine.
   D. enzyme.
   E. genetic material.

Answer: **B**

Why: Collagen is a fibrous protein found in the dermis, connective tissues, tendons, and ligaments. It is sometimes referred to as the body's glue, providing strength and flexibility.

Review: Yes ❑ No ❑

---

108. Which of the following glands are located on the sides of the vaginal opening and produce mucus?
   A. Prostate
   B. Cowper
   C. Bartholin
   D. Endocrine

Answer: **C**

Why: Bartholin glands are located on the sides of the vaginal opening and produce mucus. The prostate and Cowper glands are glands associated with the male reproductive system. Endocrine glands have no ducts and secrete hormones directly into the bloodstream.

Review: Yes ❑ No ❑

---

109. When the foot is moved outward, the joint movement is:
   A. adduction.
   B. circumduction.
   C. abduction.
   D. flexion.
   E. extension.

Answer: **C**

Why: Adduction is moving toward the body or inward; circumduction is moving in a circular motion; flexion is bending a body part; and extension is straightening a body part.

Review: Yes ❑ No ❑

110. The master gland of the body is the:
A. adrenal.
B. pituitary.
C. pineal.
D. thyroid.

Answer: **B**

Why: The pituitary gland is an endocrine gland located at the base of the brain. It is called the "master gland" because of the number of hormones it secretes and the functions it serves.

Review: Yes ❑ No ❑

---

111. A fracture of the radius characterized by bending of the bone with the skin left intact is referred to as:
A. greenstick, closed.
B. greenstick, open.
C. comminuted, closed.
D. comminuted, open.
E. Colles, closed.

Answer: **A**

Why: A greenstick fracture is an incomplete break or bending of the bone with the skin left intact and unbroken. This type of fracture frequently involves the radius bone and is common in children.

Review: Yes ❑ No ❑

---

112. Spermatozoa normally fertilize the female ovum in the:
A. ovary.
B. cervix.
C. uterus.
D. fallopian tube.

Answer: **D**

Why: Fertilization of the female ovum normally occurs in the fallopian tube after the ovum, the egg, has been released from the ovary where it is produced. The cervix is the neck of the uterus, the structure that houses and nourishes the growing fetus and placenta.

Review: Yes ❑ No ❑

---

113. The glomerulus is a cluster of blood capillaries found in the:
A. renal pelvis.
B. calyx.
C. loop of Henle.
D. bladder.
E. nephron.

Answer: **E**

Why: The renal pelvis is a cavity in the kidney where urine collects. A calyx is one of the points forming the renal pelvis. The loop of Henle is the bottom of the paperclip-shaped segment of the nephron.

Review: Yes ❑ No ❑

---

114. The disorder characterized by uncontrollable episodes of falling asleep is:
A. narcolepsy.
B. epilepsy.
C. Bell palsy.
D. Parkinson.

Answer: **A**

Why: Epilepsy is an abnormal electrical activity of the brain resulting in seizure. Bell palsy is a condition of unilateral facial muscle paralysis. Parkinson disease is a chronic progressive neurologic condition characterized by fine tremors and muscle weakness and rigidity.

Review: Yes ❑ No ❑

---

115. The regulation of body temperature is controlled by the:
A. pancreas.
B. thalamus.
C. pituitary.
D. medulla oblongata.
E. hypothalamus.

Answer: **E**

Why: The pancreas produces juices that metabolize sugar, the thalamus serves as relay for sensory input, the pituitary is the master gland, and the medulla oblongata controls heart rate, respiration, and blood pressure.

Review: Yes ❑ No ❑

116. Which of the following substances is NOT a neurotransmitter?
A. Acetylcholine
B. Norepinephrine
C. Epinephrine
D. Aldosterone

Answer: **D**

Why: Acetylcholine, norepinephrine, and epinephrine are neurotransmitters. Aldosterone is a hormone that regulates sodium and potassium levels.

Review: Yes ❑ No ❑

---

117. Cranial nerve I, the olfactory nerve, is related to the sense of:
A. sight.
B. smell.
C. sound.
D. taste.
E. touch.

Answer: **B**

Why: The olfactory nerve transmits smells from the nasal mucosa to the brain. The sense of sight, sound, taste, and touch are controlled by other cranial nerves. See Box 6-4.

Review: Yes ❑ No ❑

---

118. A blood cell that carries oxygen and has no nucleus is a/an:
A. leukocyte.
B. platelet.
C. erythrocyte.
D. thrombocyte.

Answer: **C**

Why: The erythrocyte is a red blood cell that contains hemoglobin that carries oxygen. The RBC has no nucleus. Platelets and thrombocytes are responsible for clotting. Leukocytes are white blood cells that do not carry oxygen and do have a nucleus.

Review: Yes ❑ No ❑

---

119. During respiration, exhaled air contains primarily:
A. oxygen.
B. nitrogen.
C. carbon dioxide.
D. carbon monoxide.
E. nitrous oxide.

Answer: **C**

Why: During the respiratory cycle, primarily oxygen is inhaled, or breathed in, and carbon dioxide is exhaled, or breathed out. Carbon dioxide is the waste product of respiration.

Review: Yes ❑ No ❑

---

120. A condition causing a backflow of stomach acid through an incompetent esophageal sphincter is called:
A. GERD.
B. SAD.
C. CVA.
D. IDDM.

Answer: **A**

Why: GERD stands for gastroesophageal reflux disease.

Review: Yes ❑ No ❑

7

Professional Communication

REVIEW TIP

Take this time to evaluate your review process and progress. Is your environment comfortable and conducive to studying? Are you spending the time as you initially planned? Are you staying focused and motivated (especially after the "killer" A&P chapter)? Is your study group (if you have one) productive? Are you asking family, friends, and employers for assistance and encouragement? Revise your plan if necessary, but DO NOT PROCRASTINATE. Remember why you are taking the exam!.

Communication is the process of forming and transmitting a message **(encoding)** to a receiver who interprets that message **(decoding)** and, in most cases, transmits a message back to the original sender, repeating the process (Fig. 7-1).

Every phase of health care requires communication, whether it involves patients, their families and friends, physicians, coworkers, other members of the health care team (such as hospital personnel), vendors, attorneys, governmental agencies, or other entities.

Many of the serious errors that result in patient harm are associated with faulty communication. Other consequences of miscommunication include malpractice suits, anger, distrust, and stress. Communicating in a professional, culturally sensitive manner helps ensure that messages are properly sent and correctly perceived by the recipient, and that the recipient responds appropriately to the sender. A leading principle of communication in health care is *confidentiality*. The majority of information in this chapter addresses communication between the patient and the health care provider.

COMMUNICATION GOALS

All communication has goals, either conscious or subconscious, that a person must understand to correctly formulate a message. Sometimes there is more than one goal per message. Some examples of communication goals are to:

- Obtain information
- Provide information
- Develop trust
- Demonstrate caring
- Relieve stress

STAGES OF DEVELOPMENT

Although there are several theories on what is called behavioral development, the stages are generally divided into specific age groups. There are distinct processes that normally should occur in each of these stages of development. When communicating with people of various

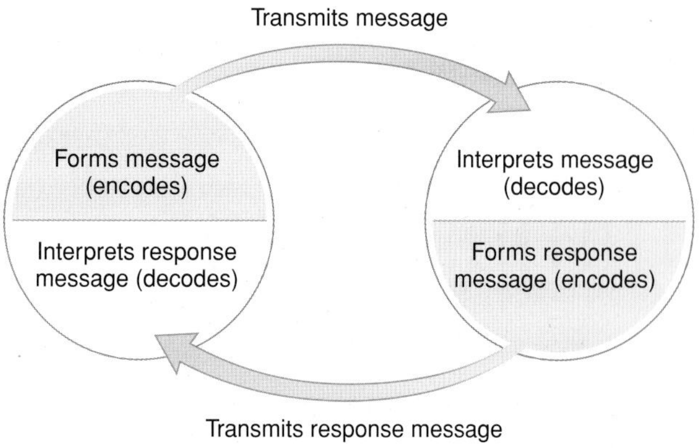

Figure 7-1 The communication process.

ages, keep in mind the behavior pertinent to each group. Familiar psychologists, Piaget and Erickson, described general stages of development, which are listed in Table 7-1).

TYPES OF COMMUNICATION

- Formal—a style associated with decorum, etiquette, and a person's recognized role
- Informal—a style associated with an easygoing, open role and relationship
- Verbal—word-of-mouth communication; may be formal or informal
  - Face-to-face
  - Telephone
  - Television
  - Audio technology (compact discs, tapes)
- Written—communication using the printed word; may be formal or informal
  - Medical records
  - Letters
  - Memorandums
  - E-mail
  - Books
  - Reports
  - Posters
  - Faxes
  - Bulletin boards
- Nonverbal—communication using body language and other nonwritten or nonoral methods
  - Open—receptive, positive appearance (e.g., the recipient leaning forward to listen)
  - Closed—nonreceptive, negative appearance (e.g., the recipient standing with frown on face and folded arms)
  - Indicators—signs that imply open or closed communication
    - Facial expressions, such as a smile or frown
    - Voice tone (e.g., soft or shrill)
    - Gestures, including sign language (e.g., extending hand for handshake or shaking a finger at a person, indicating anger or disapproval)
    - Body stance and posture, such as standing straight with arms at side or slouching with arms folded

Table 7-1 General Stages of Development

Stage	Focus	Issue
Infant/Toddler	Learns through comfort	Trust versus mistrust
Preschooler	Language acquisition	Active imagination and personifies objects
School Age	Begins to process abstract concepts	Developing sense of self-worth
Adolescent	Role integration	Self image
Adult	Career and family relationships	Commitment

COMMUNICATION BARRIERS

- Noise
- Inadequate listening
- Withdrawal or lack of attention
- Lack of privacy
- Embarrassment
- Cultural differences
  - Concepts of health and illness (e.g., only visiting the physician in the case of illness; not seeking preventive care)
  - Folk beliefs and practices (e.g., the belief that burying the umbilical cord when it falls off will help the child develop normally)
  - Childrearing traditions (e.g., "a fat baby is a healthy baby")
  - Religion (e.g., Jehovah's Witnesses prohibit blood transfusions)
  - Politeness (e.g., in some Native American cultures, it is taboo to make eye contact with another person)
  - Who speaks for whom (e.g., in some cultures, the husband speaks for his wife at the health care facility)

- Family ties (e.g., all members of family and extended family expected to stay with ill person)
- Death and dying traditions (e.g., required rites, blessings, or ceremonies)

■ Educational differences
■ Language barriers
■ Physical and developmental impairments
■ Pain or discomfort
■ Prejudice (holding a negative or positive opinion or bias concerning an individual because of his or her affiliation with a specific group; this includes gender bias)
■ Stereotyping (believing that all members of a culture, subculture, or group are the same)
■ Emotions
■ Criticizing, lecturing
■ Substance abuse

DEFENSE MECHANISMS

People commonly react to injury and illness with anxiety and, often, defensive behavior. **Defense mechanisms** are psychological behaviors that protect a person from guilt and shame. Some uses of the mechanisms are considered normal. Overuse or exaggerated use may become pathologic.

■ Compensation—overemphasizing certain behaviors to accommodate for real or imagined weaknesses (e.g., giving a child expensive gifts to make up for not spending time with him or her)
■ Denial—refusal to accept unwanted information or unpleasant circumstances (e.g., the parent who will not consider that his or her child is using drugs despite very clear indications to the contrary)
■ Displacement—transferring negative feelings, sometimes hostility, to something or someone unrelated to a negative situation (e.g., being rude to the medical office receptionist because your insurance company does not have you listed on the physician's roster)
■ Introjection—identifying and assuming characteristics or feelings of another (e.g., the expectant father who has food cravings similar to his pregnant partner)
■ Projection—placing blame or accusing another for actions or feelings committed by the person himself or herself (e.g., the patient blaming the health care provider for continued illness when the patient was noncompliant with the care plan)
■ Rationalization—justifying thoughts or actions whether right or wrong (e.g., spending money on a luxury item because you've had a bad day)
■ Regression—escaping an unpleasantness by returning to an earlier stage or behavior in life (e.g., a child who reverts to baby talk when scolded to distract the parent's anger)
■ Repression—dealing with a difficult situation by true temporary amnesia (e.g., a witness to a crime who cannot remember the crime or who he or she is)
■ Sublimation—redirecting unacceptable thoughts or behaviors to acceptable ones (e.g., the alcoholic who goes from drinking every night to attending Alcoholics Anonymous meetings every night)
■ Suppression—purposefully forgetting an unpleasant situation or avoiding it (e.g., victims of childhood sexual abuse who do not remember the molestation until, perhaps, an incident in adulthood triggers the memory)

HEALTH CARE IMPLICATIONS

Every communication within the health care setting has the potential for affecting a patient's outcome, physically and emotionally, positively or negatively. The relationship, good or bad, between the patient and the health care provider is predominately the result of their interactions. Other considerations when communicating with patients are as follows:

■ Real or unrealistic expectations of patient or health care providers
■ Feelings
■ Challenges
- Obtaining knowledge
- Interpreting and understanding each other
- Accurately exchanging information
- Accepting differences
- Making reasonable accommodations

THERAPEUTIC COMMUNICATION

The health care team should strive to make every interaction with the patient an understanding and caring one. The encounter should promote healing or acknowledgment in cases of serious disease or disability and provide some level of comfort. Therapeutic communication is:

■ Confidential
■ Respectful
■ Professional (friendly and capable but not too informal)
■ Empathetic (sympathetic but not enabling)

- Nonjudgmental
- Tolerant and supportive
- Accepting
- Reassuring
- Mindful of the patient's individuality
- Honest and open
- Sensitive and tactful
- Positive in attitude and body language

ENHANCING COMMUNICATION

The health care provider should continually strive to develop and practice better communication techniques. To promote positive and effective communication, especially in the health care setting:

- Provide a quiet, private, safe, and comfortable environment
- Listen carefully with no interruptions
- Provide feedback (paraphrasing, mirroring, repeating, restating to ensure understanding)
- Ask open-ended questions (such as "Tell me about your pain"), not questions that can be answered with yes or no or one word
- Seek clarification (who, what, how, how much)
- Use silence to allow patients to add more information
- Demonstrate open body language
- Exhibit a confident demeanor
- Focus (stay on important topics)
- Observe boundaries (e.g., remaining at a friendly but professional distance, not discussing intimate parts of patient's life or health care provider's life that do not pertain to the pertinent health care issue; not allowing rambling; not giving advice)

SPECIAL COMMUNICATION NEEDS AND STRATEGIES

- Sight-impaired patients
  - Speak in a normal tone of voice
  - Describe surroundings and locations of structures
  - Explain what you are going to do and what you are doing
  - Alert patient before touching him or her
  - Explain unusual noises associated with a procedure
  - Notify patient of anyone who is entering the room or if you are leaving the room
  - Allow touching of instruments and use models when appropriate
  - Facilitate return demonstrations as needed
  - Obtain feedback
  - Encourage questions
- Hearing-impaired patients
  - Touch the patient gently on an arm or shoulder to get his or her attention
  - Address the patient directly
  - Determine level of hearing loss and what assistive devices are used by patient
  - Increase voice volume, if appropriate, but do not shout
  - Speak distinctly and more slowly, using short sentences with slight pauses
  - Eliminate as much background noise as possible
  - Offer notepads or other non–hearing communication devices
  - Use pictures and captioned videos as appropriate
  - Facilitate return demonstrations as appropriate
  - Obtain feedback
  - Encourage questions

Box 7-1 addresses the telecommunication device for the deaf, which allows office personnel to communicate with hearing-impaired patients over the telephone.

- Non–English-speaking or limited English-speaking patients
  - Attempt to acquire some knowledge of culture to avoid negative communication (refer to "Cultural differences" in the section "Communications Barriers")
  - Provide an interpreter if possible (some insurance companies will arrange or cover the cost; some social agencies dealing with refugees and immigrants provide help)
    - Research culture to determine if there are any restrictions regarding who may act as an interpreter (e.g., in some cultures, interpreter must be of the same sex as patient)

Box 7-1

Telecommunication Device for the Deaf (TDD)

Many of the larger medical practices maintain a TDD. This equipment allows the office to call a hearing-impaired patient and to type a message that is electronically transmitted to the receiver's TDD and vice versa. If the office does not have a TDD, the office's telephone carrier may be contacted to send a TDD-facilitated message to the patient. E-mail is another effective communication technology for contacting hearing-impaired patients.

- Determine whether patient is bringing an interpreter (children and young adolescents should not be used)
- Speak directly to the patient even when using an interpreter
- Speak in a normal tone but at a slightly slower pace
- Use simple, short sentences
- Avoid slang or idioms
- Observe patient's body language as questions are asked and answered
- Use visual aids, such as pictures, hand gestures, or demonstrations
- Provide forms, educational materials, and office signs in various languages, if possible
- Use dual dictionaries of English and the patient's language

■ Pediatric patients
- Always state the truth
- Position yourself at the same height as the child
- Use vocabulary appropriate to the child's developmental age
- Incorporate dolls, pictures, and other toys to enhance communication or obtain cooperation
- Allow children to handle safe medical equipment
- Expect child to regress emotionally during illness
- Maintain a calm voice and demeanor, even if the child is "acting out"

■ Adolescent patients
- Treat the adolescent with respect
- Avoid being judgmental
- Always state the truth
- Expect adolescents to demonstrate resentment in illness, especially in chronic illness
- Allow privacy from parents during assessment and treatment, if desired by the patient
- Maintain a calm voice and demeanor even if the adolescent is "acting out"
- Do not assume, regardless of the patient's age, that he or she possesses the correct terminology and knowledge related to body functions, especially those related to the reproductive system
- Consider typical teenage preferences and behaviors when providing self-care instructions
- Obtain feedback
- Encourage questions

■ Geriatric patients
- Accommodate for hearing, sight, or other impairments

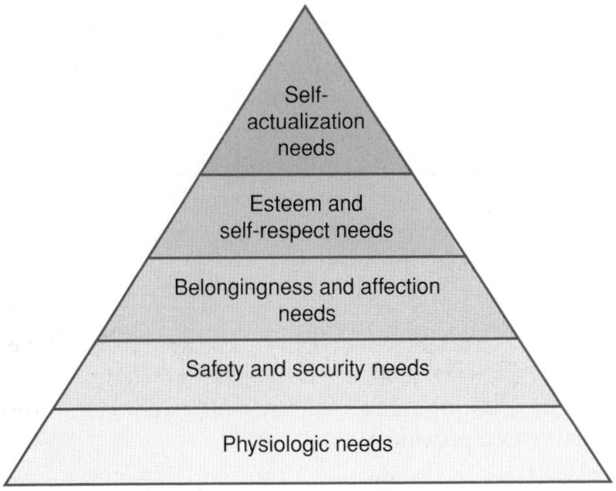

Figure 7-2 Maslow's hierarchy of human needs. (Reprinted with permission from Molle EA, Durham LS. Lippincott Williams & Wilkins' Administrative Medical Assisting. Philadelphia: Lippincott Williams & Wilkins, 2004.)

- Ensure patient's comfort and privacy
- Maintain an unrushed environment
- Use feedback strategies often
- Facilitate staying focused on pertinent topics
- Include the patient in the conversation even if a caregiver is providing the information

MASLOW'S HIERARCHY

Abraham Maslow, an American psychiatrist, theorized that people are motivated by their needs and that those needs are a progression from basic survival to reaching one's pinnacle, or self-actualization. Dr. Maslow ordered these needs in a hierarchy and listed them in a pyramid formation (Fig. 7-2). Generally, a person cannot progress from one level to the next until all needs are met in the lower levels.

The implications of **Maslow's hierarchy** for health care providers are substantial. Your communication with the patient will be more effective if you determine where that person is on Maslow's hierarchy. For example, a patient who does not have the money and other resources (e.g., transportation, child care) to visit a physician when he or she is sick will not be motivated to listen to advice regarding preventive health care or nutritional diets that are more expensive than a current high-fat, high-carbohydrate diet. Effective therapeutic communication recognizes the stage on the Maslow hierarchy pyramid, provides empathy and understanding, and then strives to discover a motivating factor within that level. The health care provider in this example can explain that if the patient ignores the treatment plan, the potential for a life-threatening illness increases, which may result in leaving his or her children without support.

STAGES OF DEATH AND DYING

Another progression in human life involves the **stages of death and dying**. Elizabeth Kübler-Ross is credited as being the first to formally outline these stages. The patient and the patient's family and close friends all experience the continuum. Communication is more effective when the stage is recognized and appropriate accommodations are made.

- Denial—refusing to accept that death will soon occur or has occurred
- Anger—lashing out at a deity, family and friends, and health care providers
- Bargaining—attempting to gain time through negotiating, pleading with a deity, with health care providers to do more, and with self
- Depression—withdrawing, feeling low in spirits
- Acceptance—resigning to the situation, preparing (if time permits), and feeling tranquil

Sudden death is thought to be more difficult. The involved parties do not have the time for a distinct progression through the stages and are unprepared; their reactions are often chaotic.

TERMS

Communication Review

The following list reviews the terms discussed in this chapter and **other important terms that you may see on the exam**.

communication the process of forming and transmitting a message to a receiver who interprets that message and, in most cases, transmits a message back to the original sender, repeating the process

compensation a defense mechanism in which a person overemphasizes certain behaviors to accommodate for real or imagined weaknesses

culture customary beliefs, traits, social forms, and behaviors associated with a religious, ethnic, or other group

decoding receiving and interpreting a message

defense mechanisms psychological behaviors that protect a person from guilt and shame

denial a defense mechanism in which a person refuses to accept unwanted information or unpleasant circumstances

diplomacy the art of handling people with tact and genuine concern

displacement a defense mechanism in which a person transfers negative feelings, sometimes hostility, to something or someone unrelated to a negative situation

encoding forming and sending a message

feedback paraphrasing, mirroring, repeating, or restating to ensure understanding

introjection a defense mechanism in which a person identifies and assumes characteristics or feelings of another

Maslow's hierarchy a progression of a person's needs from basic survival to reaching one's pinnacle, or self-actualization, identified by Abraham Maslow

nonverbal communication using body language and other nonwritten or nonoral methods; nonverbal communication may be formal or informal, open or closed

prejudice holding a negative or positive opinion or bias regarding an individual because of his or her affiliation with a specific group

projection a defense mechanism in which a person places blame or accuses another for actions or feelings committed by himself or herself

rationalization justifying thoughts or actions whether right or wrong

regression a defense mechanism in which a person escapes an unpleasantness by returning to an earlier stage or behavior in life

repression a defense mechanism in which a person deals with a difficult situation by true temporary amnesia

stages of death and dying articulated by Elizabeth Kübler-Ross, a progression of feelings and behaviors that patients, families, and close friends experience when death is imminent or has occurred; these behaviors include denial, anger, bargaining, depression, and acceptance

stereotyping believing that all members of a culture, subculture, or group are the same

sublimation a defense mechanism in which a person redirects unacceptable thoughts or behaviors to acceptable ones

suppression a defense mechanism in which a person purposefully forgets an unpleasant situation or avoids dealing with it

REVIEW QUESTIONS

All questions are relevant for the CMA (AAMA), RMA (AMT), and CMAS (AMT) exams.

1. Which of the following is the best example of nonverbal communication?
   A. Clarification
   B. Feedback
   C. Body language
   D. Messages

Answer: **C**

Why: Nonverbal communication refers to a way of exchanging messages without using words. Body language uses types of behavior or gestures and facial expressions to send a message without saying anything.

Review: Yes ❑ No ❑

---

2. When a person generalizes the behavior or characteristics of all members of a particular culture, race, or religion, it is referred to as:
   A. empathizing.
   B. stereotyping.
   C. discriminating.
   D. bias.
   E. Rationalizing.

Answer: **B**

Why: Bias occurs when personal values or opinions affect the way you treat others. Discriminating is the act of treating certain people unfairly or without respect because of their cultural, social, or personal values or beliefs. Empathizing means that you emotionally identify with what another person is feeling or experiencing. Rationalizing is the process of explaining on the basis of reason or logic.

Review: Yes ❑ No ❑

---

3. Three elements necessary for basic communication include:
   A. message, sender, receiver.
   B. message, feedback, body language.
   C. clarification, sender, feedback.
   D. sender, receiver, body language.

Answer: **A**

Why: The message is the information that is to be relayed either verbally or nonverbally. There must be someone sending and someone else receiving the message. Clarification is the process of making a message clearer or more understandable to the receiver. Feedback refers to the responses returned from either the sender or the receiver about the message.

Review: Yes ❑ No ❑

---

4. To have proper verbal communication with a patient, you should use:
   A. a monotone voice so the patient will listen better.
   B. elaborate medical terminology to impress the patient.
   C. negative body language to get the patient's attention.
   D. sarcastic remarks to get the patient's attention.
   E. conversation at the patient's educational level.

Answer: **E**

Why: A monotone voice occurs when a person is speaking without changing the pitch or key of the voice and is likely to cause the listener to lose interest in the conversation. Medical terminology is confusing for most laypersons; using such terminology will not lead to a patient understanding your message. Negative body language can make others uncomfortable and may cause them to ignore, turn away, or walk away from a conversation. Sarcastic remarks are rude and disrespectful and should not be part of any professional conversation.

Review: Yes ❑ No ❑

5. Communicating with someone who is grieving the loss of a loved one is difficult when the person refuses to acknowledge the loss. This type of behavior is referred to as:
   A. sympathy.
   B. mourning.
   C. denial.
   D. depression.

Answer: **C**

Why: Sympathy is sharing someone else's feeling, especially during a difficult situation, such as the death of a loved one. When a person is experiencing the loss of a loved one, he or she is in a period of mourning. Depression is a feeling of low spirits and being withdrawn. Denial is the inability or refusal to accept reality—in this case, the loss of a loved one.

Review: Yes ❑ No ❑

---

6. To communicate with a sight-impaired patient, it is important to:
   A. transport the patient in a wheelchair to avoid an accident.
   B. use positive body language.
   C. raise your voice to make your conversation louder.
   D. tell the patient each time before you touch him or her.
   E. give directions in writing to ensure understanding.

Answer: **D**

Why: Always talk to the patient and explain procedures before touching or performing any procedures on him or her. If a patient is sight-impaired, it does not necessarily mean that the person is totally blind. The patient may be capable of walking safely without a wheelchair, but transporting the patient does not facilitate communication. It may be difficult for the patient to see you clearly, so body language is not going to be easily seen by the patient. The patient may not be deaf or hard of hearing, so raising your voice is not necessary. Written instructions are difficult for a sight-impaired patient to read and will not be an effective method of communication.

Review: Yes ❑ No ❑

---

7. To communicate with a hearing-impaired patient, it would be advisable to:
   A. not call the patient at home, because of the hearing impairment.
   B. keep at a normal distance from the patient, but talk much louder and shout if necessary to be heard.
   C. write everything down instead of talking to the patient.
   D. speak slowly and distinctly to the patient.

Answer: **D**

Why: If a patient is hearing-impaired, it does not necessarily mean that he or she is completely deaf. It is appropriate to call this patient at home to confirm appointments. It is impolite to shout at a patient; therefore, it is appropriate to get closer to a hearing-impaired patient when having a conversation. It would not be necessary to write everything down, but you may want to write down the most important things you want the patient to remember. The key to communicating with a hearing-impaired individual is to speak slowly and clearly.

Review: Yes ❑ No ❑

---

8. Which of the following is an example of an open-ended question you would ask a patient?
   A. Did you follow the doctor's instructions?
   B. What time did you take your medication?
   C. Which insurance plan are you covered by?
   D. Will you tell me about your pain?
   E. What day can you come in for a follow-up appointment?

Answer: **D**

Why: An open-ended question is one that requires more than a single-word answer or a yes-or-no answer. This is a way to get patients to open up and talk or express their thoughts. All of the choices require only a single-word answer, except for choice D, which requires the patient to describe the pain he or she is experiencing.

Review: Yes ❑ No ❑

9. When communicating with a difficult, challenging patient, you should:
   A. exhibit a diplomatic attitude.
   B. display an attitude of authority.
   C. make sure the patient knows the office is correct.
   D. always ask the patient to put any complaints in writing.

Answer: **A**

Why: Diplomacy is the art of handling people with tact and genuine concern. Do not display an attitude of authority, because this may make a patient or client angry. Patients have rights in the physician's office, and the office may not always be correct. It is not appropriate to ask any patient to put his or her complaint in writing. Suggesting a patient "put it in writing" may be an invitation to a lawsuit. It is best to discuss concerns as they surface at the office.

Review: Yes ❑ No ❑

---

10. Which of the following is an example of behavior that demonstrates open nonverbal communication?
    A. Frowning eyes and mouth
    B. Folded arms across chest
    C. Leaning forward to listen
    D. Staring at the floor
    E. Sighing frequently during conversation

Answer: **C**

Why: Body language is a form of nonverbal communication. Open nonverbal communication is a positive, receptive way of communicating. The recipient usually leans forward to listen and makes direct eye contact with the person who is sending the message. Closed nonverbal communication is expressed through negative expressions such as frowning, folding arms, not making direct eye contact, and sighing during the conversation. These expressions reveal that an individual is not receptive to the communication.

Review: Yes ❑ No ❑

---

11. When an individual is overemphasizing certain behaviors to accommodate for real or imagined weaknesses, he or she is:
    A. regressing.
    B. compensating.
    C. projecting.
    D. rationalizing.

Answer: **B**

Why: To regress, or to go backward, is to escape an unpleasant event or situation and to return to an earlier stage or behavior in life. Projecting is placing blame or accusing someone else for something you have done. Rationalizing means reasoning or justifying one's behavior.

Review: Yes ❑ No ❑

---

12. Maslow's hierarchy of human needs is based on the concept that:
    A. affection is the most important basic need for all people.
    B. a safe environment is placed above all other needs as the number one requirement of all persons.
    C. physiologic needs are the most basic but are necessary for a person to progress any further toward reaching self-actualization.
    D. esteem must always come from those around us.
    E. security is the most basic and important need.

Answer: **C**

Why: The physiologic needs are air, food, water, rest, and comfort. Without these basic foundational needs being met, a person cannot reach any higher levels on Maslow's hierarchy of human needs. Affection is important but not a basic need for all persons. A safe and secure environment is only achieved after the basic needs are met. Esteem needs are needs to feel self-worth. Esteem can be self-generated or can come from others who admire a person.

Review: Yes ❑ No ❑

13. When communicating with pediatric patients, you should:
    A. not allow children to handle safe medical equipment.
    B. use medical terminology so the child does not understand the procedure.
    C. not lie to a child but state the truth.
    D. talk louder and make sure the child understands that you are the adult.

Answer: **C**

Why: Children are capable of understanding many things, and the truth should always be told to them. If you lie to a child that a procedure will not hurt and then it does, the child may not trust health care workers in the future. It is proper to allow children to handle safe equipment to help them feel comfortable. You should not use language the child does not understand and should not display an attitude of being an adult disciplinarian.

Review: Yes ❑ No ❑

---

14. The receiving and interpreting of a message is known as:
    A. decoding.
    B. feedback.
    C. encoding.
    D. acceptance.
    E. sending.

Answer: **A**

Why: Feedback is repeating or restating a message to ensure understanding. Encoding is the forming and sending of a message and does not involve receiving and interpreting. Acceptance means to resolve or be resigned to a situation, to accept the outcome. Sending is the process of carrying or transmitting a message.

Review: Yes ❑ No ❑

---

15. Psychological behaviors that protect a person from guilt and shame are:
    A. therapeutic techniques.
    B. defense mechanisms.
    C. cultural differences.
    D. language barriers.

Answer: **B**

Why: Therapeutic techniques include any activity that aids in a patient's recovery. Cultural differences are those traits specific to an ethnic culture or race. A language barrier is caused when people cannot communicate because they speak different languages.

Review: Yes ❑ No ❑

---

16. When communicating with a non–English-speaking patient, it is appropriate to:
    A. ignore the customs or taboos of the patient's culture.
    B. only communicate with the patient if accompanied by someone who speaks fluent English.
    C. raise your voice to increase understanding.
    D. use gestures to demonstrate information.
    E. use negative body language.

Answer: **D**

Why: You should always take into consideration the customs of the patient's culture so that you do not unintentionally offend him or her. If an interpreter is available, this person may be able to better communicate the information to the patient. The interpreter may be a family member who is not fluent in English but who knows enough to relate the messages to the patient. It is not appropriate to raise your voice just because the patient does not speak English. Using gestures will help demonstrate what you are trying to convey to a non–English-speaking patient. Using negative body language is inappropriate and rude.

Review: Yes ❑ No ❑

17. **Prejudice** is a term that means:
    A. your personal values are not the same as others.
    B. you hold an opinion or bias concerning an individual because of his or her affiliation with a specific group.
    C. you recognize the fear and discomfort that a patient is feeling.
    D. you refuse to acknowledge something.

Answer: **B**

Why: All people are free to have their own personal values, which may not be the same as those of others, but when you hold an opinion or bias concerning an individual because of his or her affiliation with a specific group of people, this constitutes prejudice, which is also a form of stereotyping. Empathy means that you recognize the fear and discomfort a patient is feeling; denial is refusing to acknowledge something.

Review: Yes ❑ No ❑

---

18. To encourage further comments from a patient, the interviewer can repeat what the patient has said using open-ended statements that require the patient to respond. This technique is called:
    A. summarizing.
    B. reflecting.
    C. listening.
    D. focusing.
    E. encoding.

Answer: **B**

Why: Summarizing is restating information in a condensed format. Listening is the act of giving attention to the person who is talking and understanding what is being said. Focusing is the technique of staying on the same topic or subject during a conversation and not deviating onto other topics. Encoding is the forming and sending of a message.

Review: Yes ❑ No ❑

---

19. A patient who is withdrawn, weeping, and isolated from others may be experiencing:
    A. anger.
    B. denial.
    C. depression.
    D. empathy.

Answer: **C**

Why: Anger is lashing out at others. Denial is the refusal to accept a situation, and empathy is feeling the same as another feels in a situation.

Review: Yes ❑ No ❑

---

20. Maintaining a professional relationship with the patient means that you should:
    A. become personally involved with the patient.
    B. become socially interactive with the patient.
    C. disclose private, personal information about the physician.
    D. give the patient your private phone number in case of emergency.
    E. deliver patient care that allows you to continue to provide objective medical care.

Answer: **E**

Why: It is appropriate to be friendly with patients, but you should not become personally or socially involved with patients. Private or personal information about the physician should never be disclosed to patients. It is also inappropriate to disclose your private phone number or address to a patient.

Review: Yes ❑ No ❑

---

21. Proper flow of communication occurs in the following order:
    A. message, response, clarification, feedback.
    B. response, clarification, feedback, message.
    C. feedback, message, clarification, response.
    D. clarification, message, response, feedback.

Answer: **A**

Why: To ensure proper communication, there must first be a message or information to send. Clarification and feedback come after the message has been sent. A response cannot be given to something not yet received.

Review: Yes ❑ No ❑

22. The progression of a person's needs from basic survival to reaching one's pinnacle or self-actualization is known as Maslow's:
    A. rationalization.
    B. self-realization.
    C. hierarchy.
    D. mechanism.
    E. triangle.

Answer: **C**

Why: A hierarchy is a system of ranking or grading things from least to greatest or small to large. Maslow's hierarchy ranks a person's needs from basic needs for survival to a rank of fulfillment of oneself or one's capabilities.

Review: Yes ❑ No ❑

---

23. To avoid breaching confidentiality, you should:
    A. use the office intercom to notify another coworker of the name of a caller on the phone.
    B. only discuss patient problems during the office lunch hour.
    C. communicate in writing, not verbally, to coworkers about patients.
    D. avoid discussing patient problems in the office hallway.

Answer: **D**

Why: Patients' names should not be announced over an intercom. Patient information should never be discussed outside the office, such as in a restaurant during lunch. At the office, patients should only be discussed in a private area, not in the hallway. Written messages are not appropriate for all communication in the office. The written message is not efficient; paper still needs to be either discarded properly or stored in a confidential area.

Review: Yes ❑ No ❑

---

24. Communication techniques that are used when interviewing a patient include:
    A. reflecting and summarizing.
    B. language barriers.
    C. stereotyping.
    D. bargaining and acceptance.
    E. criticizing.

Answer: **A**

Why: Reflecting and summarizing are communication techniques that allow the interviewer to encourage more conversation from the patient and clarify information for accuracy. Language barriers exist when the people who need to communicate do not speak or understand the same language. Stereotyping is the belief that all members of a culture or group are the same. Bargaining and acceptance are stages of dealing with grief. Criticizing is the act of judging and analyzing to find fault with something.

Review: Yes ❑ No ❑

---

25. To set the stage for successful communication, you should:
    A. ask closed-ended questions instead of open-ended questions because they are less time-consuming and more efficient.
    B. sit at the patient's level, eye to eye, and maintain eye contact with the patient if culturally appropriate.
    C. avoid using any body language such as appropriate facial expressions.
    D. discourage any additional comments from the patient because the physician will question the patient again during the examination.

Answer: **B**

Why: You should sit at the level of the patient and maintain good eye contact during the interview. This creates an atmosphere of focus on the patient. The use of facial expression and open body language will also add to a positive communication environment. Asking closed-ended questions and not encouraging additional comments will cause the patient to shut down and not express what is actually going on with his or her health. It may be more difficult for the patient to talk to or discuss anything further with the physician.

Review: Yes ❑ No ❑

26. Which of the following is an issue that becomes predominant during the adolescent stage of development?
    A. Commitment
    B. Self-worth
    C. Mistrust
    D. Imagination
    E. Self image

Answer: **E**

Why: According to noted behavioral psychologists, the predominant issue for the adolescent group is self image. Commitment is an adult issue. Mistrust is an infant or toddler issue. School-age children have issues with developing a sense of self-worth, and preschoolers develop imagination as a form of communication.

Review: Yes ❑ No ❑

8
Patient Education

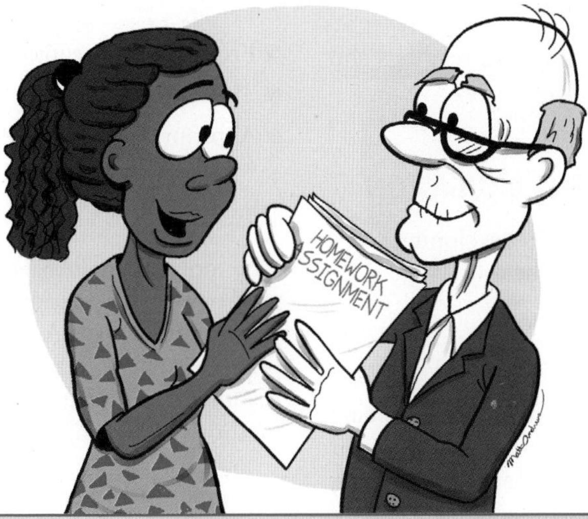

REVIEW TIP

Study the chapter on communication (Chapter 7) before you begin this chapter. The information supplied in that chapter also applies to patient education and should be integrated with the material presented here. Pick a topic pertinent to the medical office where you work or the field in which you are interested in working and develop a patient education plan. Ask your peers, supervisors, and physicians to critique it and provide input.

The emphasis on patient education in the health care setting continues to grow. The **Joint Commission** and the **National Committee for Quality Assurance (NCQA)**, both of which accredit health care organizations, have multiple patient education standards and requirements. The result is that more responsibility in this area is placed on the medical practice. Federal and state governments, health plans, insurance companies, hospitals, physician offices, other health care agencies, and the public spend millions of dollars each year publishing patient information pamphlets, videos, DVDs, and other instructional pieces. Better-informed patients tend to be more compliant with care and more apt to participate in preventive services. The intended outcome is improved health. Patient education frequently contributes to quality improvement in health care outcomes (see Chapter 4).

PURPOSE OF PATIENT EDUCATION

- Maintain and promote health
- Prevent illness
- Restore health
- Cope with impaired function

TOPICS FOR PATIENT EDUCATION

The role of the medical assistant or medical administrative specialist includes educating patients. A few of the many topics encountered in patient education are:

- Medication administration
- Medical equipment use and care

- Diet restrictions and modifications
- Prediagnostic test or procedure instructions
- Postdiagnostic test or procedure instructions
- Physical exercises
- Activity modification
- Preventive health schedules (e.g., immunizations, well-woman exams)
- Rehabilitative modalities
- Other resources, such as indigent food programs
- Health warning signs
- Self-exams (e.g., for testicular and breast cancer)
- Health monitoring (e.g., blood pressure readings and glucose testing)

CONSIDERATIONS FOR PATIENT EDUCATION

Several areas must be considered when developing plans for patient education. These include the following.

DOMAINS OF LEARNING

Domains of learning are the areas of a person's being that affect his or her capacity to learn. The educator should be aware of the person's domains of learning when formulating the teaching plan. The domains are:

- Cognitive (knowledge, comprehension)
- Affective (values, attitudes, opinions)
- Psychomotor (mental and physical abilities, sensory skills)

FACTORS INFLUENCING PATIENT EDUCATION

In addition to domains of learning, other factors, both internal and external to the patient, influence the teaching plan and the likelihood that the patient will comply or not comply with the plan. Some of these factors are:

- Motivation (refer to Maslow's hierarchy in Chapter 7)
- Goals
- Adaptation to illness
- Age
- Developmental age
- Impairments (e.g., hearing, sight)
- Pain
- Language
- Cultural or religious barriers
- Socioeconomic barriers
- Ability of the educator to convey information

ENVIRONMENT CONDUCIVE TO LEARNING

After accounting for the domains of learning and other factors influencing patient education, the health care provider must also consider the learning environment. A person is less likely to assimilate information in a chaotic environment than in one that is conducive to learning. Selecting and preparing the environment is part of the teaching plan. An environment conducive to learning is:

- Quiet
- Comfortable
- Private
- Free from interruptions
- Trusting
- Appropriate for any needed equipment or materials

TEACHING AIDS AND MODALITIES

The tools and materials selected by the educator to provide patient instruction are important to the success of the teaching plan. As an example, you do not want to provide only written material to a person who has a low reading level. Many types of instructional tools and methods are available. They include:

- Pamphlets and other written material
- Braille materials
- Hearing devices
- Videos, compact discs, DVDs, slides, tapes
- Oral presentations and discussions
- Demonstrations/return demonstrations
- Anatomic models, dolls
- Posters and other illustrations
- Record-keeping logs and journals
- Support groups
- Referral programs
- Family participation
- Feedback

COMMON SOURCES OF MATERIALS AND INFORMATION FOR PATIENT EDUCATION

Sources of patient educational materials are plentiful. Some sources will provide material at no cost; other sources may charge to cover their cost or to make a profit. In some cases, the insurance company will assume the cost. Use only credible sources with medically known and professionally accepted authors, advisors, and reviewers. All materials used or proposed should be approved by the physician or appropriate supervisory person in the medical office. Sources include:

- Professional organizations, such as the American Medical Association (AMA)
- Government agencies, such as Centers for Disease Control and Prevention (CDC)
- Nonprofit organizations, such as the American Diabetes Association (ADA)
- Commercial publishers of books and videos or DVDs
- Internet websites
- Computer programs designed to individualize information
- Libraries (public, private, and medical)
- Educational and medical supply companies for models, compact discs, and videos (catalogs are usually available)
- Insurance and health care companies (these frequently publish informational materials for members)

EDUCATIONAL PLAN

After arming yourself with the tools required for educating a patient, you are ready to begin creating the individual **patient educational plan.** The Joint Commission and NCQA standards recommend a **multidisciplinary**, or team, approach to developing the plan. Some plans are simple, such as explaining to the patient that he or she needs to reschedule an appointment, the importance of keeping that appointment, and, perhaps, escorting him or her to the scheduler, who will then arrange the required appointment. Educating a parent on how to obtain and use a small-volume nebulizer requires a more complex plan. This process could be multidisciplinary, involving the insurance company to approve rental or purchase of equipment and a medical supply company to provide the equipment. Teaching a patient about diabetes may include referring the patient to a diabetes educator. Even simple plans tend to be multidisciplinary, involving other members of the health care team. The steps of the plan are:

1. Identify the purpose and topic.
2. Assess the patient's individual needs and abilities (domains of learning).
3. Develop the plan. (Who will do the teaching? What will be taught and what materials are needed? Where will the teaching occur? How will it be done?)
   - Review the plan with the physician or the supervisor as appropriate.
   - Include appropriate patient support personnel and medical team members.
4. Implement the plan.
5. Evaluate the patient's understanding of your plan.
   - Use feedback from the patient to evaluate the effectiveness of your teaching.
   - Revise or repeat instruction if needed.
6. Provide a form of written instruction for the patient to take home (frequently patients sign documents that confirm that they have received and understood information).
7. Document the education provided in the patient's medical record.
8. Reevaluate effectiveness using follow-up visits, letters, e-mails, or telephone calls per office policy and procedure.

OTHER CONSIDERATIONS

Some offices compile pertinent standardized information in packets that may contain videos, DVDs, calendars, compact discs, and even bound books. For instance, an obstetrics office may offer information on fetal development, diet and exercise during pregnancy, or what a pregnant woman can expect in each trimester. Your responsibility may be to discuss with a patient the information contained in a particular packet and to elicit and answer any questions that arise. Each patient should be considered individually, and emphasis should be placed on areas of need for that patient. If a patient is overweight, for example, more time should be spent discussing diet. Accommodations must be made for special-needs patients and those with high-risk pregnancies.

The medical record documentation should note whether a prenatal packet was given and explained and any areas of special emphasis. These entries should include the date, the time, and your signature. Some medical practices have forms with check-off boxes, which are signed by you and by the patient. The medical record, in addition to providing information for the patient and members of the health care team, is a legal document that can protect the health care provider from liability if documentation is complete and thorough.

Accrediting bodies, governmental agencies, and contracted insurance plans also audit medical records to determine the extent and appropriateness of patient education at the medical practice. Failure to provide adequate patient education might be a reason for not obtaining full accreditation or for an insurance company not renewing a contract with a medical office.

TERMS

Patient Education Review

The following list reviews the terms discussed in this chapter and **other important terms that you may see on the exam.**

affective relating to a person's values, attitudes, opinions; a domain of learning

cognitive relating to knowledge and understanding; a domain of learning

domains of learning areas of a person's being that affect learning; the three domains are as follows: cognitive (knowledge, comprehension), affective (values, attitudes, opinions), and psychomotor (mental and physical abilities, sensory skills)

motivation a circumstance or a tangible item that drives a person into action

multidisciplinary a team approach involving different fields of knowledge and expertise

National Commission for Quality Assurance (NCQA) a national accrediting body for health care organizations

noncompliant failure or refusal to comply or do something as asked

patient educational plan a design (may be multidisciplinary) to provide education to a patient on a specific topic that includes identification of the topic, assessment of the patient's domains of learning, formulation of the actions, implementation of the actions, and evaluation of the plan's effectiveness

psychomotor relating to a person's physical and mental capabilities and sensory skills; a domain of learning

The Joint Commission (formerly the Joint Commission on the Accreditation of Healthcare Organizations or JCAHO) a national accrediting body for health care organizations

REVIEW QUESTIONS

All questions are relevant for the CMA (AAMA), RMA (AMT), and CMAS (AMT) exams.

1. The process of acquiring information from a patient to determine health care needs and abilities is called:
   A. assessment.
   B. evaluation.
   C. documentation.
   D. planning.

Answer: **A**

Why: Assessment is the gathering or acquiring of information. Evaluation is the process that indicates how well a patient is adapting or progressing. Documentation is the writing or recording of a patient's needs and progress and the physician's evaluation notes. Planning is the using of this information to fulfill the patient's needs.

Review: Yes ❑ No ❑

---

2. Properly written patient educational materials should:
   A. be narrative paragraphs rather than outlined information.
   B. not include charts or diagrams.
   C. include complex medical terms and phrases.
   D. focus on key points.
   E. be lengthy and use sophisticated words.

Answer: **D**

Why: Narrative paragraphs are usually not as easy to read or comprehend as outlined materials. Charts and diagrams are very valuable in the education process because they are visual. Medical terms and phrases usually confuse the layperson not familiar with medical language. Patient information materials should not be lengthy but should only include necessary information. Presenting information in the simplest way possible will help ensure the patient understands it.

Review: Yes ❑ No ❑

---

3. The best way to reinforce verbal instructions for a patient is to:
   A. explain the directions using pronounced body language.
   B. provide the patient with written instructions.
   C. reassure the patient using constant therapeutic touch.
   D. ask the patient to call you in a couple of days to see if there are any questions.

Answer: **B**

Why: Before leaving the office, it is best if the patient has written instructions that will act as a reminder. This is the best way to reinforce what has been discussed with the patient.

Review: Yes ❑ No ❑

---

4. As the best way to document that a patient received written instructions to take home, you should:
   A. have the receptionist file a note in the patient's chart.
   B. write an entry in the patient's chart stating that the patient received the materials.
   C. have the patient sign a document, to be placed in the patient's chart, verifying receipt of the materials.
   D. have the patient answer questions about the materials to see if he or she read the information.
   E. conduct a follow-up phone call to the patient.

Answer: **C**

Why: Placing a note or entry in a patient's chart or having a patient answer questions does not provide documented proof that the patient received educational materials. If the patient signs a document for the file verifying receipt of the materials, there is definite documentation that the event happened.

Review: Yes ❑ No ❑

5. An environment conducive to learning is characterized by:
   A. privacy.
   B. interruptions.
   C. noise.
   D. chaos.

Answer: **A**

Why: An environment that is conducive to learning is quiet, free of interruptions, and private. A patient is more likely to concentrate on the information you are providing in this kind of a place than in one that is noisy and full of activity.

Review: Yes ❑ No ❑

---

6. When evaluating a patient's progress in a patient educational program, if you discover noncompliance, this means that the patient is:
   A. following the instructions exactly as they were provided.
   B. not progressing as quickly as expected.
   C. refusing to follow prescribed orders.
   D. having a reaction to prescribed medication.
   E. progressing quickly and healing properly.

Answer: **C**

Why: Noncompliance means that the patient is refusing to follow prescribed orders. A compliant patient follows instructions exactly as they were provided. Not all patients progress at the same rate, even given the same treatment plan. Some have quick results, whereas in others, it may take longer to notice change or progress in their health. If a patient is having a reaction to a medication, this implies compliance. Because the drug does not agree with the patient, this is a case of incompatibility.

Review: Yes ❑ No ❑

---

7. When developing written patient educational materials, it is most important to consider:
   A. the patient's cognitive level of understanding.
   B. the patient's gender.
   C. incorporating more complex medical terminology in the information.
   D. including as many topics as possible in the same written brochure.

Answer: **A**

Why: The cognitive level of understanding means the level at which a person is knowledgeable or comprehends information. It is important to develop patient educational materials at a basic level the reader can understand. It is not necessarily important to consider the patient's gender when developing written patient educational materials. Using complex language or placing too many diverse topics in one document may be confusing for the patient.

Review: Yes ❑ No ❑

---

8. To provide patient education for a patient who is blind, which of the following formats of training materials would be most helpful?
   A. Posters
   B. DVDs
   C. Braille materials
   D. Pamphlets and brochures
   E. Internet websites

Answer: **C**

Why: Braille is a form of writing that blind people usually can understand. It is a writing system that uses raised dots to represent each letter of the alphabet. The other materials listed are not options for use in training someone who is blind.

Review: Yes ❑ No ❑

---

9. A team approach to patient education that includes different fields of knowledge and expertise is referred to as a(n):
   A. joint venture.
   B. multidisciplinary plan.
   C. quality assurance.
   D. accommodation.

Answer: **B**

Why: Multidisciplinary means that people from different areas of specialty or knowledge are involved together to assist patients in education. The front and back office personnel work together with other trained professionals to provide the specific information necessary to educate the patient.

Review: Yes ❑ No ❑

10. The first step in development of a patient educational program is to:
A. document the educational plan in the patient's chart.
B. identify the purpose and topic of the educational program.
C. elicit patient feedback for documentation.
D. evaluate effectiveness of the educational plan.
E. decide the format for the materials to be developed.

Answer: **B**

Why: To design an appropriate patient educational program, you must first establish the reason or purpose of the educational program. This is the main objective of the education. You cannot gather feedback or document in the patient's chart unless you first know what the educational program is. Evaluating the effectiveness is also not possible until the program has been implemented. The format for the materials should be selected after the purpose has been established.

Review: Yes ❑ No ❑

---

11. When asked to provide dietary information for a patient, an organization that could provide the most valuable materials is the:
A. Centers for Disease Control and Prevention.
B. American Academy of Family Physicians.
C. National Dairy Council.
D. American Lung Association.

Answer: **C**

Why: The National Dairy Council is the organization that developed a nutritional guide that complements MyPyramid, the guide to basic nutrition and food group categories. The other organizations specialize in other areas of health.

Review: Yes ❑ No ❑

---

12. Patient educational materials are best implemented when the:
A. patient is sent packets of materials in the mail.
B. physician tells the patient to contact a professional organization to answer questions about the materials.
C. patient is given the materials as he or she exits the office.
D. patient's family is not involved.
E. materials are discussed with the patient.

Answer: **E**

Why: If a patient is simply handed materials or is sent materials in the mail without any discussion or opportunity to ask questions, there is no assurance that the patient understands the information. Therefore, it is best to discuss the materials with the patient and answer any questions before the patient leaves the office.

Review: Yes ❑ No ❑

---

13. A national accrediting body for health care organizations that has established standards and requirements for patient education is the:
A. CDC.
B. AMA.
C. FDA.
D. NCQA.

Answer: **D**

Why: The NCQA (National Committee for Quality Assurance) is a national organization that establishes standards for practice in health care facilities. Among these standards are requirements for informing and educating patients on health care issues. The CDC is the Centers for Disease Control and Prevention, the AMA is the American Medical Association, and the FDA is the Food and Drug Administration.

Review: Yes ❑ No ❑

---

14. The cognitive domain of learning refers to:
A. attitude.
B. physical abilities.
C. sensory skills.
D. attitudes and opinions.
E. comprehension.

Answer: **E**

Why: Cognitive refers to having knowledge or comprehending information. Mental and physical abilities and sensory skills are types of psychomotor learning. Attitudes and opinions are factors of affective learning.

Review: Yes ❑ No ❑

15. The process used to carry out the agreed teaching plan in patient education is called:
    A. assessment.
    B. evaluation.
    C. implementation.
    D. documentation.

Answer: **C**

Why: Implementation means carrying out or providing the means for accomplishing. Assessment, evaluation, and documentation are other processes necessary in the patient education process.

Review: Yes ❑ No ❑

---

16. The overall purpose of patient education is to:
    A. meet with patients one-on-one.
    B. improve patient health.
    C. provide excessive information.
    D. involve patients in community activities.
    E. comply with accrediting agencies.

Answer: **B**

Why: Patients who are better informed about their health are more likely to comply with the physician's treatment plan. This ultimately will help prevent disease and promote improvement in the patient's health.

Review: Yes ❑ No ❑

---

17. A patient who needs information about drug addiction could receive education and help from an organization that specializes in:
    A. prescription medications.
    B. preventive health.
    C. substance abuse.
    D. nutrition management.

Answer: **C**

Why: Substance abuse refers to excessive use of and dependency on legal or illegal drugs. This could include prescription drugs or illegal "street" drugs. Alcohol is also categorized as a substance that is frequently abused.

Review: Yes ❑ No ❑

---

18. If a diabetic patient is reluctant to learn how to give himself or herself insulin injections, the first thing you should do is:
    A. notify the patient's physician for further assistance.
    B. recommend that the patient see an endocrinologist.
    C. ask the patient to return to the office only when ready to comply with the instruction.
    D. refer the patient to a diabetic support group or a social worker who specializes in diabetes.
    E. volunteer to give the patient the injections.

Answer: **A**

Why: You must only perform duties under the direct supervision of the physician and should only inform the physician of the problem with the patient. It is the physician who is responsible for determining what the next step will be in this patient's care. The physician may actually refer the patient to another person who specializes in this type of problem. You should never go beyond the level of patient education approved by the physician.

Review: Yes ❑ No ❑

---

19. Of the following, which patient is the least likely to respond to learning objectives?
    A. A patient who has reached the level of esteem and self-respect on Maslow's hierarchy of needs
    B. A patient who perceives the information as important to his or her health
    C. A patient who perceives the health care team as condescending
    D. A patient who has the same culture and ethnic background that you have

Answer: **C**

Why: The word **condescending** means "regarding another as being lower in status or knowledge than you." This attitude will discourage the patient from working with you. All the other answers are a positive indication that the patient will be receptive to the education or instruction. It is especially helpful if the medical assistant and the patient come from the same cultural and ethnic background. It gives them something in common.

Review: Yes ❑ No ❑

20. Of the following, which is the most important for the person who is performing patient education?
    A. Producing patient brochures
    B. Using technical words when instructing
    C. Documenting in the patient record whatever teaching is performed
    D. Learning other languages to facilitate job performance
    E. Assuring the patient considers you his or her friend.

Answer: C

Why: Although all of the answers might be helpful, if documentation does not occur, it is as if nothing happened. Documenting events is the most important task to properly monitor and evaluate the progress of the patient.

Review: Yes ❏ No ❏

---

21. One of the factors that helps the most in promoting patient learning is:
    A. the height and weight of the patient.
    B. the patient's gender.
    C. a positive emotional outlook.
    D. the patient's insurance company.

Answer: C

Why: The patient's height, weight, gender (sex), and insurance company usually have no effect on the patient's learning. If the patient has a positive emotional outlook, more than likely, he or she will also approach the patient education as a positive event.

Review: Yes ❏ No ❏

---

22. To ensure that a patient follows up with appointments for evaluation of the prescribed plan of treatment, you should:
    A. assign a project or homework for the patient to complete between appointments.
    B. ask the patient to call the office to schedule a follow-up appointment when it is convenient.
    C. provide the patient with a written appointment slip with the date and time of his or her next session.
    D. call the patient a week in advance to confirm the appointment.
    E. have the physician contact the patient if the appointment is missed.

Answer: C

Why: It is always best to provide the patient with something in writing as a reminder. Asking the patient to call the office or even calling the patient a couple of days in advance is not as effective as handing the patient a written appointment slip before he or she leaves the office. Assigning a project or homework is inappropriate, although, depending on the patient education program, you may ask the patient to keep a journal of progress to report on during return visits. It is not appropriate to have the physician contact a patient because of a missed appointment.

Review: Yes ❏ No ❏

---

23. A way to evaluate the patient's understanding of educational information is to:
    A. document in the patient's medical record that he or she received the materials.
    B. design a colorful brochure.
    C. ask for feedback from the patient.
    D. assess the patient's individual needs and abilities.

Answer: C

Why: To find out if the patient understands the information, ask for feedback. Documenting receipt of the materials does not ensure the patient understands them. Designing a brochure and assessing the patient's needs are done before the evaluation process.

Review: Yes ❏ No ❏

24. When providing patient education, you should:
    A. encourage questions from the patient.
    B. use only written materials for training.
    C. discuss training materials with the patient in the hallway so you do not occupy an exam room when the physician needs to use it.
    D. use the same method of training with all patients.
    E. present the materials at a level much higher than the patient's cognitive level.

Answer: **A**

Why: You should encourage the patient to ask any questions about the educational materials. Using only written materials may not be appropriate for all patients. You should always discuss training materials in a private exam room to maintain the patient's confidentiality. Varying the type of presentation is needed to accommodate different patients. It is important to understand the patient's level of comprehension so the training is meaningful for the patient.

Review: Yes ❑ No ❑

---

25. One factor that is a positive contribution to the patient's learning process is:
    A. just keeping quiet and only listening.
    B. maintaining noncompliance to directions or instructions.
    C. having family support.
    D. possessing a know-it-all attitude.

Answer: **C**

Why: A patient who has a good support system from his or her family will probably take the learning more seriously and have better progress with his or her health needs. If the patient is quiet and does not ask questions, learning may be hindered. Noncompliance means the patient does not do what is asked. A know-it-all attitude may cause the patient not to listen to instructions and then not know what he or she is to do later.

Review: Yes ❑ No ❑

---

26. The patient's mental and physical abilities are referred to as:
    A. psychosomatic.
    B. psychomotor.
    C. psychological.
    D. psychosocial.
    E. psychiatric.

Answer: **B**

Why: Psycho- refers to mind or mental capacity. *Motor* refers to a person's ability to perform physical functions such as body movement.

Review: Yes ❑ No ❑

---

27. The domain of learning that includes values, attitudes, and opinions is referred to as:
    A. cognitive.
    B. congenital.
    C. aberrant.
    D. affective.

Answer: **D**

Why: Cognitive refers to knowledge and comprehension. Congenital means born with, and aberrant means wandering from the norm.

Review: Yes ❑ No ❑

Unit 3

Administrative Practice

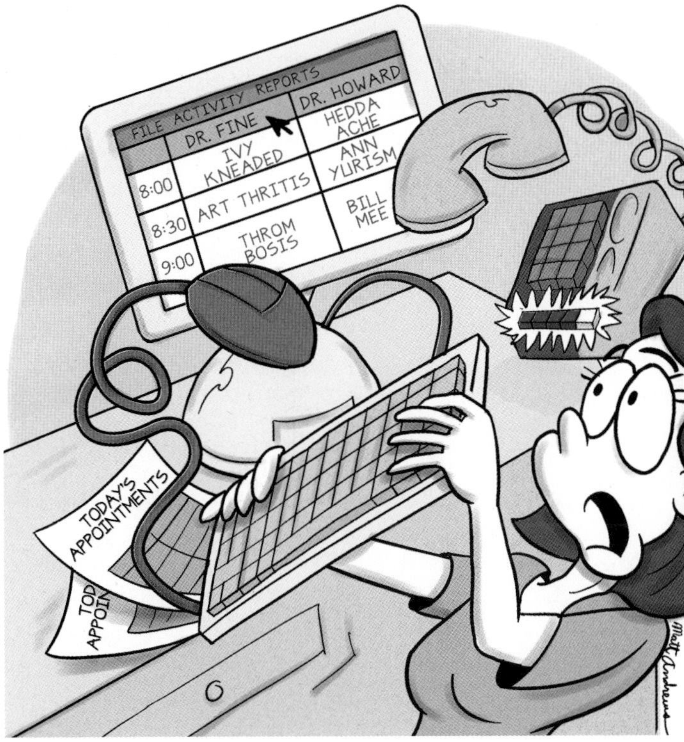

9

Administrative Technologies

REVIEW TIP

Complete the chapters on Communication (Chapter 7) and Patient Education (Chapter 8) before beginning this chapter. Many of the principles discussed in those chapters also apply to administrative techniques. This chapter lends itself to lunchtime reading and other "learning moments." Carry the review book with you and open it when you have a free moment.

Chapter 1 explained that this is a review book, not a text for primary learning. Many textbooks describe the telephone with its features (e.g., hold and transfer buttons), explain how to place long-distance calls, identify time zones, and discuss other operational functions. Although these areas are necessary for you to know in practice, they have a very low probability of appearing on the national exams. The telephone information included in this chapter has "exam probability."

The wired telephone and the cellular telephone are the most common but not the only methods of electronically transmitting messages and information. Advancing communication technology is found in all aspects of health care. This chapter also covers some of the technologies found in the medical office, such as computers and facsimile machines.

TELEPHONES

Despite the increasing use of advanced technology, the telephone remains the number one technologic method for patients and health care providers to communicate with each other. Although the medical office also relies on the phone for real-time communication with insurance companies, pharmacies, medical supply companies, and hospitals, the primary emphasis of this chapter is telephone communication between the medical office and the patient. The use of specific skills and guidelines helps ensure that telephone communication is effective.

TELEPHONE VOICE QUALITIES

- Enunciation—speak clearly
- Pronunciation—say words correctly
- Volume—use normal voice level
- Speed—use normal rate of conversation
- Inflection—change voice pitch to avoid a monotonous tone that implies boredom
- Facial expression—put a "smile" in your voice by having a pleasant look on your face while speaking even though the caller cannot see you
- Courtesy—speak politely, without irritation or impatience
- Attention—focus on the caller and listen

MEDICAL OFFICE CALLS

- Attempt to answer by the third ring
- Use standard office greeting

- Greet caller (e.g., "Good morning").
- Provide name of facility.
- State your name.
- Inquire "How may I help you?"

■ Use standard closing
- Thank the patient for calling.
- Allow caller to hang up first.

■ Direct multiple incoming calls
- Obtain permission of the first caller to be placed on hold. Explain that you have another incoming call. Allow time for the patient to respond before placing him or her on hold.
- Ask the second caller to wait; allow time for response before placing him or her on hold.
- Attempt to respond to callers within 30 seconds.
- Provide options if the hold will be longer.
- Thank the caller for waiting.

■ Screen calls
- Know who and where to refer patients for appropriate assistance.
- Manage physician's time by referring necessary calls only and taking messages for other calls.

■ Route calls
- Tell caller to whom you are forwarding the call.
- Provide the forwarding phone number to which you are transferring the call in case of disconnection.
- Inform the patient that if the party does not respond, the patient may leave a voice mail message (if available). Suggest the patient include a time when he or she is available for a return call.

■ Know the office policy regarding calls that should be directed to the physician
- Forward calls from other physicians, hospital staff, and patients to whom the physician indicated he or she would like to speak directly (e.g., close colleagues).
- Provide the patient's medical record (chart or file) for the physician when transferring a call or leaving a message if he or she does not have access to the EMR.
- Assure a patient who insists on speaking only to the physician, when the physician is unavailable, that the physician will return the call; if possible, provide a time range during which the call will be returned.
- Inform callers who will not identify themselves that you need their name and number to have the physician return the call.

■ Record message
- Use carbonized message pad, e-mail, or other methods that allow the message to be forwarded but saved.
- Maintain a copy of the message in the patient's medical record if that is office policy.
- Record the caller's name (confirm spelling), date, time, reason for call, phone number of caller, and convenient time to return call.
- Inform the caller who will return the call and give an approximate time the call will be returned.
- Initial and forward the message to the appropriate person with the patient's medical record, if needed.

■ Deal with emergencies
- Notify the physician immediately.
- Activate the emergency medical system (EMS/911); if telephone system allows, keep the caller on one line while you notify 911.
- Instruct caller to hang up and activate EMS himself or herself, if the office phone system does not have at least two lines.
- Provide EMS or emergency facility with information, including advance directives and other important details.
- Follow up with the emergency facility.

■ Manage difficult callers
- Keep your voice at a normal level and remain calm with angry callers.
- Determine the problem and notify appropriate staff to help the patient.
- Follow up to ensure the problem was addressed.
- Ensure that the physician or the administrator is aware of irate callers or callers with unresolved problems.
- Attempt to obtain identity of threatening callers and notify the physician or the administrator immediately.

MEDICAL ASSISTING AND MEDICAL ADMINISTRATIVE SPECIALIST CALLS

All health care providers *must* stay within the scope of practice for their role. The same principles apply to the phone to other communication technologies. Remember, only the physician or mid-level provider diagnoses, provides medical advice, or says anything that may be construed as such. The following are telephone calls that a non-physician may handle if he or she is the designated person in that office:

- Appointments (scheduling, rescheduling, canceling, reminding, recalling)
- Patient financial statements, insurance, fees, and service questions
- Prescription refills verified by the physician
- Diagnostic testing and other procedural preparations as written
- Satisfactory test results if reviewed and approved by physician following Health Insurance Portability and Accountability Act (HIPAA) guidelines
- Routine and satisfactory progress reports from patient if office policy allows
- Reinforcement of patient educational plan
- General information regarding office policies, locations, or appointment preparation
- Schedule procedures at other facilities
- Record diagnostic and other procedural results telephoned from health care facilities (within the continuity of care or with patient consent)
- Activate answering service
- Retrieve messages from answering service or voice mail

Telephone Confidentiality

The HIPAA confidentiality standards, expected in all health care activities, also apply to the telephone.

- Give information only to authorized persons. (*Note:* Spouses, friends, parents of adults, or adult children of patients are not generally authorized unless specifically approved by the patient in writing.)
- Verify that you are giving information to an authorized person (e.g., the patient's insurance carrier).
- Ensure telephone conversations are not overheard or that messages are not seen by unauthorized persons.
- Avoid discussing telephone conversations except in carrying out medical assisting duties with authorized persons.
- Avoid leaving information on the patient's voice mail; only state the name of the office and the phone number. Ask the patient to return the call, and leave the name of the party he or she should request.

OTHER TECHNOLOGIC DEVICES

In addition to the telephone, you may use or come in contact with other technologic devices. It is your responsibility to keep up with advances. At this book's press time, the national exams contained basic questions on the components of the computer and issues related to facsimiles (faxes). The exams will continue to incorporate new technologies.

COMPUTERS

The **computer** is an electronic device programmed to take in, store, retrieve, and process data (Fig. 9-1).

- Hardware—the central processing unit, motherboard, hard drive, disk drive, keyboard, and monitor of the computer
  - Motherboard—the fiberglass plank of the computer that contains the central processing unit, memory, and other circuitry
    - Central processing unit (CPU)—circuit on a microchip that processes data; microprocessor
    - Random access memory (RAM)—main memory bank of a computer located on the motherboard; the more RAM the computer has, the more data and the faster the data manipulation; memory is measured in bytes (e.g., megabytes—one million bytes; gigabytes—one billion bytes)
  - Hard drive—a box containing the computer's programs and data files
  - Keyboard—a set of typewriter-like keys that plugs into the computer and allows input of data

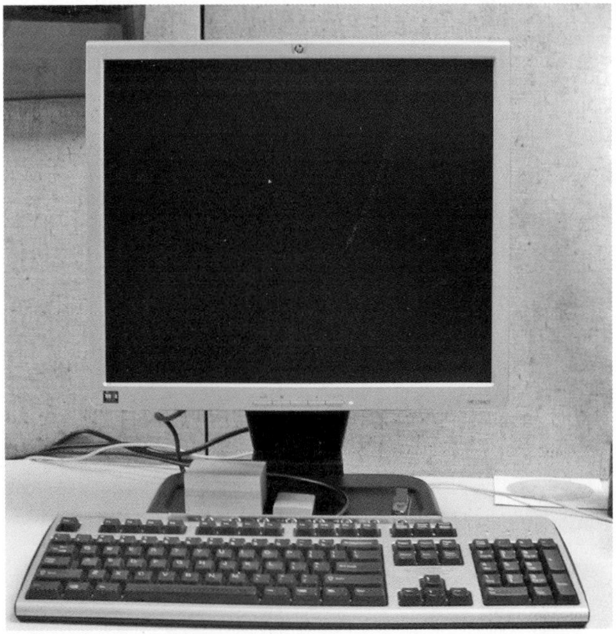

Figure 9-1 Basic components of a computer.

- Monitor—visual display terminal that allows data to be seen on a television-like screen
- Disk drive—a device that allows information to be accessed from a floppy disk or compact disc

■ Accessories
- Mouse—a device that plugs into the computer and allows the user to control the cursor (pointer) as viewed on the monitor
- Modem—a device connecting the computer to a telephone line and allowing data to be transmitted over telephone wires

■ Software—computer programs that tell the computer what to do

■ Floppy disks—diskettes; magnetic discs that can be inserted in the disk drive; they allow for storage of data outside the computer and for transmission of data into and out of the computer

■ Compact disc (CD)—a disc that can be inserted into a CD-ROM (compact disc read-only memory) drive and read by a laser beam, allowing storage of data, including audio and visual programs, outside the computer and transmission of the data into and out of the computer (Fig. 9-2)

■ ZIP drive—a drive that allows several megabytes of data to be saved to a special disc; can be internal or external to the computer

■ Digital video disc (DVD)—a high-density optical disc the contents of which can be displayed on a computer or television screen

■ USB (universal serial bus) drive—small, lightweight, removable data storage device; also called *USB stick*, *USB key*, *memory stick*, flash drive, or *thumbdrive* (Fig. 9-2)

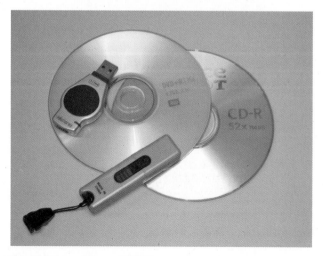

Figure 9-2 Compact discs and USB drives

Common File Formats

A file format is a mechanism used by the computer to save and retrieve specific computer information, such as text or photographs.

■ DOC—document files (DOCX is a more current version, but the general recommendation is to save files in DOC for ease of opening from all senders)

■ GIF—Graphics Interchange Format

■ JPEG—Joint Photographic Experts Group

■ RTF—rich text file

■ PDF—portable data format

Common Computer Networks

A computer network is the ability of two or more computers to communicate.

■ LAN (local area network)—a router is used to connect computers, generally of a single organization and all its sites

■ WAN (wide area network)—using telephone systems, coaxial cables, or satellites, connects the computers of a geographic area; the Internet, which contains the World Wide Web (www), is the largest example of a WAN

Other Common Computer Terms

■ **Blog**—a type of website, generally maintained by an individual who posts regular commentary or other material such as graphics or video

■ **Electronic social network**—a group of people interconnected by the web for the purpose of interacting on a specific topic or multiple topics of common interest such as Facebook and Twitter

■ **HTML** (HyperText Markup Language)—the language used to transfer documents on the Internet

■ **HTTP** (HyperText Transfer Protocol)—how messages are formatted and sent over the Internet

■ **Browser**—software that locates and displays web pages on the computer; an example is Internet Explorer

■ **Search engine**—an extensive program allowing searches for information and websites by using key words; examples are Yahoo and Google

■ **Spreadsheet**—values arranged in columns and rows that may be electronically manipulated using formulas or other processes

■ **URL** (Uniform Resource Locator)—identifies the global address and domain to access web pages

■ **Website**—a collection of screens with text, images, videos, or other digital information with a common domain

- **Word processing**—one of the most common computer applications used to create, edit, and produce text documents

Common Computer Uses in the Medical Office

The uses of computers in the medical office continue to grow. The following are the more common applications.

- Appointment and procedure scheduling
- Patient statements
- Day sheets
- Financial ledgers
- Requisitions
- Payroll and other personnel functions
- Reports
- Correspondence
- Online patient registration
- Electronic medical records
- Insurance billing and claims
- Research using the Internet
- Digital imaging
- Patient educational materials
- Patient reminder and recall notifications
- Staff training
- Inventories
- Electronically operated patient tests and procedures
- Website information regarding the practice

Computers and Confidentiality

The health care standards for confidentiality and release of patient information also apply to computers (Fig. 9-3). Computer-specific requirements and guidelines have come about through standard practice or HIPAA. One of the significant components of HIPAA is the filing of Medicare claims through a secure electronic database exchange. To ensure compliance:

- Require authorized persons to use an exclusive "electronic signature" or password to view patient records
- Change passwords frequently
- Ensure computer screens are not in view of unauthorized persons
- Turn off computers when not in use
- Install privacy filters on monitors to prevent passersby from seeing the screen
- Protect computers from illegal access with appropriate security devices such as firewalls

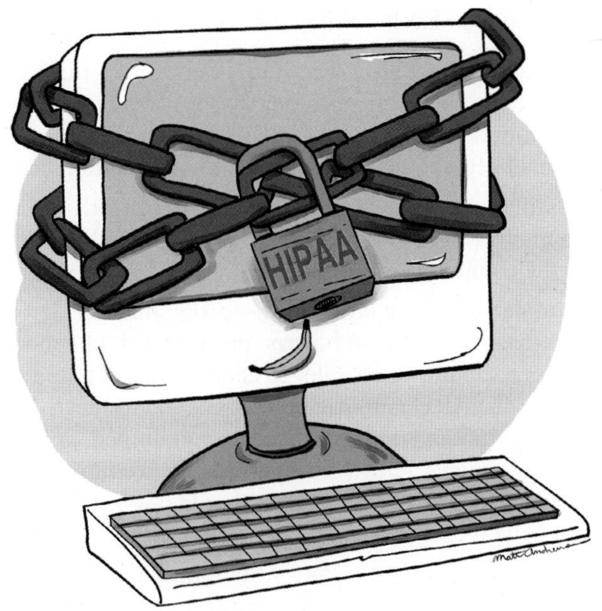

Figure 9-3 HIPAA standards also apply to computers.

- Shred confidential copied materials when no longer in use

MEDICAL TRANSCRIPTION AND EQUIPMENT

Transcription is basically a written copy of dictated or recorded information. Although generally done by a person specifically trained in this field, medical transcription may be the duty of the medical assistant or the medical administrative specialist. Common information transcribed for the medical office is:

- Patient history and physicals
- Admission and discharge notes
- Surgery and other procedural reports
- Consultations
- Correspondence

The equipment used includes:

- Transcription machine with earpieces and foot pedals
- CDs or audiocassettes
- Computer and monitor
- Keyboard
- Specific software (e.g., medical terminology spell check, pharmacology reference)

The important standard for medical transcription is if a word or phrase is not clear, NEVER guess. Always go back to the person who dictated the information for clarification. Correct spelling is absolutely necessary.

Other Common Electronic Devices

- Facsimile machine (fax)—an electronic machine that sends copies of documents over telephone wires (fax confidential information only to secured areas; fax cover sheets should include a confidentiality statement)
- Scanner—software-required device that reads documents (text, graphics, photos) and transfers the image to the computer
- Automated routing unit (ARU)—programmable device that answers calls and plays prerecorded telephone messages to prompt a caller to choose options based on needs; the ARU automatically directs the caller to the chosen option; some ARUs are programmed to telephone patients and leave appointment reminders or other messages (these messages should not be left without patient consent)
- Electronic mail (e-mail)—a system of communicating electronic messages, images, and sounds via the computer through a modem and the Internet (e-mails should not be sent to patients without their consent)
- Cellular telephones (cell phones)—portable, wireless telephones; their use should be restricted in health care facilities because they may interfere with electrical medical devices or the noise may impede patient care; medical assistants should not use personal cell phones during working hours
- Personal digital assistant (PDA)—a palm-sized, handheld, wireless computer that may be synchronized with other computers; an example is a Palm Pilot
- Pagers—battery-operated devices that alert a person to a message left through a telephone or wireless source; pagers may also display other information, such as news bulletins
- Digital camera—a camera that uses a memory card instead of film, allowing pictures to be viewed, altered, or printed through a computer

TERMS

Administrative Techniques Review

The following list reviews the terms discussed in this chapter and other important terms that you may see on the exam.

automated routing unit (ARU) programmable device that answers calls and plays prerecorded telephone messages to prompt a caller to choose options based on needs; the ARU automatically directs the caller to the chosen option; some ARUs are programmed to telephone patients and leave appointment reminders or other messages

blog a type of website, generally maintained by an individual who posts regular commentary or other material such as graphics or video

browser software that locates and displays web pages on the computer; an example is Internet Explorer

cellular telephones (cell phones) portable wireless telephones

central processing unit (CPU) a circuit on a microchip that processes data; a microprocessor

compact disc (CD) a disc that can be inserted into a CD-ROM drive and read by a laser beam, allowing storage of data, including audio and visual programs, outside the computer, and transmission of data into and out of the computer

compact disc read-only memory (CD-ROM) a computer drive that reads CDs using a laser beam

computer an electronic device that is programmed to take in, store, retrieve, and process data

diction the style of speaking and enunciating words

digital camera a camera that uses a memory card instead of film, allowing pictures to be viewed, altered, or printed through a computer

digital video disc (DVD) a high-density optical disc, the contents of which can be displayed on a computer or television screen

disk drive a device allowing information to be accessed from a floppy disk

electronic mail (e-mail) a system of communicating electronic messages, images, and sounds via the computer through the Internet

electronic social network a group of people interconnected by the web for the purpose of interacting on a specific topic or multiple topics of common interest

enunciation speaking clearly

facsimile machine (fax) an electronic machine that can send copies of documents over telephone wires

floppy disks diskettes; magnetic discs that can be inserted in the disk drive; they allow storage of data outside the computer and transmission of data into and from the computer

hard drive a box containing the computer's programs and data files

hardware the central processing unit, motherboard, hard drive, disk drive, keyboard, monitor, and mouse of the computer

HTML (HyperText Markup Language) the language used to transfer documents on the Internet

HTTP (HyperText Transfer Protocol) how messages are formatted and sent over the Internet

inflection changing voice pitch to avoid a monotonous tone implying boredom

keyboard a set of typewriter-like keys that plugs into a computer and allows input of data

LAN (local area network) uses a router to connect computers, generally of a single organization and all its sites

modem a device connecting the computer to a telephone line and allowing data to be transmitted

monitor visual display terminal (VDT) that allows data to be seen on a television-like screen

motherboard the fiberglass plank of the computer that contains the central processing unit, memory, and other circuitry

mouse a device that plugs into the computer and allows the user to control the cursor viewed on the monitor

pagers battery-operated devices that alert a person to a message left through a telephone or wireless source; pagers may also display other information, such as news bulletins

personal digital assistant (PDA) a palm-sized, hand-held wireless computer that may be synchronized with other computers; an example is a Palm Pilot

photocopy a duplicate copy of a written document

pronunciation saying words correctly

random access memory (RAM) main memory bank of a computer located on the motherboard: the more RAM, the more data and the faster the manipulation; memory is measured in bytes

scanner software-required device that reads documents (text, graphics, photos) and transfers the image to the computer

scanning a process of transferring a written document or image into an electronic version using computer hardware called a scanner

search engine an extensive program allowing searches for information and websites by using key words; examples are Yahoo and Google

software computer programs that tell the computer what to do related to that topic (e.g., word processing)

spreadsheet values arranged in columns and rows that may be electronically manipulated using formulas or other processes

transcription a written copy of dictated or recorded information

URL (Uniform Resource Locator) identifies the global address and domain to access web pages

USB (universal serial bus) drive small, lightweight, removable data storage device; also called USB stick, USB key, memory stick, flash drive, or thumbdrive

WAN (wide area network) using telephone systems, coaxial cables, or satellites, connects the computers of a geographic area; the largest example of a WAN is the Internet

website a collection of screens with text, images, videos, or other digital information with a common domain

word processing one of the most common computer applications used to create, edit, and produce text documents

ZIP drive a drive that allows several megabytes of data to be saved to a special disc; can be internal or external to the computer

REVIEW QUESTIONS

All questions are relevant for the CMA (AAMA), RMA (AMT), and CMAS (AMT) exams.

1. When assigned to answering the telephone in a physician's office:
   A. some callers are angry and it is acceptable to hang up.
   B. you should be able to determine which calls are routine, non-emergent, or emergent situations.
   C. it is routine to give family members who call normal results of laboratory findings.
   D. when many phone calls are coming into the office at one time, it is appropriate to immediately put all calls on hold and then return to each one in the order received.

Answer: **B**

Why: Hanging up on an angry patient will likely exacerbate the problem. You should try to address the caller's concern or find someone who can. All calls coming into a physician's office should be answered promptly and first determined whether they are an emergency. Only after it is known that the call is not an emergency should you place the caller on hold. HIPAA and standards prohibit giving out medical information over the telephone unless under the direction of the physician and only to authorized individuals.

Review: Yes ❑ No ❑

---

2. The style of speaking and enunciating words is referred to as:
   A. diction.
   B. pronunciation.
   C. expression.
   D. conversation.
   E. inflection.

Answer: **A**

Why: Diction is the act of articulating words distinctly as you speak so that you are clearly understood. Pronunciation is the manner of pronouncing or speaking words using phonics (speech sounds that make up a language). Expression is the use of feeling or character when speaking to help convey the spoken word. Conversation is an exchange of words, ideas, or thoughts. Inflection means to change voice pitch to avoid a monotonous tone.

Review: Yes ❑ No ❑

---

3. When answering phones during a busy time of day, it is only appropriate to place a caller on hold after you ask the following:
   A. May I have your phone number so I can call you back?
   B. Will you please hold?
   C. Are you a regular patient at this office?
   D. We are busy now; will you call back later?

Answer: **B**

Why: It is appropriate to place a caller on hold only after you have asked the caller's permission to be placed on hold. If it is an emergency, the caller will usually state that he or she cannot hold and needs immediate attention.

Review: Yes ❑ No ❑

---

4. Which of the following is a phone call that ordinarily does not require the party to speak directly to the physician?
   A. A pharmacist calls to verify information written on a prescription form.
   B. A patient calls complaining of shortness of breath, sweating, and heart pounding after taking new medication.
   C. A referring physician calls to relate information of an abnormal electrocardiogram on a patient.
   D. A nurse from the local hospital emergency room calls for orders on a patient just admitted.
   E. One of the physician's family members calls to talk with the physician about an emergency.

Answer: **A**

Why: You would refer to the prescription information written by the physician in the patient's medical record and communicate the information to the pharmacist. All the other responses would require intervention by the physician.

Review: Yes ❑ No ❑

5. The transmission of a hard copy of a written document through a phone line is called a(n):
   A. electronic mail.
   B. facsimile.
   C. photocopy.
   D. scan.

Answer: **B**

Why: The facsimile (usually shortened to *fax*) is an electronic machine that sends written images over telephone wires. Electronic mail is used in conjunction with the Internet via the computer. A photocopy is a duplicate copy of a written document. Scanning is a process of transferring a written document or image into an electronic version using computer hardware called a scanner.

Review: Yes ❑ No ❑

---

6. The primary purpose of screening telephone calls is to:
   A. manage the physician's time by referring only necessary calls.
   B. place patients on hold as soon as they contact the office.
   C. decrease the number of telemarketing calls to the office.
   D. intercept personal calls.
   E. increase the physician's patient load.

Answer: **A**

Why: You will screen phone calls to determine which calls must be forwarded to the physician and which can be handled by you.

Review: Yes ❑ No ❑

---

7. The physician has asked you to contact a patient to schedule a return office visit to discuss laboratory results. The patient is not available when you call. It is appropriate to:
   A. leave a message with the person answering the phone indicating that the patient should contact the office for laboratory results.
   B. contact the patient's workplace to leave a message for the patient to contact the physician's office to go over some blood test results.
   C. try to reach the patient later but also send a letter with the information.
   D. call the person who is listed as the emergency contact on the patient's information sheet.

Answer: **C**

Why: If a patient cannot be reached by phone, it is not appropriate to leave a message regarding test results with anyone other than the patient. Because this is not an emergency situation, a letter can be sent to the patient—but you should also try to reach the patient by telephone later.

Review: Yes ❑ No ❑

---

8. When assigned to work in the reception area of the office, you should attempt to answer all incoming telephone calls:
   A. after assisting all other calls on hold.
   B. by the third ring.
   C. by the fourth ring.
   D. by the fifth ring.
   E. in between rooming patients.

Answer: **B**

Why: It is usually impossible to answer all phone calls on the first or even second ring. All efforts should be made to answer calls by the third ring.

Review: Yes ❑ No ❑

---

9. Which of the following is an appropriate standard opening for an incoming call to the physician's office?
   A. Will you please hold?
   B. Who's calling please?
   C. Good morning, Dr. Smith's office.
   D. 555-2456, may I help you?

Answer: **C**

Why: The first thing a caller should hear is a pleasant greeting and the name of the facility.

Review: Yes ❑ No ❑

10. When transferring a patient call to the physician, you should:
    A. interrupt the physician in an exam room to forward the information about the caller.
    B. not forward the call, but ask the caller to call back later when the physician is finished with all patients for the day.
    C. inform the patient that the physician will be upset if interrupted.
    D. inform the patient that there will be an office visit charge for the call.
    E. have the patient's medical record available for the physician.

Answer: **E**

Why: The physician will want to have the patient's medical record available in the event questions arise during the conversation that require information from the medical record. It is inappropriate to tell the patient the physician will be upset with the call, and you should not interrupt a physician while in an exam room unless the call is an emergency. Offices typically do not charge patients for phone calls.

Review: Yes ❑ No ❑

---

11. After a caller has been placed on hold, you should make every attempt to respond to the caller within:
    A. 10 seconds.
    B. 30 seconds.
    C. 1 minute.
    D. 5 minutes.

Answer: **B**

Why: If a caller needs to be placed on hold, it is recommended that you check back with the caller at least every 30 seconds. Even if you are still busy with another patient, at least the caller will be encouraged to continue holding.

Review: Yes ❑ No ❑

---

12. When dealing with a difficult caller, you should:
    A. forward the call to the physician.
    B. forward the call to the office manager.
    C. tell the caller you will hang up if he or she continues to be difficult.
    D. determine the problem and the appropriate staff member who can help the caller.
    E. put the caller on hold until he or she hangs up.

Answer: **D**

Why: When a caller is difficult to deal with, it will further exacerbate the situation if you also become angry or difficult. Keep your voice at a normal level and remain calm while you try to determine what the problem is and who can best help the caller.

Review: Yes ❑ No ❑

---

13. When a patient calls with a list of symptoms, including fever, chills, and body aches, that have lasted for the past several days, you should:
    A. offer the patient an appointment to see the physician.
    B. tell the patient to stay home in bed and to take aspirin and fluids.
    C. inform the patient that there is a lot of flu going around.
    D. tell the patient that the physician does not see patients unless they have been ill for at least a week and that it is probably a flulike illness that will pass.

Answer: **A**

Why: A patient with those symptoms may actually have the flu, but it is not within your scope of practice or responsibility to diagnose. The patient should be offered an appointment to see the physician to make an appropriate diagnosis.

Review: Yes ❑ No ❑

14. When placing calls to patients to confirm appointments, the calls should be made:
A. the morning of the day of the appointments.
B. only to patients who were not given appointment cards.
C. one week before the appointment.
D. only to those patients who you know missed their last appointment.
E. in an area where you cannot be overheard by other patients.

Answer: **E**

Why: All patients should be contacted the day before their appointment, and the calls should be made from a place where other patients cannot overhear the call. Even if patients are given appointment cards, a reminder call is usually made.

Review: Yes ❑ No ❑

---

15. An electronic device that takes in, stores, retrieves, and processes data is a:
A. disk drive.
B. monitor.
C. computer.
D. floppy disk.

Answer: **C**

Why: A disk drive is a device located on the computer that allows information to be accessed from a floppy disk or CD-ROM. A monitor is used to visually display the data, and the compact disk is a device used to store data outside the computer. The computer is the entire electronic device that takes in, stores, retrieves, and processes the data.

Review: Yes ❑ No ❑

---

16. A computer program that tells the computer what to do is the:
A. disk drive.
B. modem.
C. software.
D. mouse.
E. keyboard.

Answer: **C**

Why: The disk drive is located on the computer and allows information to be accessed from a DVD or CD-ROM. A modem connects a computer to a telephone line and transmits data via that line. The mouse is the device that plugs into the computer and controls the cursor as viewed on the monitor. A keyboard is a set of typewriter-type keys that allows for input of data.

Review: Yes ❑ No ❑

---

17. The federal government enacted a standard practice for confidentiality and release of patient information as it applies to computers. This information is found in the federal register under the abbreviation:
A. HCFA.
B. HIPAA.
C. HHS.
D. HRSA.

Answer: **B**

Why: HIPAA stands for Health Insurance Portability and Accountability Act, which is the name of the federal guidelines for confidentiality and release of patient information in all forms, including electronically. HCFA is the Health Care Financing Administration; HHS is the Department of Health and Human Services. HRSA is the Health Resources and Services Administration.

Review: Yes ❑ No ❑

---

18. When you are focusing on the conversation of the telephone call and ignoring outside distractions, you are:
A. expressing yourself.
B. actively listening.
C. practicing diction.
D. demonstrating time management.
E. maintaining confidentiality.

Answer: **B**

Why: To actively listen to a conversation, you must not interrupt the speaker and you must ignore what is going on around you so that you can concentrate on the conversation.

Review: Yes ❑ No ❑

19. When routing a caller to another person, you should:
   A. forward the call immediately, not wasting time to talk to the caller.
   B. tell the caller you do not forward calls and ask the caller to call back when the person is available.
   C. place the caller on hold for up to 5 minutes while you locate the person to whom you need to transfer the caller.
   D. provide the phone number or extension to which you are transferring the caller, in case the call is disconnected.

Answer: **D**

Why: Before forwarding a call, you should inform the caller that you are going to forward the call and provide the phone number or extension in case the call is disconnected. If the person you need to forward the call to is unavailable, you can give the caller the option of calling back or leaving a message, but you would not tell the caller that you do not forward calls. You should not place a caller on hold for more than 30 seconds without checking in to see whether he or she is still willing to hold.

Review: Yes ❑ No ❑

---

20. To comply with the HIPAA requirements when using a computer, you should remember to do the following EXCEPT:
   A. change passwords frequently.
   B. protect computers from illegal access with appropriate security devices.
   C. ensure computer screens are not in view of unauthorized persons.
   D. keep the computer on at all times to save time turning it on.
   E. turn off the computer when not in use.

Answer: **D**

Why: When not in use, the computer should be turned off. This will help maintain security of the computer and prevent illegal use or its being viewed by unauthorized persons.

Review: Yes ❑ No ❑

---

21. Which of the following is a necessary quality for a good telephone voice?
   A. Maintaining a monotonous tone
   B. Using a rapid rate of conversation
   C. Focusing on surrounding activity in the office while on the phone with a caller
   D. Speaking clearly and saying words correctly

Answer: **D**

Why: Proper telephone voice qualities include changing the pitch to avoid a monotone voice. Use a normal rate of conversation and actively listen to the caller without allowing the activity around you to interfere with your ability to concentrate on the conversation.

Review: Yes ❑ No ❑

---

22. When an unidentified caller insists on speaking with the physician, the medical assistant should:
   A. hang up.
   B. tell the caller that the physician is with a patient and you need a name and a number so the call can be returned.
   C. put the caller on hold until he or she hangs up.
   D. transfer the call immediately to the physician.
   E. transfer the call to a coworker.

Answer: **B**

Why: Explain that the physician is not available to take the call but that you will forward the name and number so that the physician can return the call later. Most people will be willing to give their name and number if they know the physician will call them back.

Review: Yes ❑ No ❑

23. The proper way to deal with an emergency call is to:
   A. ask the caller to hold while you call the local emergency room for instructions.
   B. ask the caller to come to the office immediately.
   C. keep the caller on the line while contacting the emergency medical system on another line if the office has multiple phone lines.
   D. give the caller the number of the physician who is on call when his or her physician is not available.

Answer: **C**

Why: You would not want to waste time having the patient come to the office or contact the physician on call. In a true emergency, the patient should be instructed to activate 911/EMS (emergency medical system), or the physician's office should contact EMS for the patient, if possible.

Review: Yes ❑ No ❑

---

24. Telephone calls that the medical assistant or medical administrative specialist may handle include the following EXCEPT:
   A. refilling prescriptions verified by the physician.
   B. providing a patient with laboratory test results just received from a lab.
   C. scheduling procedures at other medical facilities.
   D. answering patient financial statement questions.
   E. confirming the time of an appointment for a patient.

Answer: **B**

Why: If the laboratory results were just received from the lab and have not been reviewed and approved for release by the physician, the medical assistant must not release the test results.

Review: Yes ❑ No ❑

---

25. To maintain telephone confidentiality, the medical assistant or medical administrative specialist must:
   A. give information only to authorized persons.
   B. discuss telephone conversations anywhere in the office.
   C. give information to the patient's employer if he or she contacts the office to inquire about the patient's absence from work.
   D. give information to family members with or without authorization because of their relationship to the patient.

Answer: **A**

Why: The medical assistant or medical administrative specialist should only give patient information to those who are authorized to receive the information. This does not include the patient's employer or relatives unless the patient has given permission to release the information. Always discuss information in the office in an area where patients or unauthorized persons cannot hear the conversation.

Review: Yes ❑ No ❑

---

26. Which of the following is not a device used to save computer data?
   A. HTTP
   B. USB drive
   C. DVD
   D. ZIP
   E. CD-ROM

Answer: **A**

Why: HTTP (HyperText Transfer Protocol) is how messages are formatted and sent over the Internet. All of the other devices listed are devices used to save data.

Review: Yes ❑ No ❑

27. Yahoo is an example of an Internet:
    A. browser.
    B. search engine.
    C. LAN.
    D. CPU.

Answer: **B**

Why: A search engine is an extensive program allowing searches for information and websites by using key words. Yahoo is an example of an Internet search engine. A browser is software that locates and displays web pages on the computer. LAN means local area network; CPU is a central processing unit; and a scanner is a device that reads documents (text, graphics, photos) and transfers the image to the computer.

Review: Yes ❑ No ❑

---

28. A patient history processed on the computer would most likely be saved in what type of file?
    A. RTF
    B. JPEG
    C. GIF
    D. DOC
    E. spreadsheet

Answer: **D**

Why: Word documents such as patient histories are most frequently saved in document files (DOC). Graphic images are saved in GIF format; photographic images are commonly saved in JPEG files. RTF, rich text file, can be used to save written documents; however, it is not commonly used.

Review: Yes ❑ No ❑

Note: This question is an example in which two answers are correct but one answer is a "better" choice or is more common. Your clue is the phrase "most likely." The exams will contain questions of this nature.

---

29. Equipment needed for medical transcription is a:
    A. copy machine.
    B. facsimile machine.
    C. telephone.
    D. computer.
    E. mouse.

Answer: **D**

Why: Transcription is a written copy of dictated or recorded information. A copy machine, facsimile machine, or telephone cannot transform oral information into a written format. The computer is the only instrument listed that can do this. This process can take place without the use of a mouse, although a mouse may be used minimally. The computer is the BEST answer.

Review: Yes ❑ No ❑

---

30. The correct spelling of heavy, uncontrolled bleeding is:
    A. hemmorrhage.
    B. hemorrhage.
    C. hemmorage.
    D. hemorhage.

Answer: **B**

Why: A medical terminology spell check in use while performing medical transcription would indicate that choice B (hemorrhage) is the correct spelling.

Review: Yes ❑ No ❑

10

Appointment Scheduling

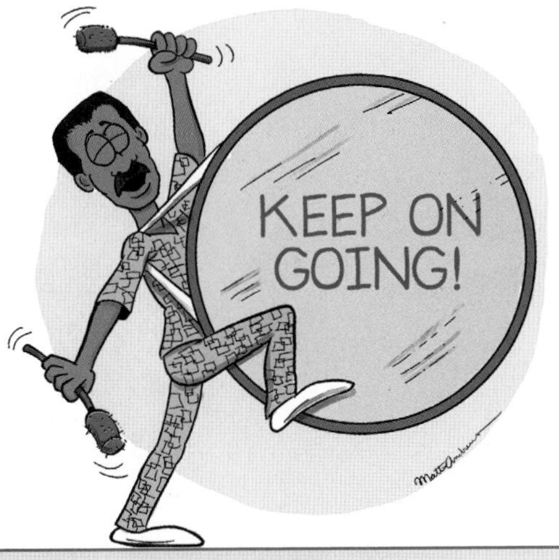

REVIEW TIP

Keep energized! This review process, even if it seems grueling, is a relatively short period of time with an end in sight. Go outside and enjoy a walk or run or just sit on a park bench and clear your head. Call someone you can count on to be cheerful. Read some jokes or inspirational pieces. To regain your focus and energy, do something that usually makes you feel good.

The goal of appointment scheduling is to maintain a smooth office flow while accommodating the needs of the medical practice and the patient. The type of scheduling used depends on the following:

- Nature of practice
- Patient population needs
- Doctor's preferences and habits
- Available facilities and staff

TYPES OF SCHEDULING

The exam questions will require you to identify the different types of scheduling. These types include:

- Open hours (tidal wave, open booking)—no appointments needed; first-come, first-served
  - Used primarily in urgent care centers
  - Eliminates broken appointments
  - Limits medical records and procedures preparation
  - Prohibits control of number of patients arriving at one time
  - Needs triage system
- Clustering (group procedures, categorizing)—similar procedures scheduled on predetermined days or in predetermined time blocks, such as new patient exams, sports physicals, and immunizations; they are designated when the appointment book matrix is developed
  - Increases efficiency and speed for procedures
  - Theoretically, allows better utilization of equipment and staff

Box 10-1

Comparison of Double Booking, Wave, Modified Wave, and Time-Specific Schedules

Double Booking

9:00	Susan F. Garcia 602-1234 Ref John S. Habib 602-2345 S/R
9:15	Tony McCall 456-3456 CPE Jane P. Morgan 564-4567 CPE
9:30	Taylor Roberts 324-6789 Inj Michael Sanchez 324-7890 NP
9:45	Joseph Armat 567-1234 Ref Selena Green 765-7890 F/U

Wave

9:00	Susan F. Garcia 602-1234 Ref John S. Habib 602-2345 S/R
	Tony McCall 456-3456 CPE Jane P. Morgan 564-4567 CPE
10:00	Taylor Roberts 324-6789 Inj Michael Sanchez 324-7890 NP
	Joseph Armat 567-1234 Ref Selena Green 765-7890 F/U

Modified Wave

9:00	Susan F. Garcia 602-1234 Ref
9:15	John S. Habib 602-2345 S/R
9:30	Tony McCall 456-3456 CPE
9:45	Jane P. Morgan 564-4567 CPE
10:00	Taylor Roberts 324-6789 Inj
10:15	Michael Sanchez 324-7890 NP
10:30	Selena Green 765-7890 F/U

Time-Specific

9:00	Susan F. Garcia 602-1234 Ref.
9:15	John S. Habib 602-2345 S/R
9:30	Tony McCall 456-3456 CPE
9:45	⇓
10:00	Jane P. Morgan 564-4567 CPE
10:15	⇓
10:30	Taylor Roberts 324-6789 Inj

- Select scheduling (Box 10-1)
  - Double booking—two or more patients scheduled at the same time
    - Used by practices with short visits or a high no-show rate
    - Increases patient waiting time
    - Reduces physician downtime
  - Wave—a specific number of patients, usually four, scheduled at the beginning of the same hour
    - Reduces physician downtime
    - Allows specific procedures, such as a routine ECG, to be performed prior to the physician seeing the patient
    - Intended to start and finish each hour on time
    - Increases waiting for patients seen later in the hour
    - Creates issues of who is seen first if more than one person arrives at the same time
  - Modified wave—hour-long blocks broken down to smaller time increments (usually 10 or 15 minutes each) and individual patients scheduled within those increments
    - Intended to start and finish each hour on time
    - Decreases patient waiting time compared with wave scheduling
    - Avoids issues of who should be seen first
  - Time-specific (streaming)—patient given an appointment based on length of time needed and on available time; this is the most common scheduling method
- Other scheduling considerations
  - Physician or office delay—keep patients informed of waiting time; offer opportunity to reschedule or wait
  - Time allotment for visits and procedures—established criteria indicate the time required for the common procedures and visits in a practice (e.g., a complete physical exam may be 45 minutes, suture removal may be 15 minutes); new patients are usually allotted more time than established patients
  - Emergencies—office criteria for handling urgent medical situations in the office and on the telephone, including involvement of the emergency medical system and poison control centers
  - "Walk-ins"—patients who come to the office without an appointment expecting to be seen; urgency and available appointment time should be considered
  - Referrals—urgency of referrals should be communicated by the referring physician, and appropriate medical records, including diagnostic results, should be sent to the consulting physician
  - Repeat appointments—schedule patients for a series of appointments (e.g., dressing changes, antibiotic administration) at the same time on the same day of

the week, if possible; this reduces the incidence of missed appointments

- Flexible hours—varied hours on certain days; may include evenings and weekends
- Buffer zone—periods during the day with no appointments scheduled to accommodate emergencies and to allow the physician to catch up if running late
- Sales representatives—the norm has become to give sales representatives, such as with pharmaceutical companies, a designated appointment or to have a specific day or time of the day set aside for these visits
- Other visitors—attorneys, and other nonmedical professionals may request to meet with the physician to function as expert witnesses or perform other consulting-type services; appointments are scheduled to accommodate the physician and the practice; these services are generally billed

Table 10-1 Appointment Abbreviations

Abbreviation	Definition
Cons	Consultation
CPE	Complete physical exam
F/U	Follow-up
Inj	Injection
NP	New patient
NS	No-show
Ref	Referral
S/R	Suture removal
US	Ultrasound

EQUIPMENT AND MATERIALS

- Appointment book—specially designed calendar-type book used to schedule appointments
  - Remains open and conforms to desk or counter space size
  - Conforms to Health Insurance Portability and Accountability Act (HIPAA) privacy standards; not able to be seen by unauthorized people
  - Accommodates practice (e.g., it has an adequate number of lines for the number of physicians)
- Daily log—separate from the appointment book; a ledger-type book listing the day's appointments and used for cross-referencing financial entries, data collection on types and number of procedures, and total patients seen
- Worksheet—copy of daily patients by list or medical assistant assignment; used to prepare rooms and equipment; it is shredded at the end of the day in compliance with HIPAA privacy standards
- Computer appointment scheduling—software that replaces the hard-copy appointment book
  - Commercial or custom software can be used (it may also incorporate financial and claims procedures)
  - Legal, HIPAA, and other standard appointment guidelines must be met

PROCEDURE

- Developing the matrix—preparing the appointment book or computer to show what times are available and unavailable for appointments
  - Block off times when appointments are not routinely scheduled, such as lunch or monthly staff meetings
  - Fill in physician's time away from the office, such as for hospital rounds, out-of-office procedures, or meetings
  - If the cluster method of scheduling is used, mark days and times that are reserved for special procedures (e.g., if Mondays are reserved for sports physicals, the top of the day's matrix would be marked "sports physicals" and times would be blocked in the increments designated by the practice for each physical)
- Scheduling
  - Begin with the first appointment available that has the time required for the specific visit
  - Consider patient and practice needs, such as fasting for blood work, preparation for procedures, or who does specific procedure
  - Obtain patient's full name and telephone number
  - Note reason for visit, using standard abbreviations (Table 10-1)

PATIENT PREPARATION

At the time the appointment is made:

- Verify that the office accepts the patient's insurance
- Inform the patient of any copay and other office financial policies
- Instruct the patient to bring his or her insurance card and any necessary insurance forms, medical records, and immunization records
- Request that a new patient allow time before an appointment to complete registration material in the office
- Provide directions to office
- Mail preregistration material if it is office policy to do so

- Obtain prior approval from the insurance company if required
- Explain any necessary preparations for procedures both verbally and in writing
- Confirm date and time of appointment at the end of conversation

PROCEDURES OUTSIDE OF THE PRACTICE

Depending on the type of practice, it may be necessary to schedule hospitalizations and procedures to be performed outside of the medical office. The following are guidelines:

- Inpatient scheduling for an illness or procedure that requires a hospital stay:
  - Ensure insurance requirements, such as prior authorization, are met
  - Check patient's availability for expected length of stay (LOS)
  - Check physician's availability for procedure
  - Know appropriate diagnosis (ICD-9 code) and procedure (CPT code)
  - If surgery or procedure, schedule with appropriate department within the hospital
  - Schedule the admission or reservation with the hospital Admissions Department (separate from scheduling the procedure to assure a bed is available on the appropriate unit afterward)
  - Provide patient preparation information and materials if appropriate
- Outpatient scheduling for a procedure that does not require a hospital stay:
  - Ensure insurance requirements, such as prior authorization, are met
  - Check patient's availability
  - Check physician's availability for procedure
  - Know appropriate diagnosis (ICD-9 code) and procedure (CPT code)
  - Schedule with appropriate facility
  - Provide patient preparation information and materials if appropriate

APPOINTMENT REMINDERS

- Appointment cards—given at the time the appointment is established
- Tickler file—an index system with cards placed in chronologic order, usually by week or month; used as reminders for items that need attention in the future, such as immunizations
- Reminder mailings—cards or computer-generated forms mailed to the patient informing him or her that an appointment is coming up or to remind the patient to call and schedule an appointment if the patient is due for a procedure (e.g., annual well-woman check)
- Telephone calls—made by the office the day before the appointment is scheduled; **leave messages only with prior patient permission** (usually obtained during initial registration)
- E-mail—sent with patient's permission
- Recall notices—cards or computer-generated forms sent to inform the patient that he or she missed a scheduled appointment or that he or she is overdue for a procedure (e.g., immunizations)

PATIENT FLOW ANALYSIS

Patient flow analysis is a periodic study conducted by the medical practice to assess the efficiency of scheduling and staff and, ideally, resolve identified problems. It generally measures the following times:

- Sign in
- Scheduled appointment
- Placement in treatment room
- Physician presentation
- Discharge

The times are then evaluated and compared with established norms and benchmarks. Some insurance companies require or recommend a patient flow analysis at intervals or may conduct one as a follow-up to member complaints or other issues. In addition to participating in the process, the role of the medical assistant and the medical administrative specialist may be to report the findings and make recommendations. Changes should not be initiated without the approval of the physician or practice manager.

LEGAL ISSUES

- Treat the appointment book and daily log as legal documents; they may be subpoenaed
- Maintain HIPAA standards by ensuring confidentiality with appointment information; if the system is computerized, screens should be protected from view, passwords changed frequently, and required firewalls in place if the system is part of a network
- Document no-shows and cancellations that are not rescheduled in the patient's medical record and in the appointment book and log

TERMS

Appointment Scheduling Review

The following list reviews the terms discussed in this chapter and other important terms that you may see on the exam.

buffer zone period in the day with no scheduled appointments, intended to accommodate emergencies and allow the physician to catch up if running late

clustering (group procedures, categorizing) similar procedures are scheduled on predetermined days or in predetermined time blocks

daily scheduling log ledger-type book listing day's appointments; used for cross-referencing financial entries, data collection on types and number of procedures, and total patients seen

double booking scheduling two or more patients at the same time

length of stay (LOS) the time the patient is in or is expected to be in the hospital

modified wave scheduling method that uses hour blocks broken down into smaller time increments; individual patients are scheduled within those increments

open hours (tidal wave, open booking) scheduling method with no appointments needed; first-come, first-served

patient flow analysis a periodic study conducted by the medical practice to assess the efficiency of scheduling and staff and, ideally, resolve identified problems

recall notice cards or computer-generated forms sent to inform the patient that he or she missed a scheduled appointment or that he or she is overdue for a procedure

reminder mailings cards or computer-generated forms mailed to the patient informing him or her that an appointment is coming up or to remind the patient to call and schedule an appointment if the patient is due for a procedure

tickler file an index system with cards placed in chronologic order, usually by week or month; used as reminders for items that need attention in the future, such as immunizations

time-specific (streaming) patient is given an appointment time based both on length of time needed and on available appointments; this is the most common scheduling method

wave scheduling a specific number of patients, usually four, at the beginning of the same hour

worksheet a copy of daily patients by list or by medical assisting assignment, used to prepare rooms and equipment; it must be shredded at the end of the day to ensure compliance with the Health Insurance Portability and Accountability Act (HIPAA)

REVIEW QUESTIONS

All questions are relevant for the CMA (AAMA), RMA (AMT), and CMAS (AMT) exams.

1. When setting up the appointment book by crossing off all times that will not be used for patient visits, this is known as setting up the:
   A. schedule.
   B. calendar.
   C. matrix.
   D. time frame.

Answer: **C**

Why: The matrix is the configuration of the appointment book after all the unavailable times are crossed out. These office times exclude vacations, meetings, lunch hour, and hospital visits.

Review: Yes ❑ No ❑

---

2. Which of the following is a guideline that applies to using the appointment book?
   A. Erase any missed appointments from the book after it has been documented in the patient's chart.
   B. Discard all used appointment books.
   C. Always allow 1 hour per day for emergency appointments.
   D. Write or print clearly and make corrections neatly.
   E. Leave open one morning and one afternoon each week for any emergencies.

Answer: **D**

Why: The appointment book is considered a legal document and could be subject to subpoena. Always write or print clearly and make any corrections neatly. Missed appointments or canceled appointments are not erased from the book. Draw a single line through the entry and note the reason why the appointment was canceled or whether it was rescheduled. Used appointment books are not discarded but retained according to office policy, usually for the same period as patient records are retained. Most offices do not keep time available for emergency appointments; if an emergency arises, the office will try to prioritize the patient into the physician's schedule. In the event of a life-threatening emergency or serious injury, the patient may be referred to the local emergency room.

Review: Yes ❑ No ❑

---

3. Of the following situations, which one constitutes a higher level of urgency and should be considered an emergency appointment?
   A. A patient needing an employment physical so that he or she can start a new job the next morning
   B. An 8-year-old child who sprained an ankle on the school playground that morning
   C. A 55-year-old man with difficulty breathing
   D. A patient who ran out of medication and needs her blood pressure checked so she can refill her medication

Answer: **C**

Why: Of the scenarios listed, none of them appears to be life-threatening *except* for someone who is experiencing difficulty breathing. Although all of these scenarios may seem like emergencies, especially to the patient, the only true emergency would involve a patient who is having difficulty breathing. The other cases can be handled as immediate status.

Review: Yes ❑ No ❑

4. The process of double booking in appointment scheduling means that:
   A. two or more patients are scheduled at the same time.
   B. one patient is scheduled but two appointment times are used.
   C. when two physicians are practicing in the same office, there are two appointment books used.
   D. at least four patients are scheduled for the same time at the beginning of the same hour.
   E. four patients are scheduled every 2 hours.

Answer: **A**

Why: Double booking schedules two patients at the same time and the patients are seen in the order in which they arrive at the office. This is used in practices in which physician visits are short.

Review: Yes ❑ No ❑

---

5. If the physician is delayed in arriving at the office for appointments, you should:
   A. immediately reschedule the patients.
   B. cancel the remaining appointments for the day.
   C. offer the waiting patients an opportunity to reschedule.
   D. offer to refer the patients to another physician's practice.

Answer: **C**

Why: When the physician is delayed, the you should keep patients informed of the approximate waiting time and offer to reschedule appointments.

Review: Yes ❑ No ❑

---

6. When making an appointment over the telephone for a new patient, it is important to secure the following information:
   A. patient's place of employment.
   B. patient's date of birth.
   C. patient's copay amount.
   D. patient's home address.
   E. patient's insurance provider.

Answer: **E**

Why: The patient's date of birth, place of employment, home address, and copay information can be obtained at the time of the appointment. It is important to know the patient's insurance company to ensure that the physician's office participates with the provider; if not, the patient can be informed of the payment procedures.

Review: Yes ❑ No ❑

---

7. When a specific number of patients, usually four, is scheduled at the beginning of the same hour, this is known as:
   A. modified wave scheduling.
   B. wave scheduling.
   C. cluster scheduling.
   D. group scheduling.

Answer: **B**

Why: In wave scheduling, the patients are seen in the order in which they arrive at the office. This reduces physician downtime but may increase waiting time for patients, who have to wait their turn if more than one patient arrives at the same time.

Review: Yes ❑ No ❑

---

8. When setting a series of repeat appointments for a patient, it is best to:
   A. have the patient call back no later than the end of the current week to schedule the return appointment.
   B. offer at least three alternative times for the return appointment.
   C. set the appointments at the same time on the same day of the week to enhance patient compliance.
   D. ask the patient to show up at a convenient time and you will work him or her into the schedule.
   E. vary the appointment times each week.

Answer: **C**

Why: Setting the return appointments at the same time and on the same day of the week will help the patient remember the appointments. It is easier to manage a schedule when there is consistency.

Review: Yes ❑ No ❑

9. The most critical aspect of the appointment book is that:
   A. the physician's personal time out of the office should not be reflected in the appointment book.
   B. when using the wave method of scheduling, always schedule one patient each hour regardless of the nature of the visit.
   C. allow at least 1 hour for lunch each day.
   D. the book is treated as a legal document, because it may be subpoenaed.

Answer: **D**

Why: The appointment book is a legal document and should be treated as any other legal document with regard to entries and corrections. It is important to build a matrix for scheduling that includes any time the physician will not be in the office. Multiple patients are scheduled per hour when using wave scheduling. The lunch break is determined by the practice and may actually be shorter or longer than 1 hour.

Review: Yes ❑ No ❑

---

10. The most common type of scheduling is:
    A. time-specific scheduling.
    B. wave scheduling.
    C. clustering.
    D. modified wave.
    E. tidal wave.

Answer: **A**

Why: Time-specific scheduling is the method of giving each patient an appointment time based on the length of time needed and what open time is available. Wave and modified wave scheduling are also used frequently but are not as common as time-specific scheduling. Clustering is the process of scheduling similar procedures on specified days or times. Tidal wave scheduling accommodates patients on a first-come, first-served basis.

Review: Yes ❑ No ❑

---

11. The abbreviation used in scheduling to designate a patient who has never been seen in the office before is:
    A. F/U.
    B. CPE.
    C. NS.
    D. NP.

Answer: **D**

Why: NP means new patient. F/U means follow-up, which would be used for a patient who is returning for an appointment. CPE means complete physical exam. NS is used to designate a patient who is a no-show.

Review: Yes ❑ No ❑

---

12. The reason for documenting a failed appointment in a patient's file is to:
    A. allow for scheduling another patient in that time slot.
    B. note all missed appointments in the event further action needs to take place.
    C. be able to erase the patient from the appointment book.
    D. allow the office to not schedule further appointments for that patient.
    E. notify the patient's insurance company.

Answer: **B**

Why: The physician may need to become involved to let a patient know that repeatedly missing appointments is disruptive to the office scheduling process. Occasionally, a patient's missing too many appointments may become of legal importance if the patient does not have a good medical outcome.

Review: Yes ❑ No ❑

---

13. The type of scheduling used in a medical practice primarily depends on the:
    A. physician's preference.
    B. location of the practice.
    C. medical assistant's preference.
    D. size of the examination rooms.

Answer: **A**

Why: The physician always determines the type of scheduling used in the office practice. You may be asked for input on the decision, but ultimately, the physician makes the decision on scheduling preference. The location of the practice or size of the examination rooms has no impact on the type of scheduling the physician prefers.

Review: Yes ❑ No ❑

14. Which of the following is the least important concern when scheduling special procedures?
   A. The facilities available in the medical office at the time of the appointment
   B. The amount of time required for the procedure
   C. The patient preparation for the procedure
   D. The equipment required for the procedure
   E. The amount of the insurance copay

Answer: **E**

Why: When scheduling a patient for a special procedure, it is necessary to know what facilities are available, how much time the procedure will take, and what equipment is required for the procedure. You should also take into account any special patient preparation, especially if the procedure requires fasting.

Review: Yes ❑ No ❑

---

15. A patient calls and requests an appointment immediately. What should be the first question you ask?
   A. The doctor is booked today. Can you come in tomorrow?
   B. Is it more convenient for you to come tomorrow morning or afternoon?
   C. When was the last time you were seen in this office?
   D. What are your symptoms and how long have you had them?

Answer: **D**

Why: You should always determine whether the call is an actual emergency or not. After this is determined, you can decide how soon the patient needs to be seen.

Review: Yes ❑ No ❑

---

16. When setting a return appointment for a patient, it is best to:
   A. have the patient call back from home after the patient checks his or her calendar.
   B. have preset appointment cards to distribute to patients with a set time and day when time is available in the appointment book.
   C. offer the patient a specific time and date.
   D. tell the patient you have only one available time and day that he or she will have to make work with his or her schedule.
   E. have the patient call the morning of the day he or she can come in for the appointment.

Answer: **C**

Why: The patient should be offered a time and day and see if they would be available to come in then. If that appointment is not acceptable, you can offer an alternative. It is too open to ask the patient to decide when to come in or to have the patient call the day of the desired appointment. They are not familiar with your scheduling procedures and may be indecisive.

Review: Yes ❑ No ❑

---

17. Scheduling duties include all the following EXCEPT:
   A. setting up the matrix of the appointment book.
   B. calling patients to remind them of their appointments.
   C. documenting any missed or rescheduled appointments in the patient's record.
   D. determining the time of day the office will accept appointments.

Answer: **D**

Why: The physician determines the appointment schedule for the office. This includes setting the time of the first and last appointments of the day and the break times throughout the day.

Review: Yes ❑ No ❑

18. When calling a hospital to schedule inpatient surgery, the information not necessary to have before the call is:
    A. patient's insurance copayment.
    B. time and day requested by the physician.
    C. urgency for the procedure.
    D. type of sedation or anesthesia required.
    E. the physician's name.

Answer: **A**

Why: Inpatient surgery is scheduled with the hospital's operating room scheduler. All the information listed is important except information about insurance or billing because this is not a responsibility of the surgery department.

Review: Yes ❑ No ❑

---

19. A tickler file is a(n):
    A. appointment card that is filed in the patient's chart.
    B. file used to hold laboratory reports if they cannot be filed right away.
    C. file of patient names that have missed appointments.
    D. filing system used as a reminder of things to do by a certain date or time.

Answer: **D**

Why: A tickler file may be a simple card file box with dividers placed in chronologic order by week or by month and containing items that will need attention in the future.

Review: Yes ❑ No ❑

---

20. A "walk-in" patient is one who:
    A. is able to ambulate without assistance.
    B. has arrived late for an appointment.
    C. arrives at the office without an appointment but wants to be seen.
    D. has an emergency.
    E. lives within walking distance of the office.

Answer: **C**

Why: A "walk-in" is a patient who shows up without an appointment but wants to see the physician. Unless it is an emergency, you should ask the patient to be seated in the waiting room and check with the physician to see whether the patient can be seen that day. If not, offer to schedule an appointment for the patient.

Review: Yes ❑ No ❑

---

21. When a patient needs a return appointment to discuss laboratory or x-ray findings with the physician, you should:
    A. call the lab and tell them to have the lab results available by the day of the appointment.
    B. call the lab to find out when the results will be available and make the return visit based on that date.
    C. ask the patient to contact the lab to determine when the results will be available.
    D. tell the lab that the results need to be back to the office by the next morning.

Answer: **B**

Why: The medical office is responsible for finding out when the lab results will be returned to the office so the return appointment can be scheduled accordingly. It is not appropriate to order tests by the next day unless the physician has made that request. The patient should not contact the lab.

Review: Yes ❑ No ❑

---

22. What type of scheduling is typical of an urgent care center?
    A. Tidal wave scheduling
    B. Wave scheduling
    C. Clustering
    D. Double booking
    E. Group scheduling

Answer: **A**

Why: Tidal wave scheduling means that there are no appointments set and patients are seen on a first-come, first-served basis. Wave scheduling is a type of scheduling in which several patients, usually four, are scheduled at the beginning of the same clock hour. Grouping and clustering are the same types of scheduling, in which patients having similar procedures are scheduled to come in on specified days or at specific times. Double booking means that two or more patients are scheduled at the same time.

Review: Yes ❑ No ❑

23. Types of patient appointment reminders used by offices include the following EXCEPT:
A. postcards.
B. appointment cards.
C. telephone calls.
D. facsimile.

Answer: **D**

Why: A facsimile, also called a fax, allows the medical office to send and receive printed material over a phone line. These machines are very popular in businesses but may not be found in homes. The fax machine is not used as a method to send appointment reminders.

Review: Yes ❑ No ❑

---

24. If the physician requests that the patient return for a fasting blood glucose and follow-up appointment, the best time of day to schedule this appointment would be:
A. the first appointment after the lunch break.
B. at the end of the day.
C. the last morning appointment before the lunch break.
D. the first appointment in the morning.
E. any time 1 hour after the patient has eaten.

Answer: **D**

Why: This patient is having a fasting blood test performed, which requires the patient to have eaten nothing for several hours before the exam. By scheduling it as the first morning appointment, the patient can come to the office and have the blood drawn before eating breakfast.

Review: Yes ❑ No ❑

---

25. When a group of patients needs immunizations, the best type of scheduling for this is:
A. tidal wave.
B. clustering.
C. modified wave.
D. double booking.

Answer: **B**

Why: Clustering is a type of scheduling used when similar procedures are scheduled on specified days or at specific times. Tidal wave scheduling allows patients to walk in at any time to be seen. This type of scheduling is typically used in urgent care facilities. Modified wave scheduling is when hour-long blocks are broken down to smaller time increments (usually 10 or 15 minutes each) and individual patients are scheduled within those increments. Double booking means that two or more patients are scheduled at the same time.

Review: Yes ❑ No ❑

---

26. When conducting a patient flow analysis, it is determined that patients wait in the treatment room for approximately 15 minutes prior to the physician presenting. As a result, you would:
A. Schedule patients 15 minutes later
B. Schedule less patients in each hour
C. Report the findings to the insurance company
D. Report the findings to the physician
E. Direct the physician to spend less time with each patient

Answer: **D**

Why: The role of the medical assistant or medical administrative specialist participating in the patient flow analysis is to report the findings. Recommendations may also be made, but it is up to the physician or practice manager to make changes and approve what should be sent to the insurance company.

Review: Yes ❑ No ❑

---

27. When scheduling an outpatient procedure, it is important to know all the following EXCEPT the:
A. LOS
B. Procedure
C. Diagnosis
D. Date

Answer: **A**

Why: A patient will not be staying in the hospital following an outpatient procedure; therefore, the length of stay (LOS) is not necessary. All other information is required.

Review: Yes ❑ No ❑

28. The primary purpose of a patient flow analysis is to:
    A. Identify patients who are late for appointments
    B. Demonstrate to insurance companies that the office does a good job
    C. Determine the efficiency of the practice
    D. Fire ineffective staff
    E. Encourage the physician to see more patients

Answer: **C**

Why: The primary purpose of a patient flow analysis is to determine the efficiency of the practice. The other answer choices may result, but these would only be incidental to the primary reason for initially conducting the analysis.

Review: Yes ❑ No ❑

---

29. When scheduling an inpatient procedure, the reason for scheduling the admission separate from the actual procedure is to:
    A. Provide billing information
    B. Reserve a hospital bed
    C. Assure the patient has meals ordered
    D. Notify the insurance company

Answer: **B**

Why: A time for a surgery, for example, may be scheduled in the operating room, but that does not guarantee that a hospital bed will be available for the patient afterward. The Admissions Department is the only area that takes the reservations for the actual hospital bed. The department where the procedure is done is only aware of patients for that department, not for all admissions throughout the facility.

Review: Yes ❑ No ❑

---

30. Electronic appointment scheduling is:
    A. Only for practices with multiple sites
    B. Less personal than a manual system
    C. Difficult to learn
    D. Unlikely to require a subpoena
    E. Held to HIPAA standards

Answer: **E**

Why: Whether appointment scheduling is manual or electronic, both HIPAA and governmental requirements must be met. Electronic scheduling may be used in single-site practices as well as multiple-site practices. It is not impersonal because it requires a staff member to conduct the appointment process, and it is generally not more difficult to learn than a manual system. As mentioned earlier, the same requirements are enforced for manual or electronic systems.

Review: Yes ❑ No ❑

11

Medical Records

REVIEW TIP

Congratulations! Believe it or not, you are nearly at the halfway point of the review chapters. The road to completion becomes easier from here. Don't give up your goal to become a nationally certified health professional. Be sure to complete Chapter 4, "Law and Ethics," before beginning this one–some material involving medical records is also covered in that chapter.

The term **medical record** is used synonymously with *patient chart* or *chart*; it contains all information related to a patient's medical care. The Medical Records chapter is divided into three sections:

- Medical records management
- The individual medical record
- Documentation guidelines

MEDICAL RECORDS MANAGEMENT

The medical assistant and medical administrative specialist are usually responsible for management of the office's medical records. This responsibility involves several functions:

- Assemble—place all the forms used by the specific practice in the patient record in the prescribed order
- File—place active medical records in the secured storage area in the order prescribed by the filing system used by that facility
- Maintain—ensure all documentation is in the medical record in the proper order and that the record is in a secured area
- Retrieve—recover the medical record from the secured storage as needed and document when and where the record was taken
- Transfer—send the record to another health care provider when the proper consent for release of medical records is obtained (send copies only, not originals)
- Protect—ensure the medical record is in a secured area and kept intact and that all computer safeguards are in place for the electronic health record.
- Audit—examine medical record files to ensure accuracy, completeness, and sequence of the documents; may be an internal file audit performed by the office staff or an external file audit performed by professional auditors of an organization or agency who are not employees of the practice
- Retain—keep the medical record in a secured area for the prescribed length of time (this is state-specific); the term **conditioning** is sometimes used to describe preparation of the chart for retention: secure all loose documents, and examine the record for completeness and correct filing order of documents

- Purge—remove medical records that are beyond the time period of the statute of limitations
- Destroy—shred or otherwise destroy the medical record, ensuring no identifying factors are recognizable, when the prescribed statute of limitations is reached; maintain a file indicating when the record was destroyed

In addition to the functions associated with medical records, you must know information about the organization and handling of medical records.

- Types of files
  - Active—patient seen within 2 to 5 years (dependent on practice type)
  - Inactive—patient *not* seen within past 2 to 5 years (dependent on practice type)
  - Closed—patient not expected to return to practice, such as if the patient is deceased, has moved, or has reached age limit in pediatrics
- File equipment and storage
  - Shelving units (active files)
    - Open or closed shelving units
    - Vertical or lateral units
    - Stationary or moveable units
    - Locked units or units locked in self-contained area
  - Electronic health records, or EHR (active, inactive, and closed files)—complex Health Insurance Portability and Accountability Act (HIPAA) security issues; firewalls should be in place if located on a network or electronically transferred
    - Combination electronic and hard-copy records
    - Total electronic records
    - Floppy disk, CD-ROM
    - Microfiche (for closed or inactive records)
    - Scanned file
  - CMS (Centers for Medicare and Medicaid Services) has established a goal that by the year 2014, health care providers will have converted all paper, hard-copy records to electronic health records. This is based on published information available at the time this text was printed.
- Medical record hard-copy supplies
  - File folders—top or side identification areas with method to secure loose file forms
  - Guides—dividers
  - Labels—alphabetic or numeric color or other coding containing section names, such as progress notes or alerts
  - Outguides—folders inserted on the file shelf when a medical record file is in use; designates who took it, when, and where (may be computerized instead of hard-copy folder)
  - Long-term hard-copy storage (inactive and closed)
    - Boxed; maintained onsite
    - Boxed; maintained offsite
- Filing systems
  - Alphabetic—charts filed by the units of the patient's name: letter by letter beginning with the patient's last name (Table 11-1)
    - Unit 1—last name, letter by letter
    - Unit 2—first name, letter by letter
    - Unit 3—middle initial or middle name, letter by letter
    - Unit 4—prefixes and suffixes (e.g., Dr., Mrs., Jr., Sr., I, II, III): numbers appear first (e.g., I, II, III); Jr. follows numbers and comes before Sr.
  - Numeric—each patient is assigned a medical record number through manual or computerized means; through a manual or computerized system, numbers are cross-referenced with the alphabetic file, sometimes referred to as a *master file*
    - Consecutive numeric order—patients are assigned numbers in the order of their first visit to the practice; charts are filed in this order; used by small practices
    - Terminal digit order—patients are assigned a six-digit number; to file the charts, the numbers are divided into three groups of two digits each and read from right to left
  - Color coding—system filed in coordination with numbers or alphabet
    - Each letter or group of letters in the alphabet is designated a specific color, which makes the letters easier to locate
    - Each group of numbers in terminal digit filing is designated a color
    - In group practices, patients of the individual physicians may be designated a color in addition to the alphabetic or numeric system
  - Alphanumeric—system using a combination of numbers and letters
    - Initial filing done alphabetically by first letter of last name or subject; then numbers are assigned

Table 11-1 Alphabetic Filing by Units

Example of	Patient Name	Unit 1 (Last Name)	Unit 2 (First Name)	Unit 3 (Middle Name)	Unit 4 (Title)
Using units	John E. Smith John William Jones	Smith Jones	John John	E. William	
Two-word last names	Susan B. Saint Nicolas	Saintnicolas	Susan	B.	
Period in last name	Harry F. St. James	Saintjames (ignore period and spell out name)	Harry	F.	
Hyphens or apostrophes (considered a single unit)	Jose Garcia-Lopez Jesse Peter O'Hara	Garcialopez Ohara	Jose Jesse	Peter	
Using titles	Dr. Jose Garcia-Lopez Mary T. El (Mrs. John)	Garcialopez El	Jose Mary	 T.	Dr. Mrs. John
Jr. and Sr. (Jr. filed before Sr.)	Joseph C. Tan, Jr. Joseph C. Tan, Sr.	Tan Tan	Joseph Joseph	C. C.	Jr. Sr.
Birth order (filed in chronologic order)	Tomas Jacob Love, I Tomas Jacob Love, II Tomas Jacob Love, III	Love Love Love	Tomas Tomas Tomas	Jacob Jacob Jacob	I II III
Jr., Sr., and numbers (numbers first in chronologic order, Jr. next, Sr. last)	Roberto De Rosa, III Roberto De Rosa, IV Roberto De Rosa, Jr. Roberto De Rosa, Sr.	Derosa Derosa Derosa Derosa	Roberto Roberto Roberto Roberto		III IV Jr. Sr.
Businesses and associations	A-One Medical Supply The McMay Insurance Group	Aone Mcmay	Medical Insurance	Supply Group	 The

  - Seldom used for medical records; more frequently used for other office files

- Medical records retention (hard copy or electronic)—the length of time a medical record should be retained
  - Guidelines from federal/state statute of limitations; retention for adults is usually 7 to 10 years
  - Retention for minors is the age of majority plus the statute of limitations (7 to 10 years)
  - Guidelines may also be issued by insurance companies and accrediting and legal organizations
  - Functional storage and retrieval systems required
- Medical records destruction
  - After completion of statute of limitations and recommended guidelines
  - Total eradication (shredding, burning, deleting); safe shredding and disposal of documents may be done by an outside company specializing in those services
  - saved notation of destruction and date

THE INDIVIDUAL MEDICAL RECORD

The individual medical record is all the information related to a patient's medical care. This information may be in the form of paper (e.g., progress notes or letters), medical imaging (such as x-rays, ultrasounds), tapes (e.g., audio, visual), disks, electronic printouts (e.g., electrocardiogram tracings, fetal monitoring strips), photographs, and any other materials that tell the "story" of the patient's medical journey. The medical record material is the property of the health care provider. The information in the medical record is the property of the patient.

- Uses
  - Facilitates good medical care through continuity
  - Provides legal protection for the health care provider and the patient
  - Functions as a quality of care monitor

Box 11-1

Example of Medical Records Form or Screen Sequencing

Medical Record Sequence of Forms

1. Patient information/insurance
2. Consent for assignment of benefits
3. Problem list
4. Medical, social, and family histories
5. Progress notes
6. Immunization record
7. Medication/prescription
8. Diagnostic reports
9. Consultation/referral reports
10. Medical records
11. Correspondence, telephone notes
12. Termination summary

- Facilitates research
- Provides resource for education

■ Determination of record organization and sequence (Box 11-1)
- Type of practice
- Physician preference
- Frequency of access

■ Potentials for legal and ethical dilemmas
- Confidentiality breach (see "Confidentiality" in Chapter 4)
- Improper release of information (Box 11-2)
- Withdrawal from care; discharge of patient
- Broken appointments
- Patient noncompliance with his or her care plan
- Questionable medical records
  - Delayed filing of tests or notes
  - Incomplete information
  - Illegible entries
  - Improperly corrected entries
  - Missing information
  - Lost record

Box 11-2

Release of Medical Records

A release of medical records to insurance companies, other recognized reimbursement agencies, and health care providers within the same health care network is generally included in a general consent form and is obtained at the first office visit.

Release of medical records to other health care providers, attorneys, or others requires a Release of Medical Information form signed by the patient or the patient's legal representative, such as a court-appointed guardian.

Lawful mandatory reporting situations or subpoenas do not require consent forms (refer to Chapter 4).

DOCUMENTATION GUIDELINES

Documentation, also referred to as *charting*, makes up the medical record. A caveat, referred to as the "golden rule," is: *If it is not documented, it was not done.*

■ "Cs" of charting (a list of terms beginning with the letter "C" to help with proper documentation)
- Client's words (use quotation marks or "patient states . . .")
- Clear
- Complete
- Concise
- Chronologic or reverse chronologic order
- *Confidential*

■ Documentation inclusions
- Name of the patient, additional identifier (e.g., medical record number), and date on each page, front and back
- Dated entry for each visit and procedure
- Health care provider signature or initials and title for all entries
- Dated entry for no-shows, cancellations, or phone calls
- Dated entry for failure to follow treatment plan
- Dated entry for prescription refills
- Notations or copies of forms for outpatient and hospital visits
- Dated entry with explanation for termination of care
- Documentation of reported results and follow-up for all tests and procedures
- Acceptable error correction method (Box 11-3)

■ Charting methods
- Source-oriented medical record (SOMR)—this file is divided into sections by guides, such as a section for progress notes or diagnostic reports; may be used in conjunction with other charting methods
- Problem-oriented medical record (POMR)—the patient's problems are numbered and listed on a

Box 11-3

Paper Record Error Correction

Draw a single line through the error with black ink and write "error" or "err." above. Never white out or completely eliminate the error. Correct the error above the entry if it involves only a few words or below the entry if the error is longer. Record the date and time and sign or initial the entry with your health care provider title.

Example:

09/10/20XX 0900 urine specimen collected. Mary Smith, MA
sputum/M.S., MA

form (problem list) that is placed in the front of the chart; each visit or treatment is associated with a problem number (for example, if asthma is the primary problem it, is listed as #1 and documented as #1 throughout the chart); may be used in conjunction with other charting methods. In addition to the problem list, POMR usually contains the following:

- Database—patient profile and demographics; baseline and assessment information including chief complaint (cc) and test results
- Treatment plan—course of procedures, medications, and other instructions for the patient's care
- Progress notes—continuing narrative of the patient's improvement or lack of improvement

- SOAP documentation—format for documenting each visit using subjective information, objective information, an assessment, and a plan, in that order; may be used in conjunction with other charting methods
  - S = subjective data (symptoms the patient states that cannot be seen, heard, or measured, such as a headache)
  - O = objective data (measurable and observable signs, such as swelling)
  - A = assessment (exam and impressions)
  - P = plan (design for tests, treatments, education, follow-up)
- Reverse chronologic order—format with the most recent records filed on top: visits in 2010 would be closer to the front of the chart than visits in 2009; may be used in conjunction with other charting methods

TERMS

Medical Records Review

The following list reviews the terms discussed in this chapter and other important terms that you may see on the exam.

active medical record the chart of a patient seen within 2 to 5 years (dependent on practice type)

audit examine medical record files to ensure accuracy, completeness, and sequence of the documents

chart the patient's medical record

closed medical record the chart of a patient not expected to return to the practice, such as a patient who is deceased or has moved

conditioning preparation of the chart for retention: secure all loose documents, and examine the chart for completion and correct filing order of documents

electronic health record (EHR) patient health information maintained in an electronic format, computerized record

Health Insurance Portability and Accountability Act (HIPAA) originally enacted in 1996, contains requirements for patient confidentiality

inactive medical record the chart of a patient *not* seen at the specific medical office within the past 2 to 5 years (dependent on practice type)

medical record all patient information related to the medical care; may be in the form of paper, medical imaging, tapes, disks, electronic printouts, photographs, and any other material telling the "story" of the patient's medical history

medical records management processes of assembling, filing, maintaining, retrieving, transferring, protecting, retaining, and destroying medical records

outguides folders inserted on file shelf when file is in use; they designate who took it, when, and where it is (may be computerized instead of hard-copy folder)

problem-oriented medical record (POMR) the patient's problems are numbered and listed on a form (problem list) placed in front of chart; each visit or treatment is associated with the number of the corresponding problem (e.g., if asthma is #1, it is documented as #1 throughout chart)

reverse chronologic order format with the most recent documentation filed on top of the past documentation

SOAP documentation format for documenting each medical visit using subjective information, objective information, an assessment, and a plan, in that order

source-oriented medical record (SOMR) the patient file is divided into sections by guides, such as a section for progress notes or diagnostic reports

terminal digit order a system of filing medical records that assigns each patient a six-digit number; to file the charts, the numbers are divided into three groups of two digits each and read from right to left

REVIEW QUESTIONS

All questions are relevant for the CMA (AAMA), RMA (AMT), and CMAS (AMT) exams.

1. When adding medical records to a patient's chart, you should:
   A. file all materials in the front of the chart regardless of the type of record it is.
   B. photocopy all records and retain in a separate file.
   C. ensure that the physician has initialed all reports before they are inserted into the chart.
   D. sign all documents with the medical assistant title and file in the patient's chart.

Answer: **C**

Why: Whenever a new document or record is generated for a patient's medical record, the physician must review the record before it is filed in the chart for storage. If there is abnormal medical information, the physician will want to act on the information to ensure proper medical care for the patient.

Review: Yes ❑ No ❑

---

2. The most common method of documentation for a patient medical record is:
   A. POMR.
   B. SOMR.
   C. SOAP.
   D. SOB.
   E. DOB.

Answer: **C**

Why: The abbreviation SOAP stands for subjective, objective, assessment, plan. This is the most common method of documenting used by physicians. POMR (problem-oriented medical records) and SOMR (source-oriented medical records) are methods used in organizing the patient's chart either by the patient's problem categories or by sources of information, respectively. SOB stands for shortness of breath and is associated with a condition a patient has, not a documentation method. DOB stands for date of birth, which is a charting abbreviation.

Review: Yes ❑ No ❑

---

3. When filing numerically using the terminal digit filing method, what is the proper sequence for filing these four numbers: 381249, 831140, 105449, 943550?
   A. 381249, 831140, 943650, 105449
   B. 831140, 381249, 105449, 943650
   C. 943650, 381249, 105449, 831140
   D. 105449, 381249, 831140, 943650

Answer: **B**

Why: Terminal digit filing divides the medical record numbers into three units of two—for instance, the number 381249 is divided into 38 12 49. The last units of the above numbers are 49, 40, 49, and 50, which are filed in the order 40, 49, 50. Because there are two numbers ending in 49, the next unit determines the order of the numbers. Because 12 comes before 54, 381249 comes before 105449.

Review: Yes ❑ No ❑

4. Which of the following is a true statement regarding guidelines for alphabetic filing?
   A. When two male family members have the suffixes Junior and Senior, Senior is filed before Junior.
   B. The chart for a patient with the last name of Saint James would be filed in the J (James) section of the files.
   C. The name McMurray is filed before MacIntosh.
   D. John William Smith is filed before John Will Smith.
   E. When a last name has a hyphen, it is filed as if the hyphen were not there.

Answer: **E**

Why: Alphabetic filing guidelines dictate that Junior is filed before Senior. These guidelines also state that the name Saint James becomes one word and is filed in the S section under Saint. The John Smith names are the same except for the middle name; Will is filed before William. A name starting with Mc is filed in alphabetic order, after Mac.

Review: Yes ❑ No ❑

---

5. When a paper medical record is in use, a folder inserted on the shelf in place of the medical record file is a(n):
   A. closed file.
   B. inactive file.
   C. file label.
   D. outguide.

Answer: **D**

Why: A closed or inactive file indicates the status of the file, and a file label is affixed to a file to indicate its name. An outguide is a folder inserted on a file shelf to replace a medical record file that is in use. The outguide folder designates who took the medical file, when it was removed, and where it is.

Review: Yes ❑ No ❑

---

6. One of the "Cs" of charting includes:
   A. clear.
   B. closed.
   C. computerized.
   D. complex.
   E. conditional.

Answer: **A**

Why: The six "Cs" of charting include client's words, clear, complete, concise, chronologic, and confidentiality. These are essential guidelines of documentation.

Review: Yes ❑ No ❑

---

7. The "P" in the SOAP method of charting includes:
   A. measurable signs.
   B. physician's exam.
   C. symptoms the patient states.
   D. plan for tests and treatments.

Answer: **D**

Why: The "P" stands for the plan and includes the plan for the patient's tests, treatment, and follow-up. Measurable signs are objective ("O"), the physician's exam is assessment ("A"), and symptoms the patient states are subjective data ("S").

Review: Yes ❑ No ❑

8. If filing using reverse chronologic order, which of the following is in the correct sequence?
   A. Laboratory test results from June 2007 would be in front of those from December 2010.
   B. Office visit entries from June 2010 would be in front of visits from December 2008.
   C. X-ray exam reports from November 15, 2009, would be in front of those from December 30 of the same year.
   D. A surgical report from an operation in 2001 would be in front of a report of a procedure performed in 2009.
   E. A physician's referral report from May 15, 2009, would be in front of a report from the same physician dated May 30, 2009.

Answer: **B**

Why: Reverse chronologic order means that the most recent records are filed in front of or on top of the past record. The only example of this is item B. All the other examples would place the older reports or events first.

Review: Yes ❑ No ❑

---

9. The proper procedure to correct an error in a patient's chart is to:
   A. date and sign the correction.
   B. white out the error before writing in the correction.
   C. draw a single line through the error with red ink.
   D. always start a new line in the chart for corrections.

Answer: **A**

Why: A correction should always be dated and signed by the person making the correction. Corrections should not be covered with white out or lined out with red ink. If it is only a word or two to correct, the correction is written above the error after the error is crossed out with a single line in black ink.

Review: Yes ❑ No ❑

---

10. A system of filing made of combinations of numbers and letters is:
    A. direct filing.
    B. numeric filing.
    C. subject filing.
    D. demographic filing.
    E. alphanumeric filing.

Answer: **E**

Why: Alphanumeric filing uses letters ("alpha") and numbers ("numeric") for filing.

Review: Yes ❑ No ❑

---

11. Of the following patient names, which would come first in alphabetic filing?
    A. Fisher, Bill
    B. Fischer, William
    C. Fishar, Bob
    D. Fishare, Bill

Answer: **B**

Why: Alphabetic filing requires that each letter be considered as a unit. All these names start with the same first three letters, *F I S*. The next letter determines which name comes first in filing. *C* comes before *H*, so the name Fischer is first in filing.

Review: Yes ❑ No ❑

---

12. The "golden rule" in documentation is the following.
    A. Always sign your complete name and title.
    B. Always document in ink.
    C. If it is not documented, it was not done.
    D. Always date and time all entries.
    E. The physician must initial all chart entries.

Answer: **C**

Why: All of the answers are part of proper documentation, but the "golden rule" of documentation is: If it is not documented, it was not done.

Review: Yes ❑ No ❑

13. Determining the organization of the medical record and sequence of filing is dependent on the following factors EXCEPT:
    A. type of practice.
    B. location of practice.
    C. physician preference.
    D. frequency of access.

Answer: **B**

Why: The location of the medical practice has no bearing on how medical records will be organized or filed. The other factors listed will determine the best way to manage the patients' medical records.

Review: Yes ❑ No ❑

---

14. The database component of problem-oriented medical records (POMR) includes what information?
    A. Patient's past medical problems
    B. Treatment plan for the patient
    C. Progress notes
    D. Patient's present illness
    E. Laboratory findings from 5 years ago

Answer: **D**

Why: POMR has four components, including database, problem list, treatment plan, and progress notes. The problem list includes past medical problems, but the database includes chief complaint, present illness, patient profile, review of systems, physical examination, and laboratory reports.

Review: Yes ❑ No ❑

---

15. The term used to describe the legal length of time regarding storage of medical and business records is:
    A. statute of limitations.
    B. release of medical records.
    C. microfiche.
    D. closed records.

Answer: **A**

Why: The statute of limitations may vary from state to state. It is the legal time limit you must retain medical and business records before they can be destroyed. Most states require a minimum of 7 years from the date of the last entry. Many practices store records permanently because of the possibility of a malpractice suit.

Review: Yes ❑ No ❑

---

16. The method of filing used when documentation is placed in order based on the date of occurrence is:
    A. demographic grouping.
    B. statistical numbering.
    C. chronologic order.
    D. consecutive numeric order.
    E. alphabetic filing.

Answer: **C**

Why: The word *chronologic* means "arranged in the order of occurrence." Most charting requires the most recent reports or records to be placed in front of or on top of older information.

Review: Yes ❑ No ❑

---

17. An important rule for releasing medical records is:
    A. Release the original medical record when the patient asks for it.
    B. There is no need to obtain the patient's signature on an Authorization for Release of Medical Record form as long as the patient has given verbal authorization.
    C. Limit the amount of medical information you release over the telephone when you are not talking directly to the patient.
    D. Release a copy of the medical record, not the original.

Answer: **D**

Why: A practice never releases the original medical record, only a copy. It is required that the patient sign a form to release medical records. A verbal consent is not official authorization. Information, no matter how limited, is never given over the telephone to anyone but the patient.

Review: Yes ❑ No ❑

18. If a patient is not expected to return to the practice because he or she has moved away, the patient's record would be classified as:
    A. inactive.
    B. active.
    C. closed.
    D. transferred.
    E. released.

Answer: **C**

Why: An inactive file would be for a patient who has not been seen within the past 2 to 5 years. An active file is used for a patient who has been seen within the past 2 to 5 years. The number of years is established by each practice, with 2 to 5 being the most common range. A closed file is used for a patient who will not be expected back to the practice. This would include deceased patients and patients who have moved away. A transferred file has been sent to another practice; it is released when the file has been approved for transfer to another health care provider.

Review: Yes ❑ No ❑

---

19. The pages of the medical record contained within the patient's file are the property of the:
    A. patient.
    B. physician.
    C. insurance carrier.
    D. spouse or guardian.

Answer: **B**

Why: The health care provider, the physician, owns the medical record. The patient can request the information contained within the record, but the actual record belongs to the physician.

Review: Yes ❑ No ❑

---

20. Indexing rules for alphabetic filing include the following EXCEPT:
    A. File records according to last name, first name, and middle initial.
    B. File abbreviated names as if they were spelled out.
    C. Disregard apostrophes.
    D. Junior is filed before Senior.
    E. Treat hyphenated names as two units.

Answer: **E**

Why: A hyphenated name is treated as one unit (i.e., Jane Fisher-Smith is filed as Fisher-Smith, Jane, not as Smith, Jane Fisher).

Review: Yes ❑ No ❑

---

21. A backup file to a computer medical record is called the:
    A. file folder.
    B. outguide.
    C. disk.
    D. electronic copy.

Answer: **C**

Why: A disk of a computer record, can be used as a backup to the electronic system. A file folder is the holder of the medical records. An outguide is used to temporarily replace a medical file while it is in use. An electronic copy refers to the computerized version of the record.

Review: Yes ❑ No ❑

22. The process of gathering all chart items together and preparing them for filing by removing loose pieces of tape or paper clips and replacing them with staples is known as:
    A. conditioning.
    B. sorting.
    C. destroying.
    D. indexing.
    E. retrieving.

Answer: **A**

Why: Conditioning is the process of making sure the chart records are presentable for filing. It is inappropriate to file records that have paper clips, because they become too bulky and take up file space. Sorting the files into groups makes it easier to file records. They can be sorted alphabetically or numerically first and then placed in the appropriate space on the file shelf. Destroying is the process of shredding the medical record to permanently remove it from storage. Indexing is the process of separating business records from the patient's medical records. Retrieving is the process of recovering the medical record from the secured storage location.

Review: Yes ❑ No ❑

---

23. The federal government policy that sets standards for electronic transmission of medical information is included in the act adopted in 1996 called:
    A. OSHA.
    B. CLIA.
    C. HIPAA.
    D. CDC.

Answer: **C**

Why: HIPAA, the Health Insurance Portability and Accountability Act, was passed by the federal government and mandates that health care providers adopt policies in their medical practice that regulate the electronic transmission of patients' medical information. In addition, the act sets standards on the disclosure and release of medical records. OSHA stands for Occupational Safety and Health Administration. CLIA stands for Clinical Laboratory Improvement Amendments. CDC stands for the Centers for Disease Control and Prevention.

Review: Yes ❑ No ❑

---

24. To avoid legal and ethical issues, patients' medical records should be properly maintained, which includes all of the following EXCEPT:
    A. entry of any broken or missed appointments.
    B. letter sent to patient to notify of withdrawal of care.
    C. notation of patient's noncompliance with the treatment plan.
    D. delay in filing test results.
    E. initialing of all corrections made in a medical chart.

Answer: **D**

Why: The patient's medical record should always document missed appointments and noncompliance with the physician's treatment plan, in case of a malpractice suit brought against the physician for questionable patient care. When a physician notifies a patient of withdrawal of care, a copy of the letter sent to the patient is included in the medical record. The medical assistant or medical administrative specialist should always ensure timely filing of reports and lab results. There is a chance these records will be lost if not filed promptly. When making corrections to a chart, draw a single line through the error, write the correct information above the error, and initial the entry.

Review: Yes ❑ No ❑

25. When using the SOAP method of charting, which of the following belongs to the O section?
    A. Patient's complaint of headache
    B. Order for an electrocardiogram
    C. Blood pressure reading
    D. Physician's request to have patient return for follow-up appointment

Answer: **C**

Why: The "O" stands for "objective data." Objective data include things that are measurable and observable. A patient's blood pressure is a measurable, objective sign. The patient's complaint of headache is subjective data—something that cannot be seen or observed. The physician's request for an electrocardiogram and follow-up appointment are all part of the plan for the patient.

Review: Yes ❑ No ❑

---

26. SOMR refers to:
    A. subjective objective medical record.
    B. safe objective medical radiology.
    C. State Office of Medical Records.
    D. Secure Office for Medical Records.
    E. source-oriented medical record.

Answer: **E**

Why: The SOMR, source-oriented medical record, is a type of filing within the medical record that sorts the information by sections such as progress notes, diagnostic reports, and correspondence.

Review: Yes ❑ No ❑

---

27. When a medical record or patient file is audited, it is:
    A. purged.
    B. examined.
    C. destroyed.
    D. shredded

Answer: **B**

Why: When a file is examined for completeness, for accuracy, and to ensure the documents are in the proper order, it is being audited. Purging, destroying, and shredding are methods of cleaning out old files and appropriately discarding medical records that no longer need to be retained or maintained.

Review: Yes ❑ No ❑

12
Correspondence

REVIEW TIP

Become familiar with the various correspondence formats and materials discussed in this chapter. Look for examples in your workplace, among your own business mail, or in other available sources.

Written communication in the medical office takes many forms. E-mail, patient instructions, faxes, and various computer applications have been discussed in previous chapters. This chapter concentrates on written correspondence involving mail and transcription. The topics are generally prescriptive, which means they follow a custom or rule.

The majority of letters generated in the medical office follow a template, or form, which is recommended by the physician's attorney, insurance carrier, or professional organization. The purpose is to protect the doctor from medicolegal risk. The few original letters are usually those dictated by the physician and sent to other physicians regarding patient findings or treatment. The medical assistant or medical administrative specialist must know the correct format, materials, and process for outgoing and incoming mail.

MATERIALS

- Letterhead—quality bond stationery used for the first page of correspondence; contains the name of physician or group, address, telephone number, and e-mail address (if appropriate), usually at the top of the page; white, gray, or buff paper is most common
- Following pages—plain quality bond stationery that matches the letterhead
- Envelopes—no. 10 is the size most commonly used because it fits $8^{1}/_{2}" \times 11"$ paper folded in thirds; should be made of quality bond paper that matches the letterhead used for letters; lower-quality envelopes with clear windows may be used for patient statements that are folded to exhibit patient's address through the window
- Resources—medical offices have various books and other sources, including the Internet, to ensure that the grammar, spelling, and format for correspondence are correct. Some helpful resources are:
  - Desk dictionary
  - Medical dictionary/encyclopedia (the exams usually have questions on misspelled words; see Box 12-1)
  - Writing style books
  - *Physicians' Desk Reference* (PDR)
  - Other medical reference books
  - Date stamp—used to imprint date received on all incoming mail

Box 12-1

Frequently Misspelled Words

abscess	ischium
aneurysm	larynx
arrhythmia	ophthalmology
cirrhosis	pharynx
curettage	pneumonia
hemorrhage	rheumatic
hemorrhoids	roentgenology
humerus	sphygmomanometer
ileum	*Staphylococcus*
ilium	tonsillitis
ischemia	

LETTERS

- Styles
  - Full block—all lines begin at left margin; this is the most common style
  - Modified block—subject and complimentary closing and signature begin at the middle of the paper; other lines begin at left margin
  - Semiblock (indented modified block)—subject and complimentary closing and signature begin in the center, and the first line of each paragraph is indented five spaces; all other lines begin at the left margin
  - Simplified—the greeting and complimentary closing are omitted; all lines begin at the left margin
- Components
  - Margins—the blank space or border around the text on a business letter; the standard margin is 1 inch
  - Date—keyed 15 lines from top of page or 2 to 4 lines below letterhead; key in full date: January 1, 2010, not 01/01/2010
  - Inside addresses—the sender's address is located on the letterhead; the recipient's address referred to as the inside address, is keyed at the left margin; abbreviations in addresses should not be used except for the state
  - Salutation (greeting)—keyed at the left margin, two lines below the recipient's address, followed by a colon
  - Subject (optional)—topic of letter, keyed two lines below salutation, usually at the left margin; sometimes begins with "RE:" ("regarding")
  - Letter body—begins two lines below the salutation or the subject line; the position of the paragraph beginning depends on the style of the letter
  - Complimentary closing—two lines below the last sentence of the letter body; if the closing contains more than one word, only the first word is capitalized
  - Keyed signature—usually four lines below the complimentary closing; use titles before *or* after name, not both (e.g., Dr. James Jones or James Jones, M.D., *not* Dr. James Jones, M.D.)
  - Reference initials—two lines below keyed signature; the initials of the individual signing the letter in uppercase letters followed by a colon and the initials of the individual processing the letter in lowercase letters
  - Enclosures—two lines below the reference initials; indicates that other items are included with the letter; may simply state "enclosures," or it may be followed by a colon and the titles of the enclosed document(s)
  - Copies—"cc:" or "Cc:" (computer software often automatically capitalizes the first "C") literally means *carbon copy*, but is still used to indicate that a copy of the document is being sent to the person whose name follows the "cc:"; this notation is listed one or two lines below the reference initials; when more than one person is copied, the names are listed in alphabetic order
  - Envelope addresses
    - Start address 14 lines down from top of envelope and 4 inches from left edge when using a no. 10 envelope
    - Do not use punctuation except when using expanded zip codes
    - Use all uppercase letters

MAIL

- Classifications—different types of mailings require different postage and handling costs. Generally, the speedier the delivery is, the more expensive the postage. The following classifications are in order according to the cost (most expensive to least expensive) and the speed of delivery
  - Express Mail®—delivery guaranteed the following day
  - Registered Mail™—first-class mail insured for a named value
  - Certified Mail™—first-class mail with a verification from the postal service that it arrived at the designated address; the sender, for an additional fee, may request a signature for the correspondence indicating who received it; the sender has the option to use the United States Postal Service's (USPS) "NetPost" Internet service or to take the correspondence to the post office

- First-Class Mail®—postage generally used for office correspondence, including patient statements; weight must be 13 ounces or less
- Priority Mail®—first-class mail handling for items 70 pounds or less; usually takes 2 to 3 days to arrive
- Standard Mail™ (bulk)—postage used for magazines, periodicals, newspapers, catalogs, and flyers; requires a minimum of 200 pieces; formerly called second- and third-class mail

■ Mail payment methods
- Stamps
- Postage meter—purchased or leased printing machines or services that print postage directly onto mail pieces or labels; postage-metered envelopes do not need to be canceled and therefore save time; meter date is automatically or manually changed daily; postage meter services may be purchased online

■ Incoming mail procedure
- Stamp items with date received
- Staple or paperclip original envelope to incoming mail piece
- Stamp payment checks with endorsement
- Ensure all envelopes are empty before disposing of them
- Sort according to type
- Check clinical mail for urgency
- Distribute mail to appropriate staff
- Carry out any assigned functions related to the mail, such as posting payments

OTHER CORRESPONDENCE

Two other types of correspondence important to medical offices are memorandums and transcription. Questions on these topics may be on the national exam.

MEMORANDUMS

Interoffice correspondence is usually in the form of a **memorandum** (plural is *memorandums or memoranda*), or memo.

■ Components
- Date—the day the memo is written; placed 13 lines from top of the page, with a 1-inch side margin; left justified
- To—the parties to whom the memo is directed; two lines below "Date" line
- From—the name of the party sending the memo; two lines below "To" line
- Subject—the topic of the memo; two lines below "From" line
- Message—begins three lines below "Subject" line

■ Distribution
- Hard copy sent to individual staff members
- Hard copy posted in office
- Electronic mail

TRANSCRIPTION

Transcription is the conversion of the dictated word of the health care provider to a word-processed form. Letters and patients' medical histories and treatments are the most common transcribed documents in the medical office. Transcribed documents involving the patient become part of the patient's medical record. The rules of confidentiality apply, including when these documents may be mailed to other entities.

The transcriber should always check with the health care provider if in doubt about any portion of the document; never guess. The format used is based on the type of document and the facility preference. Accurate transcription requires the following:

■ Equipment
- Transcriber with digital counter, foot pedal, and earphones
- Word processing tools

■ Resources
- Medical dictionary/spell checker
- Drug reference book/software
- Diagnostic and procedural code sources
- Grammar book/checker

A significant amount of transcription is being replaced by the electronic medical record.

TERMS

Correspondence Review

The following list reviews the terms discussed in this chapter and other important terms that you may see on the exam.

Certified Mail first-class mail with a verification from the postal service that the mail arrived at the designated address; the sender, for an additional fee, may request a receiver sign for the correspondence; the sender has the option to use the United States Postal Office website or to take the correspondence to the post office

Express Mail next-day delivery service

full block style of letter writing with all lines beginning at left margin; most common letter style

letterhead quality bond stationery used for the first page of correspondence; contains, usually at the top of the page, the name of the physician or group, address, telephone number, and e-mail address (if appropriate); white, gray, or buff paper is most common

memorandum (plural *memorandums* or *memoranda*) memo; interoffice correspondence consisting of *date, to, from, subject*, and a message; may be hard copy or e-mail

modified block style of letter writing in which the subject, complimentary closing, and signature begin in the middle of the paper; all other lines begin at left margin

postage meter purchased or leased printing machines or services that print postage directly onto mail pieces or labels

Priority Mail faster delivery than first-class mail; usually takes 2 to 3 days

Registered Mail first-class mail insured for a named value

semiblock (indented modified block) style of letter writing with the subject, complimentary closing, and signature beginning at the center; the first line of each paragraph is indented five spaces; all other lines begin at left margin

simplified style of letter writing with the greeting and complimentary closing omitted; all lines begin at left margin

Standard Mail (bulk) postage used for magazines, periodicals, newspapers, catalogs, and flyers; requires a minimum of 200 pieces; formerly called second- and third-class mail

transcription the conversion of the dictated word of the health care provider into a word-processed form

REVIEW QUESTIONS

All questions are relevant for the CMA (AAMA), RMA (AMT), and CMAS (AMT) exams.

1. The most formal and professional style of letter format is:
   A. memorandum.
   B. semiblock.
   C. full block.
   D. indented block.

Answer: **C**

Why: The full block letter is written so that all the left margins are indented at 1 inch. This style has the most professional look.

Review: Yes ❑ No ❑

---

2. The standard business envelope is a:
   A. no. 7.
   B. no. 9.
   C. no. 10.
   D. no. 12.
   E. no. 8.

Answer: **C**

Why: A no. 10 envelope is used for standard $8^1/_2$" × 11" paper folded into thirds.

Review: Yes ❑ No ❑

---

3. The punctuation mark following the salutation of a professional business letter is a:
   A. period.
   B. hyphen.
   C. semicolon.
   D. colon.

Answer: **D**

Why: The salutation is the opening of the letter, which is followed by a colon in a professional letter.

Review: Yes ❑ No ❑

---

4. The standard margin used for a business letter is:
   A. $^1/_2$ inch.
   B. 1 inch.
   C. $1^1/_2$ inches.
   D. 2 inches.
   E. $2^1/_2$ inches.

Answer: **B**

Why: One inch is used as the standard margin for all sides of a letter. The letter appears standardized and professional.

Review: Yes ❑ No ❑

---

5. The component of a letter that indicates the purpose of the correspondence is the:
   A. subject line.
   B. enclosure.
   C. letterhead.
   D. salutation.

Answer: **A**

Why: The subject line introduces the main topic of the letter and begins with the abbreviation "RE" (short for "regarding") followed by a colon. The word "enclosure" is placed below the reference initials, indicating that there are other documents included with the letter. Letterhead is stationery with the sender's name and address at the top of the page. The salutation is the greeting of the letter.

Review: Yes ❑ No ❑

---

6. Which of the following is true regarding the date on a business letter?
   A. The date includes the month and year only.
   B. The date is not necessary on a business letter.
   C. It is proper to abbreviate the date to save space.
   D. The date is placed on the same line as the inside address on the right of the paper.
   E. The date is placed two lines below the letterhead.

Answer: **E**

Why: The date the letter is written should be placed two lines below the letterhead.

Review: Yes ❑ No ❑

7. Certified Mail is also considered or classified as:
   A. First-Class Mail.
   B. Second-Class Mail.
   C. Third-Class Mail.
   D. Express Mail.

Answer: **A**

Why: Certified Mail is sent first class, and the sender can request verification that the mail piece was delivered to the recipient. Second-Class Mail was used to send items such as magazines, and Third-Class Mail was the same as bulk mail and was typically used to send promotional materials. (These types of mail are now called Standard Mail.) Express Mail is sent with a guarantee of next-day delivery.

Review: Yes ❑ No ❑

---

8. The mail classification used to send most medical office mail is:
   A. Priority Mail.
   B. Second-Class Mail.
   C. Express Mail.
   D. First-Class Mail.
   E. Standard Mail.

Answer: **D**

Why: First-Class Mail is used for most office correspondence, including letters and postcards. Priority Mail and Express Mail expedite the delivery. Second-Class Mail is now called Standard Mail, and it is primarily used for printed matter, newsletters, bulletins, and catalogs.

Review: Yes ❑ No ❑

---

9. The style of letter in which all the lines begin at the left margin except the subject and complimentary closing is:
   A. modified block.
   B. semiblock.
   C. simplified.
   D. full block.

Answer: **A**

Why: The modified block is a style of letter that is less formal. The subject, complimentary closing, and signature lines begin at the center of the page, with all other lines beginning at the left margin.

Review: Yes ❑ No ❑

---

10. The proper style of writing the date in a professional letter is:
   A. 2010
   B. Jan. 1, 2010
   C. January 1, 2010
   D. January 1, '10
   E. January 01, '10

Answer: **C**

Why: The proper date in a professional letter should be written out fully. The month is not abbreviated, and four digits are used for the year.

Review: Yes ❑ No ❑

---

11. How many lines below the salutation should the body of the letter start?
   A. 1
   B. 2
   C. 3
   D. 4

Answer: **B**

Why: Two lines is the standard amount of space between the salutation and the body of the letter. This amount of space allows the salutation to be set apart from the body.

Review: Yes ❑ No ❑

---

12. An example of a properly keyed signature is:
   A. Dr. James Jones, M.D.
   B. Dr. Jones, M.D.
   C. James Jones, M.D.
   D. Doctor Jones, M.D.
   E. J. Jones, M.D.

Answer: **C**

Why: It is not appropriate to use both the title "Dr." and the initials "M.D." in the same title. You may use either one, but not both. The first name and the last name of the person signing the letter should be spelled out completely.

Review: Yes ❑ No ❑

13. The classification of mail that guarantees delivery the following day is:
   A. First-Class Mail.
   B. Certified Mail.
   C. Registered Mail.
   D. Express Mail.

Answer: **D**

Why: Express Mail will ensure that the delivery will arrive the next day. This service is more expensive than other types of mail classes, but offices rely on Express Mail for sending records and office correspondence that must arrive by the next day. Certified Mail and Registered Mail are used when the sender wants to have confirmation of delivery or have the mail delivered to a specific person. First-Class Mail is the most common type of delivery used for letters but has no guarantee of what day the mail will be delivered. Typically it will take 2 to 3 days for most first-class mail to reach its destination.

Review: Yes ❑ No ❑

---

14. At the bottom of a professional letter, the reference initials represent:
   A. the individual processing the letter, in uppercase letters.
   B. the individual signing the letter, in uppercase letters.
   C. the individual signing the letter, in lowercase letters.
   D. only the individual processing the letter.
   E. the individual receiving the letter.

Answer: **B**

Why: The initials for both the individual signing the letter and the person who processed the letter are indicated. The uppercase initials belong to the individual signing the letter; the lowercase initials belong to the person who processed the letter.

Review: Yes ❑ No ❑

---

15. The abbreviation "cc:" or "Cc:," when used at the end of a professional letter, means:
   A. there is an enclosure in the envelope with the letter.
   B. the letter was sent to another person.
   C. the physician requested a copy of the letter.
   D. there is a copy of another letter enclosed with this letter.

Answer: **B**

Why: The abbreviation "cc:" means *carbon copy*. With computer processing, the abbreviation "cc:" is also proper and means *correspondence copy*. This is used to indicate that a duplicate or copy of the letter has been sent. The abbreviation is placed at the bottom left margin of the letter. The name of the person follows the abbreviation (e.g., cc: James Jones, M.D.).

Review: Yes ❑ No ❑

---

16. When mail arrives at the office, the first step in processing the mail is to:
   A. record all insurance payments.
   B. distribute the mail to the appropriate staff members.
   C. review it with the physician.
   D. dispose of advertisements.
   E. date stamp each item of mail.

Answer: **E**

Why: Before anything else is done with the mail, the mail is opened and stamped with the current date. This records the date it was received by the office in case there is a question in the future about the arrival date of materials. After that, the medical assistant or medical administrative specialist can sort the mail and determine distribution of the remaining mail.

Review: Yes ❑ No ❑

17. The process of converting the dictated word of the health care provider to a word-processed form is:
    A. dictation.
    B. recording.
    C. transcription.
    D. documentation.

Answer: **C**

Why: Transcription is the process of converting the health care provider's dictated words to a word-processed form.

Review: Yes ❑ No ❑

---

18. The style of letter in which the first sentence of each paragraph is indented five spaces is:
    A. full block.
    B. modified block.
    C. semiblock.
    D. simplified.
    E. block.

Answer: **C**

Why: The semiblock style is similar to the modified block except the first sentence of each paragraph is indented five spaces. This style is less formal than the full block but more formal than a simplified letter. All of these types of letters use the block format.

Review: Yes ❑ No ❑

---

19. When a professional letter requires more than one page, the pages following the first page:
    A. are printed on embossed letterhead the same as the first page.
    B. are not numbered.
    C. do not include the date of the letter.
    D. are the same paper as the first page with no letterhead printing.

Answer: **D**

Why: A professional letter is processed on quality bond stationery with the first page containing the physician's name, address, and telephone number. All pages following the first page should contain the name of the person to whom the letter is addressed, the date of the letter, and the page number.

Review: Yes ❑ No ❑

---

20. The inside address of a professional letter is the:
    A. address of the sending group practice.
    B. recipient's address written with abbreviations to save space.
    C. physician's home address printed at the left margin.
    D. physician's office address.
    E. recipient's address written without abbreviations.

Answer: **E**

Why: The inside address is the address of the person or company to whom the letter is being sent. It should not contain any abbreviations.

Review: Yes ❑ No ❑

---

21. If there are materials included in the envelope with the letter, this should be noted:
    A. below the inside address.
    B. within the body of the letter only.
    C. two lines below the reference initials.
    D. four lines below the complimentary closing.

Answer: **C**

Why: If there are materials to be mailed with the letter, it should be noted by using the abbreviation "Enc." or the word "Enclosures" followed by the name of the document or the number if there is more than one.

Review: Yes ❑ No ❑

---

22. The classification of mail used for at least 200 pieces of promotional information is:
    A. Certified Mail.
    B. Second-Class Mail.
    C. Standard Mail.
    D. Registered Mail.
    E. Priority Mail.

Answer: **C**

Why: Standard Mail is also known as bulk mail. This is a classification used to mail promotional pieces such as flyers or brochures. There must be a minimum of 200 pieces to qualify for this class of mail.

Review: Yes ❑ No ❑

23. A postage meter is a:
    A. device used to weigh letters or packages.
    B. scale to determine the classification of mail for letters.
    C. machine that prints postage onto mail pieces or onto an approved label.
    D. machine used to scan zip codes.

Answer: **C**

Why: A postage meter is a postage-printing machine or system used in the home or office. Meters print postage directly onto mail pieces or onto an approved label that you affix to your mail piece.

Review: Yes ❑ No ❑

---

24. The keyed signature is typed:
    A. four lines below the complimentary closing.
    B. two lines before the return address.
    C. two lines after the reference line.
    D. four lines below the salutation.
    E. six lines below the salutation.

Answer: **A**

Why: The keyed signature is the typed full name of the person signing the letter. It is placed four lines below the complimentary closing to allow space for the handwritten signature.

Review: Yes ❑ No ❑

---

25. The letterhead on stationery should include the following EXCEPT the:
    A. physician's name.
    B. office address and office telephone number.
    C. physician's home telephone number.
    D. medical group's name.

Answer: **C**

Why: The physician's personal information should not appear on professional business stationery used for office correspondence. The physician's home telephone number is private and usually unlisted.

Review: Yes ❑ No ❑

13

Medical Insurance

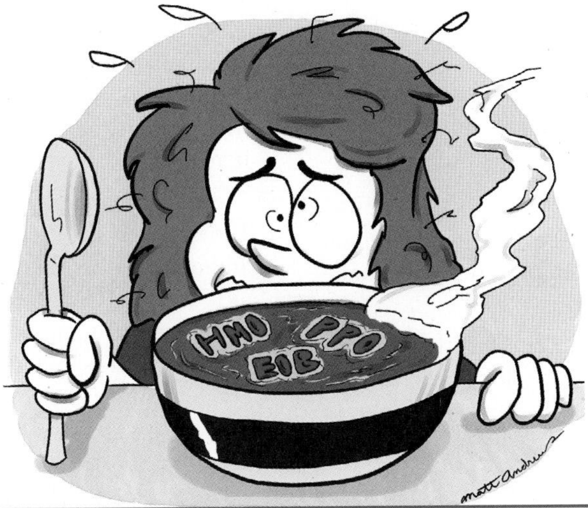

REVIEW TIP

As you read this chapter, write any definition or insurance type that requires further review on an index card or piece of paper (definition on the front, answer on the back); writing the information helps reinforce it. Go over the cards whenever you have a "learning moment" or at a set study time. This is a good exercise for study groups.

The intent of medical insurance is to provide financial protection for costs associated with sickness or injury. Because of the complex American social and health systems, the types of medical insurance and payers are varied and dependent on eligibility criteria.

Health care is one of the few services paid for by a party other than the one receiving the actual service. The insurance company or responsible governmental agency or private entity is known as the **third-party payer**—the party that pays the second party (doctor, hospital, pharmacy, etc.) for the medical bills of the first party (patient or insured individual). The term *third-party administrator* is sometimes used.

This chapter is organized differently from previous chapters. The types and sources of insurance are described with information that has "exam probability." The "Terms" section contains the remaining materials and definitions for medical insurance. *Do not skip it.*

COMMON TYPES OF MEDICAL INSURANCE PLANS

An insurance company (carrier), whether private or governmental, may offer all common plan types or a hybrid of multiple types. The medical assistant and medical administrative specialist must know not only the insurance company but also the plan covering the patient. Each plan has different costs and benefits to the patient and different payments to the health care provider.

- Health maintenance organization (HMO)—an association that provides all care to the insured person for a fixed fee, usually paid for by the insured or employer through a monthly premium; a copayment may or may not be required
- Indemnity—plan through which the insured person selects his or her own health care providers; an established

amount or percentage of care costs is paid by the insurance plan on a fee-for-service basis; usually has deductibles and limits

- Preferred provider organization (PPO)—a list of physicians, hospitals, and other health care services approved by the insurance plan to provide these services at a discounted rate
- Major medical—type of insurance that does not cover primary care, but covers costs associated with significant illness or injury (e.g., hospitalization, surgeries); premiums are lower than full-coverage insurance

SOURCES OF MEDICAL INSURANCE

- **Commercial**—for-profit companies that provide health insurance for a fee to individuals or groups; Blue Cross and Blue Shield is perhaps the most widely known
  - Eligibility
    - Individual plan—coverage provided for a person and eligible dependents when premiums are made and designated criteria are met
    - Group plan—generally associated with employment; coverage provided for employee and usually dependents; premiums may be paid by employer or shared with the employee
  - Benefits—dependent on plan selection, premiums, and eligibility criteria
- Medicare—federal insurance program established in 1965 under the Social Security Act (Title 18) and administered by the Centers for Medicare and Medicaid Services (CMS), formerly called HCFA; primarily designed for eligible citizens age 65 years and older
  - Eligibility
    - Persons and spouses of persons age 65 years or older who are eligible for Social Security benefits
    - Retired railroad workers
    - Persons receiving Social Security benefits
    - Persons with end-stage kidney disease who have contributed to Social Security
  - Benefits
    - Part A—benefit is automatic when eligibility and deductible are met; covers hospital inpatient costs, hospice, limited nursing facility stays, and home health
    - Part B—optional benefit; requires premiums, deductibles, and coinsurance; covers physician costs, outpatient services, durable medical equipment, and medical supplies
    - Part C—formerly called Medicare + Choice, now referred to as Medicare Advantage; requires participants to be covered under both Medicare Part A and Medicare Part B; allows participant to choose a Medicare Advantage plan, which is HMO-type coverage
    - Part D—optional benefit; covers approved pharmaceuticals
  - **Advanced Beneficiary Notice of Noncoverage (ABN)**—notification to the beneficiary (person insured by Medicare) of their potential liability for payment of services under certain conditions that are not covered or approved for payment by Medicare; i.e., frequency of coverage such as a maximum number of glucose tests that will be approved for payment within a specific time frame
- **Medigap**—also called Medicare Supplement Insurance; commercial medical insurance intended to cover Medicare deductible, coinsurance, and other uncovered items
- Medicaid—federal insurance program established in 1965 under the Social Security Act (Title 19) and administered by the Centers for Medicare and Medicaid Services (CMS), formerly called HCFA; eligibility, benefits, and name differ from state to state (e.g., in California, it is called MediCal); provides health coverage for the categorically needy
  - Eligibility—low-income (calculated as a percentage of poverty level, which differs from state to state) families and individuals who are citizens or, in some cases, select refugees and immigrants
  - Benefits—minimum benefits are mandated by the federal government, and other benefits are defined by the states; minimum medically necessary benefits include:
    - Primary care
    - Early, periodic screening, diagnosis, and treatment (EPSDT) for children
    - Hospitalizations
    - Outpatient services
    - Family planning
    - Skilled nursing facilities (SNFs)
    - Medi/Medi—persons eligible for both Medicare and Medicaid (dual eligibility); Medicaid is *always* the payer of last resort
- **TRICARE**—formerly CHAMPUS; offers three health care benefits plans sponsored by the federal government, primarily for spouses and dependents of service men and women
  - TRICARE Standard—program under TRICARE that automatically enrolls all eligible beneficiaries
  - TRICARE Prime—PPO-type TRICARE option with an annual deductible
  - TRICARE Extra—HMO-type TRICARE option with an annual deductible and copays

- Eligibility
  - Spouses and dependents of active military personnel
  - Military retirees, spouses, and dependents
  - Spouses and dependents of deceased active or retired military personnel
  - Former spouses of active or retired military personnel who meet requirements
  - Spouses, former spouses, and dependents of court-martialed active-duty service personnel
  - Spouses, former spouses, and dependents of retirement-eligible military personnel who lost eligibility as a result of child or spousal abuse
  - Other select individuals
- Benefits
  - Hospitalization
  - Maternity care
  - Inpatient and outpatient treatment for mental illness
  - Physician services
  - Diagnostic testing
  - Emergency services, including ambulances
  - Family planning
  - Durable medical equipment
  - Home health care

■ **CHAMPVA** (Civilian Health and Medical Program of the Veterans Administration)—a service benefit program with no premiums for select family members of specific veterans

- Eligibility
  - Spouses and dependents of military personnel with permanent, total, service-related disability
  - Spouses and dependents of military personnel who died from a service-related disability
- Benefits—the same as TRICARE Standard

■ **Workers' compensation**—medical and disability insurance that covers employees in the event of a work-related injury, illness, or death

- Eligibility
  - Federal coverage—federal employees, coal miners, and maritime workers
  - State coverage—all workers not covered by federal statutes
- Benefits
  - Medical treatment related to disability, including prostheses
  - Temporary disability payments
  - Permanent disability payments
  - Death benefits to survivors

Box 13-1

Breaking Down Relative Value Reimbursement

RBRVS = the **system** for reimbursement
RVS = the list of **procedures** with the (relative) value for each
RVU = the **component** that is multiplied by a factor to determine the (relative) value ($)

COMMON METHODS OF DETERMINING INSURANCE PAYMENT

■ Fee schedule—list of a physician's customary charges; may incorporate insurance plan–specific discounts

■ Resource-based relative value system or scale (RBRVS)—a method used to establish physician fees for specific medical services by assigning worth to a relative value unit (RVU) (Box 13-1)

- RVU—a component (e.g., time) that is multiplied by a monetary conversion factor to establish physician payment; it includes the physician's:
  - Service
  - Overhead
  - Cost of malpractice insurance
- Relative value studies (RVS)—relative values listed by health care procedure codes; allow comparison of reimbursement for different codes

■ Usual, customary, and reasonable (UCR)—a method used by insurance carriers to establish provider payments based on a fee compendium of other like providers

- Prevailing fee—the usual, customary, and reasonable fees of like providers in the same geographic area
- Copayment—a portion of the cost to the provider (usually a flat fee) owed by the insured at the time of service; may also be called *coinsurance*; routine waiving of copayment by the medical office is against federal guidelines for Medicare and Medicaid

■ Capitation—payment made to a provider based on a fixed amount per enrollee assigned to that provider regardless of services provided

■ Diagnostic-related groups (DRG)—a classification of diagnoses used to determine hospital payment for Medicare inpatients; this method does not take into account length of stay (LOS)

■ **Preauthorization/Precertification**—under some health plans, individuals are required to receive advance authorization from the insurance provider for particular medical services; usually required for referral to a physician specialist

ELECTRONIC HEALTH CARE CLAIMS

- Claims are transmitted electronically from the provider's computer to the Medicare contractor's computer
- When submitting electronic claims, the provider must use a computer with software that meets electronic filing requirements and national standards established under Health Insurance Portability and Accountability Act (HIPAA)
- Claims are reviewed by the Medicare contractor for accuracy of submission, and the entire batch of submitted claims may be denied and returned for correction even if one claim is found with an area of noncompliance with submission standards

TERMS

Medical Insurance Review

The following list reviews the terms discussed in this chapter and other important terms that you may see on the exam.

Advanced Beneficiary Notice of Noncoverage (ABN) notification to the beneficiary (insured by Medicare) of their potential liability for payment of services under certain conditions that are not covered or approved for payment by Medicare

assignment of benefits authorization for the insurance company to send insurance payments directly to the health care provider; also, an agreement with Medicare that the provider will accept the remittance as full payment

beneficiary a person eligible to receive insurance benefits

birthday rule a method used to determine the primary insurance carrier when children are covered under both parents' insurance plans; the parent whose birthday falls earliest in the calendar year becomes the primary carrier

capitation a health care insurance payment made to a provider based on a fixed amount per enrollee assigned to that provider, regardless of services provided

carrier insurance company that provides the policy and benefits

coinsurance a percentage or an established dollar amount of costs contractually assumed by the insured party

copayment a portion of the cost to the provider owed by the insured at the time of service; may be referred to as *coinsurance*

deductible an established dollar amount of actual costs of medical services that must be paid by the insured party before the insurance carrier will cover costs; usually applies every year

dependent a person covered under the primary insured's policy

diagnostic-related groups (DRG) a classification of diagnoses used to determine hospital payment for Medicare inpatients

exclusion conditions or circumstances that are not covered under the insurance plan

explanation of benefits (EOB) a claim summary indicating what services were covered, what was not covered, and why; also referred to as *remittance advice*

fee-for-service a payment made to the health care provider for each service rendered

fee schedule a list of a physician's customary charges; may incorporate insurance plan–specific discounts

health maintenance organization (HMO) an association that provides all care to the insured person for a fixed fee, usually paid for by the insured or employer through a monthly premium; a copayment may or may not be required

indemnity a plan through which the insured person selects his or her own health care providers; an established amount or percentage of care cost is paid by the insurance plan on a fee-for-service basis; usually has deductibles and limits

major medical a type of insurance that does not cover primary care but covers costs associated with significant illness or injury, such as hospitalization or surgeries; premiums are lower than full-coverage insurance

Medicaid provides health coverage for the categorically needy; a federal insurance program established in 1965 under the Social Security Act (Title 19) and administered by the Centers for Medicare and Medicaid Services (CMS), formerly called HCFA; eligibility, benefits, and name differ from state to state (e.g., in California, it is called Medi-Cal)

Medicare primarily for people older than age 65 and others eligible for Social Security; federal insurance program established in 1965 under the Social Security Act (Title 18) and administered by the Centers for Medicare and Medicaid Services (CMS), formerly called HCFA

point of service facility where the health care service took place (e.g., physician's office, emergency department)

preauthorization process of obtaining approval for a service through the individual's insurance company by establishing that it is a medical necessity

precertification process of determining whether a service is covered under the insured person's plan

predetermination a process of ascertaining the amount the insurance carrier will pay for a specific service

preexisting condition a diagnosed and treated health condition that the patient had before obtaining insurance

preferred provider organization (PPO) a plan allowing the insured person to select physicians, hospitals, and other health care services from an approved list issued by the insurance plan to provide care at a discounted rate

premium a dollar amount the insured person pays for insurance coverage

prevailing fee the usual, customary, and reasonable fees of like providers in the same geographic area

primary care provider (PCP) physician contracted through a specific insurance plan to provide or to coordinate the care of all patients assigned through the insurance carrier

quality improvement organization (QIO) formerly called a peer review organization (PRO); group of professionals that monitor health care treatments, length of hospital stays (LOS), outcomes, and other indicators for appropriateness and improvement opportunities

relative value studies (RVS) relative values listed by health care procedure codes; allows comparison of reimbursement for different codes

relative value unit (RVU) the component (e.g., time) that is multiplied by a monetary conversion factor to establish physician payment for the resource-based relative value system or scale

resource-based relative value system/scale (RBRVS) a system that calculates physician reimbursement for services using relative value units (RVUs)

Temporary Assistance to Needy Families (TANF) formerly known as Assistance to Families with Dependent Children (AFDC); the federal welfare program

third-party payer the entity (usually the insurance company) that pays the second party (doctor, hospital, pharmacy, etc.) for the medical bills of the first party (patient or insured individual); also referred to as the *third-party administrator*

TRICARE formerly CHAMPUS; health care benefit plans provided by the federal government, primarily for spouses and dependents of service men and women

usual, customary, and reasonable (UCR) a method used by insurance carriers to establish provider payments based on a compendium of other like provider fees

utilization review a process of reviewing and monitoring a provider's usage of health care resources for appropriateness and comparison with peers

waiting period the time an individual is required to wait before being eligible for insurance benefits

waiver a special policy provision that forgoes a stipulation or requirement

workers' compensation medical and disability insurance to cover employees in the event of a work-related injury, illness, or death

REVIEW QUESTIONS

All questions are relevant for the CMA (AAMA), RMA (AMT), and CMAS (AMT) exams.

1. When a patient gives written authorization for reimbursement to the physician for billed charges, this is called:
   A. coordination of benefits.
   B. capitation.
   C. assignment of benefits.
   D. copayment.

Answer: **C**

Why: Assignment of benefits is necessary if the physician agrees to wait for payment from the insurance company for billed charges.

Review: Yes ❑ No ❑

---

2. Coordination of benefits means:
   A. the patient pays a specific amount of money for medical services before the insurance pays.
   B. one insurance plan will work with other insurance plans to determine how much each plan pays.
   C. there is a flat fee paid for each service.
   D. there is a deductible required by the patient before payment from the insurance is made.
   E. each insurance company will pay an equal amount of the patient's bill.

Answer: **B**

Why: Some patients have more than one benefit or insurance plan. Usually there is a primary carrier, and the other becomes the secondary. The primary carrier determines an amount it will pay on a claim, and the secondary carrier will then determine the amount of the remaining balance that it will pay.

Review: Yes ❑ No ❑

---

3. The person who is covered by a benefits plan is the:
   A. employee.
   B. carrier.
   C. administrator.
   D. insured.

Answer: **D**

Why: The insured is the person who is covered by the insurance benefits. This person could be an employee, but this would have to involve an employer-sponsored benefits plan. An administrator and a carrier are persons involved directly with the insurance provider.

Review: Yes ❑ No ❑

---

4. A person's spouse or child who is covered under the benefits plan is called the:
   A. group member.
   B. coinsured.
   C. primary carrier.
   D. carrier.
   E. dependent.

Answer: **E**

Why: The dependent is related to the group member, the primary person covered, either as a family member or as an employee.

Review: Yes ❑ No ❑

---

5. The amount that will be paid by the insurance plan for each procedure or service is based on the:
   A. coinsurance.
   B. capitation.
   C. deductible.
   D. fee schedule.

Answer: **D**

Why: A fee schedule is a list of a physician's customary charges, which may incorporate insurance plan–specific discounts. Coinsurance refers to the portion the patient is responsible for after the benefit plan pays a percentage of the eligible benefits and the member pays the deductible. Capitation is a system of payment used by managed care plans and refers to a fixed, per capita amount for each patient enrolled over a stated period. The deductible is the amount the insured must pay each calendar year before the plan begins to pay benefits.

Review: Yes ❑ No ❑

6. A government-sponsored program that provides health benefits to low-income or indigent persons is:
A. CHAMPUS.
B. CHAMPVA.
C. Medicare.
D. Medicaid.
E. Blue Cross and Blue Shield

Answer: **D**

Why: Medicare, CHAMPUS, and CHAMPVA are all government-sponsored insurance programs, but only Medicaid determines eligibility based on income. States typically use the same criteria as their state welfare assistance programs. Blue Cross and Blue Shield is an independent health insurer.

Review: Yes ❑ No ❑

---

7. Expenses resulting from work-related illness or injury are usually covered by:
A. Medicare.
B. HMOs.
C. workers' compensation.
D. employee's health insurance.

Answer: **C**

Why: Employees in every state are covered by a workers' compensation program administered by the state. Medicare is a federal insurance program, primarily for people older than 65. An HMO is an association that provides all care to the insured person for a fixed fee. Employee's health insurance refers to an insurance program that an employee may voluntarily enroll in but that does not usually cover illness or injury determined to be work-related.

Review: Yes ❑ No ❑

---

8. The statement issued to the provider and the patient that lists the details of a payment that has been made by the insurance plan is the:
A. fee schedule.
B. coordination of benefits.
C. assignment of benefits.
D. explanation of benefits.
E. deductible.

Answer: **D**

Why: The explanation of benefits (EOB) tells how the payment was made, including the deductible and coinsurance information. The EOB statement may show several claims that have processed during a particular period. A fee schedule is a list of a physician's customary charges. Coordination of benefits occurs when a person has insurance coverage from more than one company. The primary carrier will work with other insurance plans to determine how much each plan pays. Assignment of benefits occurs when a patient gives written authorization for reimbursement to the physician for billed charges. The deductible is an established dollar amount of actual costs of medical services that must be paid by the insured party before the insurance carrier will cover costs.

Review: Yes ❑ No ❑

---

9. If a patient is diagnosed with a disease before the effective date of the insurance plan, it is a(n):
A. preexisting condition.
B. crossover claim.
C. exclusion.
D. capitation.

Answer: **A**

Why: A preexisting condition is any illness or disease that was diagnosed before the effective date of the insurance plan. A typical illness that may be considered preexisting is cancer.

Review: Yes ❑ No ❑

10. The amount of eligible charges each patient must pay each calendar year before the plan begins to pay benefits is called:
    A. coinsurance.
    B. exclusion.
    C. eligibility.
    D. capitation.
    E. deductible.

Answer: **E**

Why: It is the patient's responsibility to pay the deductible amount before the insurance benefits will pay a percentage of the allowable charges. Most deductible amounts are between $1500 and $2500 per patient per year.

Review: Yes ❑ No ❑

---

11. Medicare is a federal health insurance program for:
    A. anyone over 62 years of age.
    B. disabled workers who are at least 65 years of age.
    C. blind individuals who are at least 50 years of age.
    D. individuals 65 years of age or older who are retired and on Social Security.

Answer: **D**

Why: Medicare is available to any individual who is 65 years of age or older who is retired and on Social Security or who retired from a railroad or civil service. Blind and disabled individuals receiving Social Security benefits have no age restrictions.

Review: Yes ❑ No ❑

---

12. Medicare Part A provides coverage for:
    A. clinical laboratory services.
    B. physician's office services.
    C. hospitalization.
    D. physician's hospital services.
    E. outpatient referral fee for a specialist.

Answer: **C**

Why: Medicare Part A primarily covers the cost of inpatient hospitalization for the hospital room and board, general nursing, and hospital services and supplies. All of the physician's charges are covered under Part B.

Review: Yes ❑ No ❑

---

13. The process of determining whether a service or procedure is covered by the insurance provider is called:
    A. coordination of benefits.
    B. precertification.
    C. capitation.
    D. assignment of benefits.

Answer: **B**

Why: Contacting the insurance carrier for precertification determines whether the patient's insurance company will pay for a specific service or procedure. The patient may still be responsible for a portion of the charges after the insurance plan has paid a percentage of the charges. If the carrier does not precertify the service or procedure, the patient may be responsible for all the charges.

Review: Yes ❑ No ❑

---

14. The medical bills of spouses and children of veterans with total, permanent, service-connected disabilities are covered under:
    A. Blue Cross.
    B. HMO.
    C. workers' compensation.
    D. HCFA.
    E. CHAMPVA.

Answer: **E**

Why: The Civilian Health and Medical Program of the Veterans Administration (CHAMPVA) is a federal government–sponsored insurance that covers veterans' spouses and children. Blue Cross and Blue Shield is a private insurance company; an HMO is a type of insurance plan. Workers' compensation covers a patient who has a work-related illness or injury. HCFA is the Health Care Finance Administration (now called the Centers for Medicare and Medicaid Services, or CMS).

Review: Yes ❑ No ❑

15. The process of making a payment to a provider based on a fixed amount per enrollee assigned to that provider regardless of services provided is:
A. exclusion.
B. deductible.
C. capitation.
D. predetermination.

Answer: C

Why: Capitation is the process of paying a provider based on an established amount per person enrolled in the plan regardless of services rendered.

Review: Yes ❑ No ❑

---

16. A group of physicians who review cases for appropriateness of hospitalizations and discharges is called:
A. relative value studies.
B. preferred provider organization.
C. quality improvement organization.
D. third-party payer.
E. state medical board.

Answer: C

Why: Physicians and specialists review cases from hospitalizations to determine whether the patient's care was provided in the most cost-effective setting. Many inpatient procedures are performed on an outpatient basis to save the patient excessive charges from an inpatient stay. The quality improvement organization (QIO), formerly referred to as the peer review organization (PRO), evaluates cases to ensure the procedures are necessary and cost-effective.

Review: Yes ❑ No ❑

---

17. A health maintenance organization is best described as:
A. a group of physicians who have a contract to provide services to participating patients for a predetermined fee.
B. independently practicing physicians providing services to patients covered under all types of insurance.
C. a group of physicians who are partners in the same corporation.
D. a group of physicians who specialize in wellness.

Answer: A

Why: An HMO (health maintenance organization) comprises physicians who work under contract to provide services to the subscribers of the plan. The plan is set up on a contracted fee-for-service basis, also known as capitation.

Review: Yes ❑ No ❑

---

18. A database or list of charges for each procedure indicating the charge of the majority of physicians in a geographic area is referred to as:
A. utilization review.
B. usual, customary, and reasonable.
C. coordination of benefits.
D. explanation of benefits.
E. capitation.

Answer: B

Why: UCR (usual, customary, and reasonable) refers to the typical charges for services for physicians. Charges that exceed the UCR limit are considered unreasonable and are not eligible for reimbursement.

Review: Yes ❑ No ❑

---

19. Medicare Part B does not cover:
A. physician office visits.
B. diagnostic laboratory services.
C. hospitalization.
D. outpatient x-rays.

Answer: C

Why: Part A of Medicare covers hospital charges and services except for the physician charges that are covered under Part B.

Review: Yes ❑ No ❑

20. Health benefits policies are purchased by an individual by paying the:
    A. premium.
    B. deductible.
    C. copayment.
    D. coinsurance.
    E. exclusion.

Answer: **A**

Why: A premium is an annual amount charged by the insurance plan to enroll an individual for the health benefits of the policy. When an employee subscribes to health insurance through his or her workplace, a portion of the premium may be taken directly from each paycheck.

Review: Yes ❑ No ❑

---

21. A primary care physician, or PCP, is:
    A. only authorized to accept assignment of benefits.
    B. a specialist who accepts referral patients.
    C. not authorized to accept Medicare patients.
    D. a general practitioner who oversees patients in an HMO or PPO.

Answer: **D**

Why: A PCP may be a general practitioner, pediatrician, family practitioner, or general internist who refers patients to see specialists for services as needed.

Review: Yes ❑ No ❑

---

22. A condition or circumstance for which the health insurance policy will not provide benefits is a(n):
    A. benefit.
    B. exclusion.
    C. review.
    D. waiting period.
    E. capitation.

Answer: **B**

Why: An exclusion is any condition or circumstance that is not covered by the insurance plan. For example, some insurance plans do not cover cosmetic surgical procedures.

Review: Yes ❑ No ❑

---

23. Insurance coverage that provides a specific monthly or weekly income when an individual becomes unable to work because of an illness or injury is:
    A. workers' compensation insurance.
    B. disability income insurance.
    C. TRICARE insurance.
    D. major medical insurance.

Answer: **B**

Why: Disability income insurance provides temporary or permanent income during a period when an individual cannot work because of illness or injury. This is not to be confused with workers' compensation insurance, which provides coverage of medical costs incurred from work-related injuries or illness. TRICARE is an insurance plan for spouses and dependents of service men and women provided by the federal government. Major medical insurance covers the costs associated with significant illness or injury, but it does not provide income for an individual if he or she is unable to work.

Review: Yes ❑ No ❑

---

24. The amount of money owed by the insured to the provider at the time of service is called:
    A. capitation.
    B. exclusion.
    C. fee-for-service.
    D. indemnity.
    E. copayment.

Answer: **E**

Why: A copayment may also be called coinsurance. It refers to the amount of money that the patient is responsible to pay to the provider at the time of service. It is usually a fixed dollar amount per visit.

Review: Yes ❑ No ❑

25. When a dependent child is covered by the benefit plans of both parents, determination of the primary carrier is based on the:
A. coordination of benefits.
B. coinsurance.
C. assignment of benefits.
D. birthday rule.

Answer: **D**

Why: The birthday rule is based on which parent's birthday falls earliest in the calendar year. The insurance plan carried by that parent becomes the primary carrier.

Review: Yes ❑ No ❑

---

26. In order to be eligible for Medicare Part C, the participant must be enrolled in
A. Medicare Part B and Medicare Part D.
B. an HMO plan.
C. Medicare Part A and Medicare Part B.
D. Medicaid.
E. Medigap.

Answer: **C**

Why: Medicare Part C requires participants to be covered under both Medicare Part A and Medicare Part B. Medicare Part C allows the participant to choose a Medicare Advantage plan, which is HMO-type coverage. Enrollment in an HMO is not a criterion for eligibility for Medicare Part C. Medigap is a supplement to Medicare insurance that assists with the payment of coinsurance, copayments, or deductibles.

---

27. The Medicare part specifically designed to provide pharmaceutical coverage is:
A. Part A.
B. Part B.
C. Part C.
D. Part D.

Answer: **D**

Why: Part A primarily covers hospitalization, Part B primarily covers outpatient care, Part C is HMO-type coverage, and Part D is designed to provide pharmaceutical coverage.

Review: Yes ❑ No ❑

---

28. A hospital payment system that categorizes patients by diagnosis and treatment is referred to as:
A. ICD.
B. CPT.
C. UCR.
D. HCPCS.
E. DRG.

Answer: **E**

Why: Diagnosis-related groups (DRGs) are established by a comparison of patients with medically related diagnoses or treatments.

Review: Yes ❑ No ❑

---

29. UCR provider payments are based on:
A. what the majority of physicians in a specific geographic area charge for procedures.
B. state laws where the physician practices medicine.
C. the maximum amount paid by other insurance companies for similar procedures.
D. recommendations of the federal government.

Answer: **A**

Why: Usual, customary, and reasonable charges (UCR) are based on what the average or majority of physicians in a specific region would charge for the same or similar procedure. Any amount that exceeds the UCR rate may be considered ineligible for payment.

Review: Yes ❑ No ❑

30. When a Medicare patient is told that he or she may be responsible for payment of services not covered by Medicare, the physician's office should inform the patient and have the patient sign a form called a/an:
    A. EOB.
    B. HMO.
    C. ABN.
    D. DRG.
    E. CPT.

Answer: **C**

Why: ABN is an advanced beneficiary notice that is the formal notification to the patient that certain services may not be covered by Medicare. EOB is an explanation of benefits that were covered for services. HMO is a type of insurance plan, and DRG is a classification of diagnoses used to determine hospital payment for Medicare inpatients.

Review: Yes ❑ No ❑

14

Medical Coding and Claims

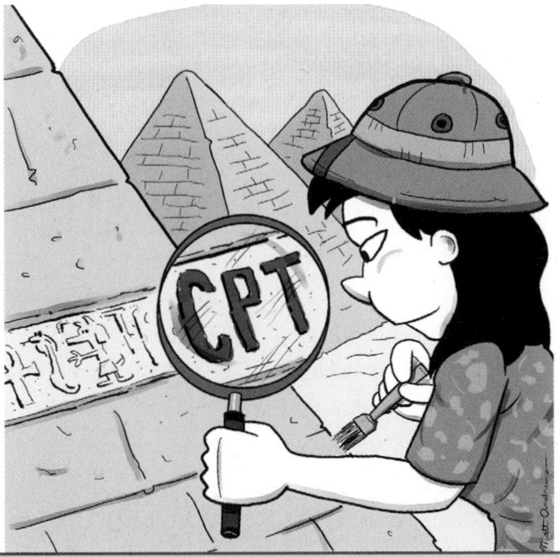

REVIEW TIP

If you are not comfortable with coding, while reviewing this chapter, use the current International Classification of Diseases, coding book, a Current Procedural Terminology (CPT) coding book, and a Health Care Procedural Coding System (HCPCS) manual that includes Level II codes. This will simplify definitions and explanations. Further explanation of these manuals and their contents is included in this chapter.

Medical coding is a process that assigns numeric and alphabetic identifiers to illnesses and injuries, medical procedures and services, drugs, and equipment. The two major coding systems are diagnosis coding and procedural coding. It is important that the diagnosis and the procedure be compatible. For example, a woman should have a pregnancy diagnosis to have a cesarean section surgical procedure. The insurance claim is the submission of these medical codes and other information for reimbursement to the health care provider.

The organization of this chapter is similar to Chapter 13. The types of coding are described with information that has "exam probability." The "Terms" section contains the remaining information and definitions. *Do not skip it.*

PROCEDURAL CODING

The systems used for coding health care professional services, supplies, pharmaceuticals, equipment, and other materials are referred to as *procedural coding*. These systems provide uniform methods for collecting data and determining payment. The American Medical Association (AMA) developed the **Current Procedural Terminology (CPT)** coding system, and the federal Health Care Finance Administration (HCFA) developed two additional levels. The CPT codes are included in the HCFA coding system and are considered Level I. Each level is described in more detail later in the chapter but is listed below to provide an overview.

- Health Care Procedural Coding System (HCPCS [pronounced "hicpics"])—a method developed by the

Box 14-1

Example of CPT Coding Process for Incision and Drainage of a Hematoma of the Skin

Follow the steps using a CPT code book.

1. Go to "skin" in index; read down to "incision and drainage," which gives you a range of codes or individual codes (e.g., 10040–10180).
2. Turn to the section with the codes suggested from the index, which will be under the "Surgery" section; "Integumentary System."
3. Read the suggested codes until you find the one that matches your procedure.
4. Read and follow any notes and cross-references (in this case, there are none).
5. Select the most descriptive and complete code, which in this case is 10140.

Health Care Finance Administration (now the Centers for Medicare and Medicaid Services, or CMS) for coding procedures and other services delivered to Medicare patients. There are three levels:

- Level I—consists of codes for procedures and professional services; the codes are the same as the CPT codes
- Level II—consists of codes for services not covered in the CPT codes: supplies, drugs, and other reimbursable equipment and materials
- Level III—consists of codes for regionally approved Medicare/Medicaid procedures or new procedures that have not been assigned a permanent CPT code

CPT CODING

CPT coding was first published by the AMA in 1966. Each procedure code contains five numeric digits. The manual is updated annually and organized into six sections representing the major clinical areas, each with a range of five-digit numbers. The actual numbers may change, but the range is reserved for that section, whether or not all the numbers are in use.

■ Sections

- Evaluation and management (E&M)—99200 to 99499
- Anesthesia—00100 to 01999
- Surgery—10000 to 69999
- Radiology—70000 to 79999
- Pathology and laboratory—80000 to 89999
- Medicine—90000 to 99199

Box 14-2

Examples of CPT Coding Modifiers

A cholecystectomy was performed by one physician, and postoperative management was performed by another.

Example 1

The physician performing the surgery would use the following:
CPT code: 47600-54
(47600 for the cholecystectomy and -54 as the modifier indicating the physician performed the surgery only)

Example 2

The physician providing postoperative care would use the following:
CPT code: 47600-55
(47600 for the cholecystectomy and -55 as the modifier indicating the physician is providing postoperative care only)

■ General steps for CPT coding (Box 14-1):

1. Identify the procedure or service to be coded.
2. Locate the term(s) in the CPT index.
3. Review term, subterms, and code numbers for descriptions that specifically match all the components of the procedure to be coded.
4. Locate codes in the body of the manual as directed by the index; do *not* code directly from the index.
5. Read and follow any notes and cross-references.
6. Select the most descriptive and complete code.
7. Select a modifier when applicable.

■ Modifier—an addition to the initial CPT code that identifies certain circumstances (Box 14-2)

- Common modifiers—identified by the initial CPT code followed by a dash and two numbers
  - -24: unrelated E&M service
  - -50: bilateral procedure
  - -54: surgical care only
  - -55: postoperative care only
  - -56: preoperative care only
  - -80: assistant surgeon
- Common HCPCS modifiers also used in CPT coding
  - -E1—upper left eyelid
  - -E2—lower left eyelid
  - -E3—upper right eyelid
  - -E4—lower right eyelid
  - -FA—left thumb

Box 14-3

Example of Coding for New and Established Patients

Coding for office or other outpatient visit of patient, which requires:

- A problem-focused history,
- A problem-focused examination, and
- Straightforward medical decision making.
- Use CPT code 99201 for a new patient.
- Use CPT code 99211 for an established patient.

    - -F1 to -F4—left fingers, digits 2 through 5
    - -F5—right thumb
    - -F6 to -F9—right fingers, digits 2 through 5
    - -TA—left great toe
    - -T1 to -T4—left toes, digits 2 through 5
    - -T5—right great toe
    - -T6 to -T9—right toes, digits 2 through 5
- E&M section—the E&M section is unique; it covers services (e.g., counseling) rather than, in most cases, actual procedures, and requires specific components based on assessment and judgment; E&M codes also specify whether the patient is "new" or "established" (Box 14-3)
- Common E&M terms
    - New patient—a person who has not received care from the physician or another physician of the same specialty in the same group practice within 3 years
    - Established patient—a person who has received care from the physician or another physician of the same specialty in the same group practice within 3 years
    - Concurrent care—similar services provided to the same patient on the same day by more than one physician
    - Critical care (definition used for coding professional services)—intensive care in acute life-threatening conditions requiring constant bedside attention by the physician
    - Counseling (definition used for coding professional services)—discussion with patient or family concerning diagnosis, recommendations, risks, benefits, prognosis, options, and necessary condition-related education
    - Consultation—services rendered by a physician whose opinion or advice is requested by another physician or agency in the evaluation or treatment of a patient's illness or suspected problem
- Components—E&M codes usually involve five components: three major and two contributory (Table 14-1)
    - Examination (major)
    - Problem severity (major)
    - Medical decision making (MDR) (major)
    - Coordination of care and counseling (contributory)
    - Time (contributory)
- Levels of care—each of the five components involves levels of care ranging from minimal to high
    - Problem focused (PF)—minimal; only involves affected body area or one organ system
    - Expanded problem focused—low; involves an affected body area or one organ system and symptoms related to other body areas
    - Detailed—moderate; involves the affected body area or areas and related body system(s)
    - Comprehensive—moderate to high or high; involves multiple systems or complex involvement of one organ system

HCPCS LEVEL II CODES

HCPCS Level II provides coding for services not covered in the CPT codes: supplies, pharmaceuticals, ambulance services, and other reimbursable equipment and materials.

The codes begin with a letter (A–V), followed by four numeric digits. A question concerning Level II codes is usually found on the exams; know the beginning letters of the main sections.

- Selected HCPCS Level II sections
    - A0000–A0999—transportation and ambulance services
    - A4000–A8999—medical supplies
    - E0100–E9999—durable medical equipment
    - J0000–J8999—drugs administered other than oral

Do not confuse HCPCS Level II codes with four-letter ICD-9 E codes for external injuries. It is important to differentiate services and materials from the diagnosis before selecting the code.

HCPCS LEVEL III CODES

HCPCS Level III provides codes for regionally approved Medicare/Medicaid procedures or new procedures that have not yet been assigned a regular CPT code. Examples might be a procedure such as a bone marrow transplant for a new use that is covered by Medicaid in one state but not in another, or an experimental drug that is covered in

Table 14-1 **Components and Levels of an Evaluation and Management Office Visit**

	Components					
	History	**Examination**	**Medical Decision Making (MDR)**	**Problem Severity**	**Coordination of Care and Counseling**	**Time**
Level 1 (minimal)	Problem focused	Problem focused	Straightforward	Minor	Consistent with the nature of the problem and the patient's or family's needs	10 min.
Level 2 (low)	Expanded problem focused	Expanded problem focused	Straightforward	Low to moderate	Consistent with the nature of the problem and the patient's or family's needs	20 min.
Level 3 (moderate)	Detailed	Detailed	Low complexity	Moderate	Consistent with the nature of the problem and the patient's or family's needs	30 min.
Level 4 (moderate to high)	Comprehensive	Comprehensive	Moderate complexity	Moderate to high	Consistent with the nature of the problem and the patient's or family's needs	45 min.
Level 5 (high)	Comprehensive	Comprehensive	High complexity	Moderate to high	Consistent with the nature of the problem and the patient's or family's needs	60 min.

limited circumstances until it is approved by the Food and Drug Administration. The Level III HCPCS code begins with a letter (W–Z), followed by four numeric digits.

DIAGNOSTIC CODING

In 1979, the **International Classification of Diseases, Ninth Revision, Clinical Modifications (ICD-9-CM)** became the primary system for coding diseases and injuries in the United States. It is published by the U.S. Department of Health and Human Services and based on the World Health Organization's ICD-9. The ICD-9-CM and the ICD-9 are considered the same, and generally, the acronyms are used interchangeably. **ICD-9** will be used throughout this text to represent the classification of diagnoses used in the United States.

The ICD-9 has multiple uses.

- Purpose
  - Track disease processes
  - Classify causes of morbidity and mortality
  - Support medical research
  - Evaluate utilization of health care resources
  - Profile physicians' services and charges
- ICD-9
  - Volumes for physician offices
    - Volume 1—tabular (numeric) listing of diseases
    - Volume 2—alphabetic listing of diseases
  - Coding digits
    - Three to five numeric digits are used for each code (three digits alone are uncommon)
    - A decimal is placed after the third digit
    - Each digit provides more specific description of the disease or condition (Table 14-2)
    - Fifth digit: identified at the beginning of the three-digit category for the disease entity (e.g., diabetes) or at the beginning of a four-digit subcategory (a further descriptor of the disease entity)
    - If listed, the fifth digit is not optional
  - Special ICD-9 codes

Table 14-2 Example of Descriptors with Five-Digit ICD-9 Codes

Code	Description
250	Diabetes mellitus
250.1	Diabetes mellitus with ketoacidosis
250.13	Diabetes mellitus with ketoacidosis type 1 uncontrolled

- E codes—supplementary classification of ICD-9 coding that denotes the external cause of an injury or poisoning rather than a disease; explains the mechanism of injury
- V codes—ICD-9 coding identifying health care encounters for reasons other than illness

- ICD tables
  - Drugs and chemicals (use E codes)
  - Neoplasms
  - Hypertension

- General steps for ICD coding
  1. Locate the term in the alphabetic index.
  2. Refer to the notes under the main heading.
  3. Read the terms in parentheses.
  4. Note indented subterms.
  5. Proceed to tabular index and instructional terms.
  6. Assign code.

The exams contain critical thinking questions that require you to differentiate among CPT, HCPCS Level II, and ICD-9 codes. Knowing how to recognize the types of codes will allow you to identify the correct one without needing to be familiar with the actual digits. Box 14-4 assists you in this process.

INTERNATIONAL CLASSIFICATION OF DISEASES, TENTH REVISION, CLINICAL MODIFICATIONS (ICD-10-CM)

In 1993, the World Health Organization published the International Classification of Diseases, Tenth Revision (ICD-10), which, at the time of this writing, is not in complete use in the United States. It is scheduled for full implementation October 1, 2013, and will replace the ICD-9-CM, the diagnosis-based system used in both physician offices and hospitals. The ICD-9 Procedural Coding System (PCS) is currently used in hospitals only and will be replaced by the ICD-10-PCS. The CPT system will continue to be used in physicians' offices for coding procedures. Documents and other materials may refer to the ICD-9 as I-9 and the ICD-10 as I-10. Another term is the General Equivalency Mapping (GEM), which is a crosswalk between the ICD-9 and the ICD-10. The CMS reports that the change from the ICD-9-CM is a result of the obsolescence of a system that is inconsistent with current medical practice. The CMS website lists the following advantages of the ICD-10:

- Improved ability to measure health services
- Increased sensitivity with grouping and reimbursement methods
- Enhanced ability for public health surveillance
- Decreased need for supporting documentation with claims

Box 14-4

Can You Recognize the Difference in Codes?

Procedural Codes

CPT or HCPCS Level 1	Five numeric digits (e.g., 99202); codes for professional services
HCPCS Level II	Letter A–V and four numeric digits (e.g., J3105); codes for nonprofessional services or materials
HCPCS Level III	Letter W–Z and four numeric digits (e.g., Z5602) (fictional); codes for regional use or temporary code for new procedures

Diagnostic Codes

ICD-9	Three to five numeric digits with a decimal after the third (e.g., 569.82); codes that identify the patient's diagnosis
ICD-9 E codes	Letter E and three to four numeric digits with a decimal after the third digit (e.g., E919.3); further describes the diagnostic code by reporting the external cause of an injury rather than a disease
ICD-9 V codes	Letter V and two to four numeric digits with a decimal after the second digit (e.g., V59.2); identifies health care encounters for reasons other than illness

Table 14-3 Example of ICD-10 with ICD-9 Comparison

General Description of Code	Number of ICD-10 Codes for General Description	Example of ICD-10 Code and Specific Description	Number of ICD-9 Codes for Description	Example of ICD-9 Code and Specific Description
Mechanical complication of other vascular device, implant, and graft	156	T82.310 Breakdown (mechanical) of aortic (bifurcation) graft (replacement)	1	996.1 Mechanical complication of other vascular device, implant, and graft

- Provides codes for comparing mortality and morbidity data
- Provides better data for:
  - Measuring patient care
  - Designing payment systems
  - Processing claims
  - Making clinical decisions
  - Identifying fraud and abuse
  - Conducting research
  - ICD-10-CM: diagnostic coding system developed for use in the United States by the CDC; consists of three to seven alphanumeric digits (Table 14-3):
    - Digit 1: alphabetic
    - Digit 2: numeric
    - Digits 3–7: alphabetic or numeric

CLAIMS

A **claim** is a bill sent to the insurance carrier for payment of professional services. The universal health care insurance form is called the **CMS 1500**. (*Note:* This has a high probability to be an exam question!) It was originally designed by HCFA, now called CMS, and is used for group and individual claims. In 1990, the form was printed in red to accommodate optical scanning.

The Health Insurance Portability and Accountability Act (HIPAA) regulations regarding confidentiality must be upheld with insurance claims as with all medical documents. Extensive firewalls and other safeguards are required for electronic claims submission.

- Claims submission types
  - Paper—processed by computer; hard copy sent to the insurance carrier through the mail (this method is becoming obsolete)
  - Electronic—processed by computer and sent to the insurance carrier through an electronic data exchange, the Internet, telephone wires, or a disk
  - Digital fax—processed by computer and faxed to the insurance company, where it is read by an optical coder and transmitted into the claims system
- CMS 1500 abbreviations: use only capital letters with no punctuation
  - SSN—Social Security number
  - EIN—employer identification number
  - PIN—provider identification number
  - NPI—national provider identifier
- Dirty claims—claims held or rejected by the insurance carrier because of problems or errors such as the following:
  - Incorrect data
  - Missing data
  - Diagnosis not supporting the procedure
  - Coding errors
  - Patient ineligible for services
  - Claim to wrong carrier
  - Coding or dates not compatible with documentation
- Common fraudulent claim terms
  - Unbundling—using several CPT codes to identify procedures normally covered by a single code
  - Upcoding—deliberately using an incorrect code to bill at a higher rate
  - Phantom billing—billing for services or supplies not provided
  - Ping-ponging—unnecessary or excessive referrals of patients to other providers and back to primary office
  - Yo-yoing—scheduling the patient for unnecessary follow-up visits
  - Gang visits—billing for individual visits when not all the patients present during the visit received services (e.g., visiting a nursing home and not providing services for all patients who are billed)
  - Split billing—billing for several visits when services were performed on one visit

- Other fraudulent claim practices
  - Falsifying medical records to justify higher payment
  - Omitting relevant information, especially additional diagnoses
  - Altering dates of service
  - Altering the diagnosis
- Appeals for disputed claims
  - Process specific to the insurance carrier
  - Five levels of CMS appeals
    - Predetermination
    - Reconsideration
    - Administrative Judge
    - Appeals Review Board
    - Federal Court Review

HIPAA AND COVERED ENTITIES

A *covered entity* is a medical office that performs any of the following procedures electronically:

- Files claims or managed care encounter forms
- Checks claims status
- Checks eligibility
- Checks certifications or authorizations
- Receives payment and remittance advice
- Provides coordination of benefits

A medical office is also considered a covered entity if any of the above procedures is conducted by a contracted service on the office's behalf. HIPAA requires covered entities to maintain confidentiality (see Chapter 9).

TERMS

Medical Coding and Claims Review

The following list reviews the terms discussed in this chapter and other important terms that you may see on the exam.

abuse an unreasonable and generally unacceptable departure from precedent and custom with one person taking advantage of another person or set of circumstances; abuse may or may not be unlawful

adverse effect a pathologic reaction to a drug that occurs when appropriate doses are given

appeal a resort to a higher authority for a decision

benign tumor a nonmalignant lesion that is not invasive or metastatic

chief complaint a patient's statement describing symptoms and conditions that are the reason for seeking health care services

claim a bill sent to the insurance carrier for payment related to patient care

clean claim completed insurance claim form submitted to a carrier without deficiencies or errors

CMS 1500 universal health insurance claim form used in the physician's office, originally designed by the Health Care Financing Administration (now called the Centers for Medicare and Medicaid Services, or CMS)

comorbidity a condition that exists along with the condition for which the patient is receiving treatment and may increase patient's length of stay (LOS) if hospitalized

concurrent care similar services provided to the same patient on the same day by a different physician

consultation services rendered by a physician whose opinion or advice is requested by another physician or agency in the evaluation or treatment of a patient's illness or suspected problem

counseling discussion with patient or family concerning diagnosis, recommendations, risks, benefits, prognosis, options, and necessary condition-related education; definition used for the coding of professional services

critical care intensive care in acute life-threatening conditions requiring constant bedside attention by the physician; definition used for the coding of professional services

Current Procedural Terminology (CPT) coding system first published by the American Medical Association in 1966; a manual, updated annually, that contains the codes for procedures and services performed by doctors and other select medical personnel

dirty claim a claim held or rejected by the insurance carrier due to problems or errors

E code a supplementary classification of ICD-9 coding that denotes the external cause of an injury rather than a disease; explains the mechanism of injury; includes drug events such as poisonings and adverse effects

eponym the name of a disease or procedure derived from the name of a place or person

established patient a person who has received care from the physician or another physician of the same specialty in the same group practice within 3 years

etiology the cause of disease

fraud intentional and unlawful deception for gain that results in harm to another person or organization

gang visits billing for individual visits when not all the patients present during the visit received services

General Equivalency Mapping (GEM) a crosswalk between the ICD-9 and the ICD-10

Health Care Procedural Coding System (HCPCS [pronounced "hicpics"]) a method developed by the Health Care Finance Administration for coding procedures and other services delivered to Medicare patients

in situ neoplasm confined to the site of origin

International Classification of Diseases, Ninth Revision, Clinical Modifications (ICD-9 or ICD-9-CM) a coding system published by the U.S. Department of Health and Human Services to classify diseases and injuries

International Classification of Diseases, Tenth Revision, Clinical Modifications (ICD-10-CM) diagnostic coding system developed for use in the United States by the CDC; consists of three to seven alphanumeric digits

International Classification of Diseases, Tenth Revision, Procedural Coding System (ICD-10-PCS) procedural coding system developed for use in the United States by the CDC; consists of seven alphanumeric digits

late effect a residual condition occurring after the acute phase is over

malignant tumor a neoplasm with invasive and metastatic properties

new patient a person who has not received care from the physician or another physician of the same specialty in the same group practice within 3 or more years

Not Elsewhere Classified (NEC) a term used in ICD-9 coding when information is not available to code the term in a more specific category

Not Otherwise Specified (NOS) a term used in ICD-9 coding for unspecified diagnosis

phantom billing billing for services or supplies not provided

ping-ponging unnecessary or excessive referrals of patients to other providers and back to primary office

point of service (POS) facility where the health care service took place (e.g., physician's office, emergency department)

primary diagnosis the symptoms, conditions, and initial impressions diagnosed as the cause for the patient seeking health care services

principal diagnosis the definitive diagnosis, obtained generally through hospitalization

split billing billing for several visits when services were performed during one visit

superbill also called an *encounter form*; a charge form custom-designed for the specific medical practice; lists the ICD-9 and CPT codes common to the services of that practice

unbundling using several CPT codes to identify procedures normally covered by a single code

upcoding deliberately using an incorrect code to bill at a higher rate

V codes ICD-9 codes identifying health care visits for reasons other than illness

yo-yoing scheduling the patient for unnecessary follow-up visits

REVIEW QUESTIONS

All questions are relevant for the CMA (AAMA), RMA (AMT), and CMAS (AMT) exams.

1. The abbreviation for the manual first published by the American Medical Association containing the codes for procedures and services performed by doctors and medical personnel is:
   A. ICD.
   B. CPT.
   C. HCPCS.
   D. DRG.

Answer: **B**

Why: The Current Procedural Terminology manual is used to determine the proper insurance codes to use when filing insurance claims for procedures and services.

Review: Yes ❑ No ❑

---

2. The coding term used for the level of care that involves multiple systems or complex involvement of one organ system is:
   A. problem focused.
   B. expanded problem focused.
   C. detailed.
   D. minimal.
   E. comprehensive.

Answer: **E**

Why: Problem focused refers to minimal care involving a specific body area or one organ system. Expanded problem focused refers to the same level of care as problem focused with the addition of symptoms related to other body areas. Detailed level of care involves the affected body area(s) and related body system(s).

Review: Yes ❑ No ❑

---

3. When a health professional has a discussion with a patient and his or her family concerning diagnosis, recommendations, risks, benefits, prognosis, and options, the specific coding component used is under the heading:
   A. consultation.
   B. critical care.
   C. concurrent care.
   D. counseling.

Answer: **D**

Why: Counseling involves meeting with a patient or the family members to discuss the patient's condition and prognosis, treatment, and concerns surrounding the treatment. This gives the patient or family member an opportunity to ask questions about the information provided by the health care practitioner.

Review: Yes ❑ No ❑

---

4. A pediatric patient comes into the office for otitis media. The physician also administers a routine childhood vaccination. What diagnostic codes would be used in this situation?
   A. 99201 and 99212
   B. 86850 and E 858.1
   C. 041.5 and J 5678
   D. 382.9 and V 03.81
   E. 99201 and V 71.5

Answer: **D**

Why: D is the correct answer because it includes an ICD-9 code, consisting of a three-digit number followed by a decimal and another digit, and a V code, an ICD-9 code that identifies health care reasons other than disease (immunization). The numbers in A are five-digit CPT codes; those in B are a CPT code and an ICD code related to external injuries (preceded by the letter E). C consists of an ICD code and a HCPCS Level III code (as recognized by the letter J and four digits); E is a combination of a CPT code and a V code.

Review: Yes ❑ No ❑

5. When a claim is deliberately coded incorrectly to increase the payment, it is referred to as:
   A. superbilling.
   B. customary coding.
   C. upcoding.
   D. bundling.

Answer: **C**

Why: When a CPT code is manipulated to increase the amount of reimbursement, it is known as upcoding. This is an unethical practice.

Review: Yes ❑ No ❑

---

6. ICD-9-CM codes that identify health care encounters for reasons other than illness or injury are known as:
   A. E codes.
   B. F codes.
   C. CPT codes.
   D. T codes.
   E. V codes.

Answer: **E**

Why: V codes are used to identify reasons other than illness or injury and to identify patients whose injury or illness is influenced by special circumstances or problems.

Review: Yes ❑ No ❑

---

7. The coding system published by the U.S. Department of Health and Human Services used to categorize diseases and injuries is the:
   A. Physician's Desk Reference.
   B. Current Procedural Terminology.
   C. International Classification of Diseases.
   D. Relative Value Study.

Answer: **C**

Why: The International Classification of Diseases, Ninth Revision, Clinical Modification manual (ICD-9-CM) is a numeric code system for diagnoses of diseases and injuries.

Review: Yes ❑ No ❑

---

8. CMS developed codes for use when specific services, materials, drugs, and procedures are not listed in the CPT code book. These are known as:
   A. RVU.
   B. HCPCS.
   C. DRG.
   D. E codes.
   E. E&M codes.

Answer: **B**

Why: HCPCS, the CMS Common Procedure Coding System, was developed to accommodate coding areas not already specified in the CPT code book. These services, materials, drugs, and procedures are provided to Medicare patients.

Review: Yes ❑ No ❑

---

9. The largest of the six major sections of the CPT manual, which contains codes from 10000 to 69999, is:
   A. medicine.
   B. anesthesia.
   C. radiology.
   D. surgery.

Answer: **D**

Why: The six sections of the CPT manual are as follows: Evaluation and Management, 99200 to 99499; Anesthesia, 00100 to 01999; Surgery, 10000 to 69999; Radiology, 70000 to 79999; Pathology and Laboratory, 80000 to 89999; and Medicine, 90701 to 99199.

Review: Yes ❑ No ❑

---

10. When a physician requests the services of another physician whose opinion or advice assists in the evaluation or treatment of a patient's illness or suspected problem, the code section used is titled:
    A. critical care.
    B. consultation.
    C. counseling.
    D. concurrent care.
    E. comorbidity.

Answer: **B**

Why: A consultation is the process of seeking the advice or opinion of another physician or specialist to aid in the diagnosis or evaluation of a patient's disease or condition.

Review: Yes ❑ No ❑

11. Of the following, which is not one of the purposes of diagnostic coding?
   A. To track disease processes
   B. To support medical research
   C. To provide increased revenue for the physician or medical practice
   D. To classify the causes of morbidity and mortality

Answer: **C**

Why: Diagnostic coding helps establish statistics and demographic information about diseases and illness. Diagnostic coding is not a mechanism to increase a physician's income.

Review: Yes ❑ No ❑

---

12. When a patient has received an external injury, which type of code is used to explain the mechanism of the injury?
   A. V code
   B. CPT code
   C. UCR code
   D. E code
   E. NOS

Answer: **D**

Why: E codes are supplemental codes that are used to code external injuries rather than diseases.

Review: Yes ❑ No ❑

---

13. Which CPT code identifies a sigmoidoscopy?
   A. 531.03
   B. 453.30
   C. 45330
   D. 685

Answer: **C**

Why: Answer C is correct because it is the only five-digit number that is characteristic of a CPT code.

Review: Yes ❑ No ❑

---

14. The CPT code used for a cholecystectomy, along with the modifier indicating that the physician provided only preoperative care, is which of the following?
   A. 47600
   B. 99201
   C. J3105
   D. 47600-V59.2
   E. 47600-56

Answer: **E**

Why: Answer E is a CPT code indicating a procedure and includes a dash and a two-digit modifier that identifies a specific circumstance. A and B are CPT codes without modifiers. C is a HCPCS Level II code, recognized by the letter J followed by four digits. D is a CPT code with an attached ICD code, which is never done.

Review: Yes ❑ No ❑

---

15. The components used to determine the level of E&M code applicable include the following EXCEPT the:
   A. comprehensive depth of the patient history.
   B. problem severity.
   C. amount of time spent with the patient.
   D. number of procedures ordered for the patient.

Answer: **D**

Why: The E&M, or Evaluation and Management, codes require assessment of the visit and judgment of the provider as to the depth of the visit, complexity of the illness, and amount of time involved in treatment of the patient.

Review: Yes ❑ No ❑

---

16. The Health Care Finance Administration is now named:
   A. Centers for Disease Control and Prevention.
   B. Department of Health and Human Services.
   C. Centers for Medicare and Medicaid Services.
   D. National Institutes of Health.
   E. American Medical Association.

Answer: **C**

Why: The Health Care Finance Administration (HCFA) has been renamed the Centers for Medicare and Medicaid Services, or CMS. This is the federal government agency that oversees the regulations and policies for Medicare and Medicaid.

Review: Yes ❑ No ❑

17. The patient's statement describing symptoms and conditions that are the reason for seeking health care services is the:
    A. adverse effect.
    B. primary concern.
    C. objective finding.
    D. chief complaint.

Answer: **D**

Why: The chief complaint is the primary reason that brings the patient to the health care provider for treatment. The insurance company requires this information to appear on the claim form.

Review: Yes ❑ No ❑

---

18. When a patient has a condition that coexists with his or her primary condition and complicates the treatment and management of the primary condition, it is referred to as:
    A. late effect.
    B. comorbidity.
    C. etiology.
    D. critical care.
    E. concurrent care.

Answer: **B**

Why: Comorbidity occurs when the patient experiences a complication in the treatment plan resulting from a condition other than the primary condition. This may actually lengthen a hospital stay.

Review: Yes ❑ No ❑

---

19. **Etiology** is a term meaning:
    A. residual condition.
    B. metastatic disease.
    C. cause of the disease.
    D. prognosis of a disease.

Answer: **C**

Why: Etiology is the study of all factors that may be involved in the development of a disease.

Review: Yes ❑ No ❑

---

20. The coding abbreviation NOS means:
    A. Not Otherwise Specified.
    B. No Objective Signs.
    C. Nonspecific Objective Symptoms.
    D. Non Organic Syndrome.
    E. Not Otherwise Classified.

Answer: **A**

Why: NOS means "Not Otherwise Specified," a term used in the ICD-9-CM coding system to indicate an unspecified diagnosis.

Review: Yes ❑ No ❑

---

21. When coding, the term describing a cancer that has not invaded neighboring tissues is:
    A. metastatic.
    B. carcinoma.
    C. in situ.
    D. benign.

Answer: **C**

Why: In situ refers to a neoplasm or new growth (tumor) that is confined to the site of origin and has not spread or metastasized.

Review: Yes ❑ No ❑

---

22. The coding abbreviation NEC is used:
    A. if information is unavailable for more specific coding.
    B. to describe external injuries.
    C. to abbreviate normal causes for the disease.
    D. when the patient is newly established.
    E. if the patient has extensive injuries.

Answer: **A**

Why: NEC means "Not Elsewhere Classifiable." This term is used in ICD-9-CM coding when information necessary to code the disease or injury in a more specific category is not available.

Review: Yes ❑ No ❑

23. The reference manual used to code a cholecystectomy is:
   A. PDR.
   B. ICD.
   C. CPT.
   D. HCFA.

Answer: C

Why: The CPT manual is the Current Procedural Terminology book that contains procedures, including surgeries. A cholecystectomy is the surgical removal of the gallbladder. If disease of the gallbladder—cholecystitis or cholelithiasis—needs to be coded, the ICD manual is used.

Review: Yes ❑ No ❑

---

24. If a patient's current injury is a fracture of the left ankle but he or she then experiences a malunion of this fracture, this is referred to as a(n):
   A. principal diagnosis.
   B. secondary complaint.
   C. adverse effect.
   D. concurrent care.
   E. late effect.

Answer: E

Why: A late effect is a problem that occurs after the original problem. A malunion of a fracture means the fracture did not heal properly.

Review: Yes ❑ No ❑

---

25. A claim that is submitted to the carrier without deficiencies or errors is called a:
   A. common claim.
   B. customary claim.
   C. managed claim.
   D. clean claim.

Answer: D

Why: A clean claim means that the completed insurance claim form contains all the necessary information without deficiencies so it can be processed and paid promptly.

Review: Yes ❑ No ❑

---

26. A physician charging an unreasonable amount for a procedure is most likely an example of:
   A. fraud.
   B. abuse.
   C. upcoding.
   D. phantom billing.
   E. unbundling.

Answer: B

Why: Abuse is an unreasonable and generally unacceptable departure from precedent and custom, with one person taking advantage of another person. Fraud is intentional deceit resulting in harm and unlawful. Upcoding is selecting a higher level of care than actually provided. Phantom billing is charging for services that were not rendered. Unbundling is billing separately for services that should have been billed under one code for the sole purpose of making more money.

Review: Yes ❑ No ❑

---

27. Phantom billing is an example of:
   A. fraud.
   B. abuse.
   C. upcoding.
   D. unbundling.

Answer: A

Why: Phantom billing is charging for services that were not provided and is an unlawful intentional deceit.

Review: Yes ❑ No ❑

---

28. All ICD-10-CM codes contain:
   A three to five numeric digits.
   B. three to five alphanumeric digits.
   C. three to seven numeric digits.
   D. three to seven alphanumeric digits.
   E. seven alphanumeric digits.

Answer: D

Why: ICD-10-CM codes contain three to seven alphanumerical digits because that is how the coding system is designed.

Review: Yes ❑ No ❑

29. The final appeal for a denied CMS claim is determined by the:
    A. Attorney General.
    B. Supreme Court.
    C. Administrative Judge.
    D. Federal Court Review.

Answer: **D**

Why: The Attorney General and the Supreme Court do not become involved in Medicare/Medicaid claims. The fourth level of appeal is with an Administrative Judge, and the final level of appeal is the Federal Court Review.

Review: Yes ❑ No ❑

---

30. The ICD-10 is scheduled for full implementation in the United States on:
    A. January 1, 2012.
    B. April 15, 2012.
    C. January 1, 2013.
    D. April 15, 2013.
    E. October 1, 2013.

Answer: **E**

Why: October 1, 2013 is the date designated by the federal government to provide organizations with enough time for implementation. October 1 is also the beginning of the federal fiscal year.

Review: Yes ❑ No ❑

15

Financial Practices

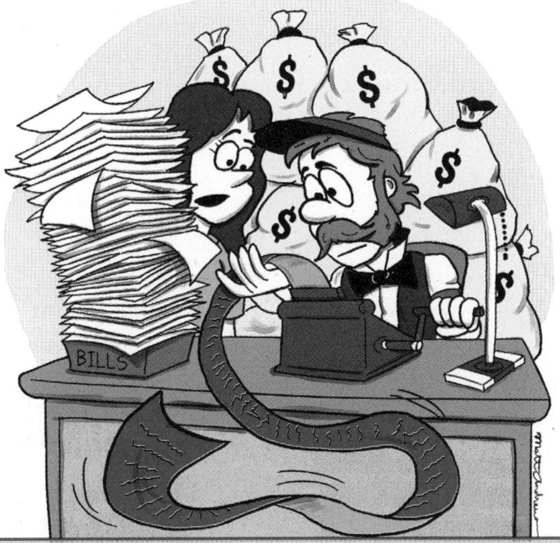

REVIEW TIP

You've worked hard and made it this far. Good work! An unknown author said, "You can be on the right track but you can still get hit if you just sit there." So keep going!

Chapters 13 and 14 described how physician fees are established and reimbursement is obtained through insurance companies using claims and coding. This chapter concentrates on the day-to-day financial practices in the medical office.

ACCOUNTS

Accounts are records of financial transactions and the resulting balances during a fiscal period, usually January 1st through December 31st. The medical office primarily deals with two types of accounts: **accounts receivable**, which is the money owed to the practice (e.g., patient bills), and **accounts payable**, which is the money the practice owes (e.g., rent, utilities, medical supplies, payroll). The following accounting functions apply to both accounts receivable and accounts payable.

- Accounting functions
  - Entries—recording of each transaction
  - Postings—transferring information from the journal (day sheet) to the accounts receivable ledger or to the individual patients' ledgers
  - Adjustments—changes made to the amount of money owed for reasons other than additional services or payments, such as fee discounts or refunds
  - Billings—records of charges sent to the patient in the form of statements to indicate balance due and to request payment; most practices bill on a monthly cycle
  - Balancing—ensuring accuracy in totals by comparing them with preestablished criteria (e.g., in accounts receivable, the total of balances from individual patient statements must equal the total of accounts receivable recorded in the journal)

- Accounts receivable
  - Components
    - Day sheet—a daily record of the services rendered, charges made, and payments received; may be a manual or a computerized system
    - Journal—a chronologic collection of the day sheets with running totals for a specific period
    - Accounts receivable ledger—a listing by individual patient names of all monies owed to the practice
    - Patient ledger—a patient statement or itemized statement that is an individual form of each patient's accounts receivable activities; often used as the patient bill
    - Charge slip—a form given to the patient to indicate the charges for the service(s); may be a copy of the superbill or the patient ledger
    - Receipt—a numbered form given to the patient indicating the payments he or she made that day
    - Pegboard system—a system of layered forms that allows all transactions to be completed at one time (Fig. 15-1); composed of day sheet, patient ledger, charge slips, receipts, and day sheet–sized board with pegs to hold forms in place
  - Age of accounts receivable—the period between when the service is rendered and the bill is paid, usually in 30-day intervals; computerized financial programs will process statements calculating the amount of money that is owed on the account for 30, 60, 90, or 120 days since the date of service; also known as **aging analysis**
  - Monthly trial balance—a list and total of all the debit and credit accounts for the medical practice; usually a two-column chart with debt listed in one column and credit listed in the other column; a monthly trial balance ensures that debits equal credits

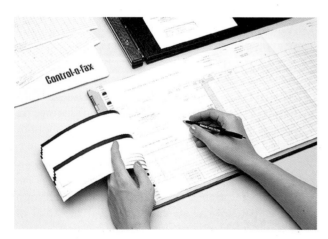

Figure 15-1 Pegboard system.

  - Collections—efforts to obtain money owed to a medical office
    - Office efforts can include payment by cash, check, or charge at time of service; payment plans with or without interest; payment through billing, by billing all patients on the same day each month or by cycling patients for billing on different days of the month based on preestablished criteria, such as billing those whose names begin with certain letters on the same day; and telephone calls and letters for aging bills
    - Collection agency—an outside company, independent of the medical practice, that is contracted by the medical practice to attempt to obtain payment of delinquent bills after internal efforts have failed; **a medical practice should not make further efforts to collect a bill after the account is turned over to the collection agency;** collection agencies are usually paid 50% of the amount collected
    - Small claims court—a less formal court setting that allows the parties to represent themselves in civil disputes involving small amounts; the amount is designated by the court and is generally less than $5,000
    - Bankruptcy—if a patient declares bankruptcy, the medical office must attempt to collect unpaid bills through the court-appointed representative
    - Deaths—unpaid bills of deceased patients **should be collected through the patient's estate**
- Accounts payable
  - Purchase order—a document sent to a vendor via mail, fax, or the Internet to purchase supplies and equipment for the medical office
  - Invoice—a bill sent from the vendor stating what was purchased and the charges
  - Materials—items received from the vendor should be verified with the invoice or packing list and purchase order
  - Bill—statements sent to the medical office requesting payment for materials or services
  - Payment—money remitted by the medical office for materials or services
  - Petty cash—a small sum of money (usually less than $200), kept separate from the cash drawer, **used for incidental expenses** (e.g., postage due)

BANKING

- Checks
  - Payee—the person to whom the check is written; the person receiving the money

- Payer—the person or organization giving the money to the payee
- Acceptable checks—cashier's check, traveler's check, certified check, personal check with proper identification, money order
- Unacceptable checks—third-party checks (except from the patient's insurance company), payroll checks, personal checks without identification if unfamiliar with the person and his or her financial history with the medical practice
- Voided check—a check written by the practice but not used because of error or other reason; write *VOID* across the front and keep with canceled checks in the proper numeric sequence
- Lost or stolen check—the bank should be notified immediately and a notation made in the checkbook
- Endorsement—signing the back of a check as the payee for the amount represented on the front of the check
    - Blank endorsement—only the signature of the payee on the back of the check (can be easily cashed by anyone)
    - Restrictive endorsement—signature of the payee with instructions, such as "for deposit only"
- Nonsufficient funds (NSF)—indicates that the checking account on which the check is written does not hold enough money to honor the amount of the check; medical offices usually add a charge to the balance to cover the associated bank charges

■ Deposits—checks and cash paid to the medical office and placed in a checking account at the bank; usually deposits are made daily

- Deposit slip—a form completed with the deposit listing all checks and cash and the total amount deposited; contains account number and other identifying information
- Check register (checkbook)—a book or computer program maintained by the office listing in chronologic order all checks written, deposits made, and an ongoing balance; used to reconcile bank statement

■ Bank statements—reports sent by the bank listing the monthly account activities, including checks written and cashed, deposits, bank charges, and balances

■ Reconciliation (balancing or trial balancing)—process of verifying that the information on the bank statement tallies with the information in the check register (Box 15-1)

■ Line of Credit—a financial agreement between a bank or financial institution and a borrower establishing the maximum amount of money the borrower can obtain through a loan; the total amount of the funds may be borrowed at one time or in increments as needed until the maximum amount has been reached

Box 15-1

Example of Main Components of Checking Account Reconciliation

1. Beginning balance	$25,000.00
2. Total deposits	+45,000.00
3. Total checks cleared	–35,000.00
4. Total checks outstanding	–10,000.00
5. Charges	00.00
Ending balance	$25,000.00

To determine the ending balance, add lines 1 and 2, and then subtract lines 3, 4, and 5 from the total of lines 1 and 2.

COMMON TAXES

The federal and state governments require medical offices to pay specific taxes. The most common and "exam probable" taxes follow.

■ Federal income tax—a specified percentage of income withheld based on total amount earned

- W-2 form—a federal tax form prepared for each office employee containing all income and deductions for the previous calendar year
- W-4 form—a federal tax form for each employee that contains the number of tax exemptions he or she claims

■ Federal Insurance and Contribution Act (FICA)—a percentage of income withheld for Social Security and Medicare

■ Federal Unemployment Tax Act (FUTA)—a percentage of each employee's income paid by employer for an unemployment fund

INCOME

The amount of money a medical practice earns is the **income** (accounts receivable). The practice also incurs expenses such as wages, taxes, supplies, equipment, and utilities (accounts payable). Certain additional deductions (e.g., bad debts) are allowed in addition to expenses. These are deducted from the total income.

■ Gross income—total amount of earned income for the medical practice before deductions

■ Net income—amount of earned income for the medical practice after deductions (Box 15-2)

Box 15-2

Example of Gross and Net Income Difference

Gross income	$250,000
Deductions & expenses	–75,000
Net income	$175,000

TERMS

Financial Practices Review

The following list reviews the terms discussed in this chapter and other important terms that you may see on the exam.

accounts records of financial transactions and the resulting balances during a fiscal period, usually January 1st through December 31st

accounts payable the money the practice owes (e.g., rent, utilities, medical supplies, payroll)

accounts receivable the money owed to the practice, such as patient bills

accounts receivable ledger listing by individual patient name of all monies owed to the practice

adjustments changes to the amount of money owed for reasons other than additional services or payments (e.g., fee discounts, refunds)

age of accounts receivable (aging analysis) the period between when the service is rendered and the bill is paid, usually in 30-day intervals; computerized financial programs will process statements calculating the amount of money that is owed on the account for 30, 60, 90, or 120 days since the date of service

asset anything of value owned by an individual or business

balancing ensuring accuracy in totals by comparing them with preestablished criteria; in accounts receivable, the total of balances from individual patient statements must equal the total of accounts receivable recorded in the journal

blank endorsement only the signature of the payee appears on the back of the check

credit value added to an account, usually in the form of payment for a debt owed to that party

currency official paper money of a country

day sheet a daily record of the services rendered, charges made, and payments received; may be a manual or computerized system

debit value subtracted from or owed by an account

endorsement signing the back of a check as the payee for the amount represented on the front of the check

entry the recording of each transaction on the appropriate forms or components

gross income the total amount of income for the medical practice before deductions

income the amount of money a medical practice earns

invoice a bill sent from a vendor stating what was purchased and what the charges are

journal a chronologic collection of day sheets with running totals for a specific period

liability obligation; debt of the individual or business

line of credit a financial agreement between a bank or financial institution and a borrower establishing the maximum amount of money the borrower can obtain through a loan

monthly trial balance a list and total of all the debit and credit accounts for the medical practice

net income the amount of income for the medical practice after deductions

patient ledger a patient statement that is an individual form of each patient's accounts receivable activities; often used as the patient bill

payee the person to whom the check is written; the person receiving the money

payer the person or organization giving the money to the payee

pegboard system a system of layered day sheets, patient ledgers, charge slips, and receipts; allows all entries to be made with one transaction

petty cash a small sum of money (usually less than $200), separate from the cash drawer, used for incidental expenses

posting transferring information from the journal (day sheet) to the accounts receivable ledger or to the individual patients' ledgers

purchase order a document sent to a vendor via mail, fax, or the Internet to purchase supplies and equipment for the medical office

reconciliation the process of verifying that the information on the bank statement agrees with the information in the check register

restrictive endorsement signature of the payee with instructions (e.g., "for deposit only")

superbill (encounter form) a provided form that has all the necessary information to file an insurance claim related to that office visit

REVIEW QUESTIONS

All questions are relevant for the CMA (AAMA), RMA (AMT), and CMAS (AMT) exams.

1. The patient's bill or statement is also referred to as the patient's:
   A. receipt.
   B. charge slip.
   C. ledger.
   D. posting.

Answer: **C**

Why: A patient's ledger is an individual form containing each patient's accounts receivable activities.

Review: Yes ❑ No ❑

---

2. The listing by individual patient names of all monies owed to the practice is the:
   A. receipt.
   B. charge slip.
   C. day sheet.
   D. accounts payable roster.
   E. accounts receivable ledger.

Answer: **E**

Why: Accounts receivable refers to the money owed to the practice by patients. These amounts are recorded in a ledger called the accounts receivable ledger.

Review: Yes ❑ No ❑

---

3. A check written from an account that does not have enough money for the amount of the check is called a(n):
   A. voided check.
   B. NSF check.
   C. blank check.
   D. third-party check.

Answer: **B**

Why: When there is not enough money in an account to cover the amount of a check, the bank account has non-sufficient funds (NSF) to cover the check.

Review: Yes ❑ No ❑

---

4. The Federal Insurance and Contribution Act was created to sponsor:
   A. unemployment.
   B. life insurance.
   C. Social Security and Medicare.
   D. workers' compensation.
   E. Medicare.

Answer: **C**

Why: The Federal Insurance and Contribution Act (FICA) requires deduction from an employee's pay to cover the cost of sponsoring Social Security and Medicare.

Review: Yes ❑ No ❑

---

5. The process of verifying that the information on the bank statement agrees with the information in the check register is:
   A. registering.
   B. accounting.
   C. reconciling.
   D. examining.

Answer: **C**

Why: Reconciliation is the process of making things right. The balance in the checkbook should equal the balance on the bank statement after adjustments have been made for outstanding checks and deposits.

Review: Yes ❑ No ❑

6. When a discount or refund is applied to an account, this is referred to as a(n):
   A. charge.
   B. adjustment.
   C. payable.
   D. receivable.
   E. withholding.

Answer: **B**

Why: When a medical practice applies a discount or refunds money to an account, it is making an adjustment to the total amount owed by the client. Another example is when a client pays his or her balance in full and then the medical practice receives an insurance payment to cover some or all of the visit; the patient should be refunded the overpayment.

Review: Yes ❑ No ❑

---

7. Activities that an office can do to assist in the collection of money owed the practice include:
   A. allowing patients to pay for services when they get paid.
   B. requiring all patients to pay cash when services are rendered and not providing any payment plans.
   C. asking patients at the time of service if they want to pay for the services by cash, check, or charge.
   D. sending billing notices to patients on a quarterly basis.

Answer: **C**

Why: Patients should be asked at the time of service what method of payment they want to use to pay for the services. This allows the office to establish that it is necessary to pay for services at the time they are rendered. If a patient is unable to pay in full, billing for the balance should be done on a monthly basis.

Review: Yes ❑ No ❑

---

8. When a patient declares bankruptcy, the medical office must:
   A. turn over the patient's balance owed to a collection agency.
   B. write off the balance of the account.
   C. sue the patient for the balance owed on the account.
   D. collect unpaid bills through the court-appointed representative.
   E. set up a loan repayment plan with interest.

Answer: **D**

Why: After bankruptcy has been declared, the office is not allowed to contact the patient directly but must attempt to collect any debt through the court-appointed representative.

Review: Yes ❑ No ❑

---

9. The form enclosed with merchandise ordered from a vendor that states the contents of the package and the amount owed is a(n):
   A. ledger.
   B. invoice.
   C. purchase order.
   D. receipt.

Answer: **B**

Why: The invoice usually accompanies the merchandise and includes the total amount due on the order. A ledger is a list of the accounts receivable activities for a patient or a company. A purchase order is a document sent to a vendor to purchase supplies and equipment for the medical office. A receipt is given as proof of payment.

Review: Yes ❑ No ❑

---

10. If a check is written but not used, what is written across the front of the check?
    A. Void
    B. Nonsufficient funds
    C. Do not use
    D. Error
    E. Reconcile

Answer: **A**

Why: The word "void" means useless or invalid. A voided check should be filed with the canceled checks for tracking purposes.

Review: Yes ❑ No ❑

11. The amount of money earned before taxes or deductions are taken out is called:
    A. net income.
    B. total income.
    C. prior earnings.
    D. gross income.

Answer: **D**

Why: The gross income refers to the entire amount of money earned by an employee or the amount of income in a business before expenses, deductions, or taxes have been subtracted.

Review: Yes ❑ No ❑

---

12. The cash kept on hand in a business practice used for incidental purchases is called:
    A. purchase order.
    B. petty cash.
    C. ancillary money.
    D. spending money.
    E. currency.

Answer: **B**

Why: "Petty" refers to a small amount. Petty cash is usually around $200 cash and is used to purchase items that are needed on a daily basis that are paid for right away. Postage stamps, coffee supplies, office supplies, and so on are often bought with petty cash.

Review: Yes ❑ No ❑

---

13. The money owed by the physician for items such as rent, utilities, and payroll is referred to as:
    A. financial responsibility.
    B. accounts receivable.
    C. business expenses.
    D. accounts payable.

Answer: **D**

Why: Accounts payable refers to the amount of money the physician or business owner needs to pay out for expenses of the business.

Review: Yes ❑ No ❑

---

14. To balance a checkbook, you must have:
    A. a copy of all the bills paid in the month to verify all checks written.
    B. paycheck stubs to prove deposits made.
    C. the monthly bank statement.
    D. a copy of all endorsed checks.
    E. day sheets.

Answer: **C**

Why: The bank sends a monthly statement that lists all deposits made, checks written and cashed, bank charges and fees, and the beginning and ending balance on the account for the month. This statement is used to compare with the check register to balance it.

Review: Yes ❑ No ❑

---

15. The signature of the payee of a check with instructions stating "for deposit only" is an example of a(n):
    A. blank endorsement.
    B. unlimited endorsement.
    C. restrictive endorsement.
    D. registered endorsement.

Answer: **C**

Why: A check that has a signature and "for deposit only" on the reverse side indicates that it can only be deposited into the account of the payee, making it a restrictive endorsement. If the payee signs the check without writing any restrictions, it can be cashed by anyone if lost or stolen.

Review: Yes ❑ No ❑

---

16. The monitoring of unpaid accounts to determine how overdue the accounts are is called:
    A. posting.
    B. calendar tracking.
    C. collections.
    D. overdue auditing.
    E. aging accounts.

Answer: **E**

Why: Aging of accounts is a way to monitor the ability of offices to collect money on unpaid accounts. Usually the practice will measure in 30-day intervals up to 120 days.

Review: Yes ❑ No ❑

17. The most common schedule of billing patients is:
   A. weekly.
   B. monthly.
   C. bimonthly.
   D. quarterly.

Answer: **B**

Why: Monthly billing is the most accepted method of billing because it is highly effective in collection of unpaid debts. Most people pay bills based on monthly income and, if budgeted properly, will schedule payments on owed accounts monthly.

Review: Yes ❑ No ❑

---

18. When the medical assistant is given the task of trying to collect payment on an account, it is appropriate practice to first:
   A. contact the client's employer.
   B. contact the client at home before 8:00 AM.
   C. leave a message on the client's answering machine about possible lawsuits or small claims court activity if he or she does not call you back.
   D. contact the client about the overdue bill through a mailed letter or notice attached to his or her bill.
   E. visit the patient at his or her home to discuss a payment plan.

Answer: **D**

Why: It is improper collections activity to contact someone before 8:00 AM or after 9:00 PM. It is also inappropriate to visit patients at their homes or to contact a client's employer. Threatening calls are a form of harassment and intimidation and should not be made. Initially, the office should try to collect the money through written correspondence. This method also provides a paper trail for tracking if further collection methods need to be tried.

Review: Yes ❑ No ❑

---

19. When a charge is made to an account, it is called a(n):
   A. posting.
   B. credit.
   C. debit.
   D. adjustment.

Answer: **C**

Why: A debit is a charge to an account and represents what is owed. Posting is the process of transferring information from a day sheet to an accounts receivable ledger or to an individual patient's ledger. A credit is the same as a payment, or applying money to an account to lower the balance owed. An adjustment is a change made to the amount of money owed for reasons other than additional services or payments.

Review: Yes ❑ No ❑

---

20. A preprinted form that has the basic office charges listed and space for the patient's current charges is an example of a(n):
   A. ledger.
   B. journal.
   C. day sheet.
   D. superbill.
   E. invoice.

Answer: **D**

Why: A superbill is usually a three-copy form that has all the necessary information for the patient to use in filing an insurance claim. It states the coding for the office visit with diagnosis and the amount charged for the services during the visit. Most superbills also have a place to put information about the patient's return or follow-up visit.

Review: Yes ❑ No ❑

---

21. An example of a debit adjustment is:
   A. applying a professional discount to the account.
   B. posting the payment made from the patient's insurance company.
   C. return of a nonsufficient fund check from a patient's bank.
   D. removing a charge from a patient's account that was placed there by mistake.

Answer: **C**

Why: A debit adjustment increases or adds to the patient's account balance. When a patient's check is not honored by the bank because there are not enough funds in the account to cover the amount, the office will apply the amount of the check back to the account. The payment is eliminated, and the patient owes the amount of the check plus an additional fee.

Review: Yes ❑ No ❑

22. When a check is received in the office, the medical assistant should first:
A. place the check in a cash lockbox.
B. endorse the check in writing or with a rubber stamp reading "for deposit only."
C. contact the bank to verify the funds are in the account.
D. enter the receipt of the check in the patient's medical chart.
E. process a receipt to send to the patient.

Answer: **B**

Why: Checks received in the office should be immediately endorsed "for deposit only" so no one would be able to cash the checks if the checks were lost or stolen.

Review: Yes ❑ No ❑

---

23. To reconcile a checking account, you must:
A. ensure that the information on the bank statement agrees with the information in the check register.
B. add to the checkbook balance any monthly fees or bank charges that are listed on the bank statement.
C. add any outstanding checks to the bank statement balance.
D. add to the bank statement the amount of interest earned on the account that month.

Answer: **A**

Why: The purpose of reconciling a checking account is to ensure that the information contained on the bank statement agrees with the information in the check register. Steps in reconciling that account include subtracting monthly fees or charges from the checkbook balance, subtracting outstanding checks from the bank statement balance, and adding the amount of interest earned to the checkbook balance.

Review: Yes ❑ No ❑

---

24. The amount of money an employee is paid after taxes are withheld is called:
A. gross income.
B. tax withholding.
C. wage.
D. net income.
E. deduction.

Answer: **D**

Why: The gross income is the amount of money earned before tax withholding. The wage is the amount of money earned by the employee, usually based on an hourly rate. Net income is known as "take home" pay after all the taxes and other deductions have been subtracted from the gross amount. A deduction is any amount of money taken out of the total income. Deductions may include state and federal taxes and insurance premiums.

Review: Yes ❑ No ❑

---

25. At the end of each calendar year, the employer is required to provide a statement to each employee of the year's total gross income and the taxes withheld. This form is the:
A. W-4.
B. W-2.
C. FICA.
D. FUTA.

Answer: **B**

Why: The W-4 form is the Employee's Withholding Allowance Certificate. The employee completes this form when employed and specifies the amount of deductions claimed for tax purposes. A W-2 form is issued to the employee at the end of each year to show the amount of money the employee earned during the year. It is required as proof of income when filing income tax. The Federal Insurance and Contribution Act (FICA) was developed to sponsor Social Security and Medicare. The Federal Unemployment Tax Act (FUTA) requires employers to pay a percentage of each employee's income to sponsor an unemployment fund.

Review: Yes ❑ No ❑

26. If a medical practice periodically had unexpected expenses and needed a loan, the practice owner could apply for:
A. additional petty cash.
B. a withholding allowance.
C. an endorsement.
D. reconciliation.
E. a line of credit.

Answer: **E**

Why: A line of credit is an established amount of money that a bank will loan a borrower. It can be used all at one time or in increments as needed. Petty cash is a small amount of cash kept on hand in the office for small purchases. Withholding allowance refers to money held out of earnings for tax purposes. Endorsement is the act of signing the back of a check as the payee for the amount represented on the front of the check. Reconciliation is the process of verifying that the information on the bank statement agrees with the information in the check register.

Review: Yes ❑ No ❑

---

27. A chart or table that includes a list and total of all the debit and credit accounts for a medical practice is a/an:
A. check register.
B. pegboard daysheet.
C. aging analysis.
D. monthly trial balance.

Answer: **D**

Why: A monthly trial balance is a chart of all the debits and credits for the practice and is used to ensure that the practice debits equal the credits. A check register is a log of all the activity of the checking account. A pegboard daysheet lists patient charges and payments made in a single day for the practice. Aging analysis is the process of determining the period between when the service is rendered and the bill is paid, usually in 30-day intervals.

Review: Yes ❑ No ❑

16

Practice Management

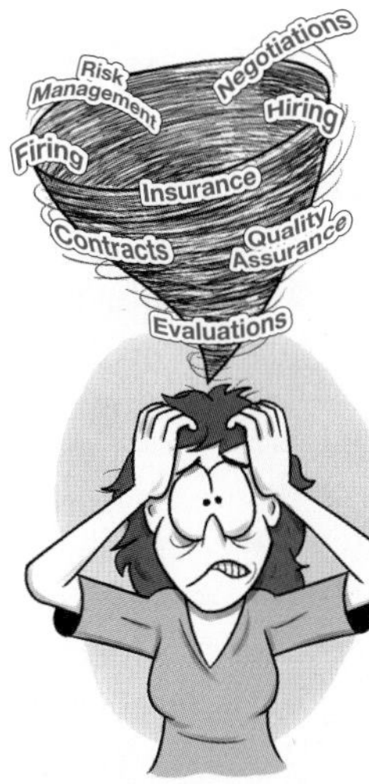

REVIEW TIP

Depending on the size of the practice, many management functions may be delegated to other departments and positions. An example is human resources. Questions involving these areas are incorporated into the role of practice management. Do not be confused if the manager where you work or completed your externship performs more or less of the functions that are included in this chapter. Also, do not be confused if the person in charge of your medical office has a different title such as practice or office administrator or executive or director. For the purposes of the national exams, the terms practice management and medical office management are used. If your medical office manager is not aware that you are preparing to take the national exam, this may be an opportunity to tell him or her and ask for any encouragement or advice that he or she may have.

Today's medical offices may be owned by a physician or corporation where the physician is not an owner but a contracted employee. One person is in charge of overseeing the day-to-day operations, the medical office manager. Depending on the size of the practice, other supervisory personnel may report to the practice manager. Each supervisor would then have staff reporting directly to him or her. Additional supervisory staff titles include clinical team leader or supervisor or manager; administrative team leader or supervisor or manager; and supervisors or managers of various departments such as human resources, laboratory, billing, and so on. In multispecialty organizations, clinical supervisors may be designated by specialty, such as pediatrics, internal medicine, and cardiology.

ORGANIZATION

Every medical office has an organizational model that may or may not be represented by a formal **organizational chart**. The chart shows the supervisory structure and reporting relationships between different functions

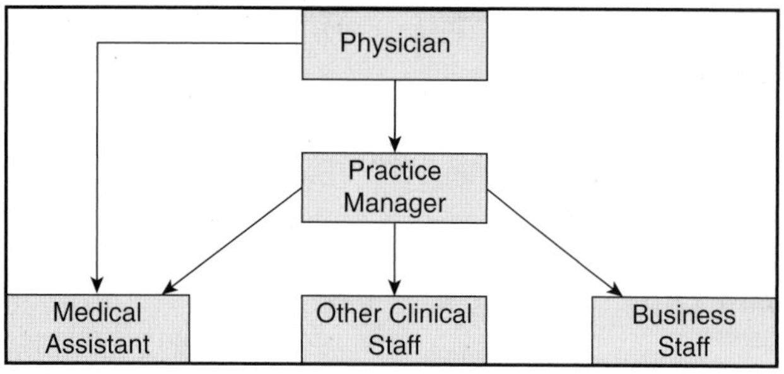

Figure 16-1 Organizational chart of physician-owned medical practice.

and positions—who is responsible for whom and what. In most states, the medical assistant is under the direct supervision of the physician and/or **midlevel providers**, such as the physician assistant or nurse practitioner, for direct patient care activities. The practice manager is usually responsible for interviewing, hiring, firing, evaluating, assuring training, and credentialing medical assistants, which are all considered administrative functions and not direct patient care functions. Figure 16-1 is a simplified organizational chart of a physician-owned practice. A physician-owned medical practice often has the legal designation of a professional corporation (PC).

Figure 16-2 shows a simplified organizational chart of a corporate-owned medical facility. The company may be for profit or nonprofit. Again, the practice manager is in charge of the day-to-day operations, with the exception of the direct patient care functions of the medical assistants, the physicians, and the midlevel providers who are accountable to the medical director. The dotted lines between the practice manager and the medical director indicate equality in rank and collaboration between the roles. The dotted line from the practice manager to the other physicians indicates collaboration. For example, the practice manager may ensure the physicians are properly credentialed. The medical director has the majority of the responsibilities for the physicians such as schedules and evaluations. The president, practice manager, medical director, and other physicians and staff are employees of the company and paid by the company. A board of directors is ultimately responsible but is not involved in the daily operations of the company.

The organizational charts reflect the **chain of command**, which demonstrates how each position is accountable to those directly superior and how the authority passes from one link in the chain to the next, or from the top to the bottom. Today's businesses, including medical offices, operate using a chain of command. It is important for employees to understand the chain of command and stay within it. Questions regarding the chain of command may be on the exam.

MANAGEMENT STYLES

Managers tend to direct or lead using a specific management or leadership style. Many names are associated with the styles, but four are most common. A manager usually gravitates to one style but may use a combination of the styles depending on the situation and group of employees:

- **Autocratic**—the manager makes all the decisions (autocratic directive); appropriate when rapid decisions must be made; an autocratic manager may make decisions but allows staff some autonomy in carrying out the work (autocratic permissive)
- **Democratic (participatory or teamwork)**—staff takes part in the decision making; democratic managers may monitor staff closely (directive) or not (permissive); should not be used when there is not enough time to get appropriate employee input; this style helps employees grow and develop
- **Bureaucratic**—the manager "goes by the book"; follows procedures exactly and generally does not like making complex decisions; best for training situations and working with precise tasks
- **Laissez-faire**—the manager provides very little leadership and gives employees lots of leeway; employees may feel insecure and lack confidence in the manager; this style works best in creative fields

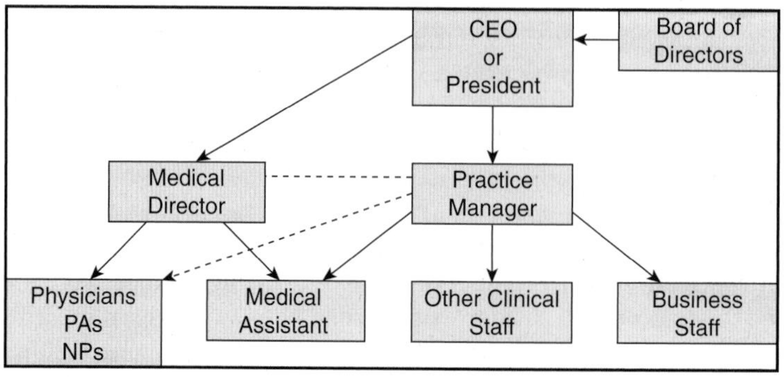

Figure 16-2 Organizational chart of corporate-owned medical practice.

COMMUNICATION

Chapter 7 discusses general communication techniques and communication with patients, persons with special needs, and coworkers. The practice management position requires excellent verbal and written communication and interpersonal skills. Some of the routine individuals and groups with whom the practice manager communicates on a regular basis are:

- Staff
- Patients
- Physicians (within the practice and in other practices)
- Hospitals
- Insurers
- Vendors
- Employers
- Contractors
- Governmental agencies
- Other regulatory and professional agencies
- Educational facilities
- Bankers
- Attorneys
- Community organizations

Communicating with each individual and group requires knowledge of the business or situation and often excellent problem-solving techniques. The role of the manager is also to assure that all communication is appropriate, respectful, timely, and Health Insurance Portability and Accountability Act (HIPAA) compliant. Many offices have policies and procedures related to communication, especially electronic communication.

STAFF COMMUNICATION

The following are communication modalities often used with staff.

- Staff meetings
  - **Agenda**—the list of meeting topics and the order in which they will be addressed (Fig. 16-3)
  - **Minutes**—the meeting record, including the date and time, who was present and absent, what was discussed, and who was responsible for any actions
- **In-service**—facilitating and communicating education and training conducted in the facility
- E-mail—a large number of offices have e-mail for each employee or group of employees
- Newsletters—provide information on what is going on in the practice, new policies and procedures or requirements, accomplishments and awards, and internal and community events; also often highlight staff members or departments

Valley Health Care: Staff Lounge
Staff Meeting Agenda
November 1, 20XX
12:00 to 1:30 p.m.
Lunch provided

Introductions	**Dan Martinez**
Staff News	**All**
Quality Assurance Report	**Susan Kuchara**
Policy and Procedure Update	**Dan Martinez**
EHR Committee Report	**Vrushti Patel**
Report from AHIMA Conference	**Shondeen Roberts**
Old Business:	
■ Extending office hours	**Dan Martinez**
■ Upcoming flu shot clinic	**Susan Kuchara**
New Business:	
■ Holiday party	**Dan Martinez**
Other	
Adjournment	

Next meeting December 2, 20XX 12:00 to 1:30 p.m.

Figure 16-3 Staff meeting agenda.

- Bulletin boards—usually located in the staff lounge; should not contain any confidential or sensitive information because janitorial staff and others outside of the practice may have access
- Communication books—becoming replaced with electronic communication; a notebook or binder with information the manager wants to inform the staff about is kept in a central location; employees may be required to initial each entry to assure it was read
- **Open door policy**—a practice giving staff the freedom to come talk with the manager any time that the office door is opened
- Suggestion box—staff submit ideas in a box with a name or anonymously

LEGAL AND BUSINESS FUNCTIONS

Another role of the practice manger is to assure compliancy with legal requirements and the standard for medical and business practices. This responsibility involves many systems and processes. Some of the more common ones are assuring that:

- Policy and procedure manuals are developed, maintained, reviewed, and updated (usually annually)
- Physicians and midlevel providers are properly licensed
- Physician and midlevel provider Drug Enforcement Administration (DEA) forms are up-to-date
- Medical assistants, phlebotomists, coders, and other personnel are properly trained and certified or credentialed according to federal, state, and professional standards
- Required licenses to operate the facility, such as local business licenses, are up-to-date
- Centers for Medicare and Medicaid Services (CMS) and accrediting approvals are in place and up-to-date
- Insurance requirements such as malpractice and liability contracts are up-to-date and reflect current values
- Contracts with health insurance companies, laboratories, attorneys, and other services necessary to conduct business are in place
- Required reporting to authorities, such as communicable diseases, is in compliance

BUDGET AND OVERALL FINANCES

A **budget** is created annually and reviewed at least monthly. The budget is the predicted expenses and revenues to operate over a given period of time. First, the manager must know the total expenses, which include such items as salaries with potential raises, rent, utilities, supplies, equipment rental and purchase, technology costs, insurance and business fees, taxes, contracted services such as janitorial support, and others. The manager reviews the commercial health care insurance and governmental agency patient care contracts and other sources of income such as sports physicals. He or she estimates the number of patients from each entity and then calculates the anticipated reimbursement or payments. This is the projected revenue. Sometimes the manager must renegotiate the contract if costs have risen. If revenues are lower than expected and the expenses are higher, the manager makes the decisions on what to cut back on, such as supplies and salaries, to balance the budget.

SCHEDULING AND TRAVEL

Ensuring that adequate staff are on duty at all times for the business to function properly is an additional aspect of the practice manager's role. Scheduling is a job that may be relegated to a supervisor or other person depending on the size of the practice but is monitored by the manager. Often physicians and other staff, such as medical assistants, travel for educational purposes with expenses covered by the practice. Planning for staffing the office when personnel are gone may be necessary. In addition to staffing, the following are some travel-related responsibilities:

- Travel and lodging accommodations; may be done through a travel agent; online websites are common; food may be paid for on a per diem basis, which means a certain money amount is designated either daily or per meal
- **Itinerary** preparation, which is the schedule of travel and events, with arrival and departure times and other specifics such as contact numbers
- Speaker accommodations for physicians or other staff presenting at conferences or other events, which may include arranging for media, creating biographies and presentation material such as PowerPoint presentations, and copying and shipping handout materials

OTHER BUSINESS FUNCTIONS

The contemporary medical office relies on technology for communication, appointment scheduling, coding, billing, diagnostic test ordering and reporting, prescription refills, and the electronic health record. These areas require highly specialized skills to install and maintain. The office manager:

- Evaluates and purchases the systems that fit the needs and budget of the practice
- Facilitates the installation and staff training
- Oversees the ongoing operations

Other managerial functions include assuring mailing and shipping services, inventory and supply purchase, and appropriate market and public relation strategies such as websites, brochures, and community events.

HUMAN RESOURCES

Human resources (HR), personnel services, or people services refers to how employees are managed by the business and deals with the following.

- Writing job descriptions, which should contain:
  - Name of organization
  - Name of position
  - Grade, if appropriate
  - Summary of position
  - Job responsibilities
  - Requirements and qualifications
  - Title of supervisor
- Recruiting staff
- Verifying qualifications and credentials
- Interviewing (Box 16-1)
- Hiring
- Terminating the employee following a process (unless the offense is very serious, and then termination may be immediate):
  - First offense: brings undesirable behavior to the attention of the staff member
  - Second offense: gives verbal or written warning
  - Third offense: gives written warning if verbal warning was previously given
  - Fourth offense: terminates the employee
- Performing staff evaluations and an improvement process as necessary:
  - Discusses the need for improvement with employee
  - Writes an improvement plan/contract with the employee
  - Provides additional training as needed
  - Follows progress at scheduled intervals
  - Terminates employee if improvement plan/contract not met
- Orienting new staff

Box 16-1

Interviewing Topics to Avoid

The U.S. Equal Employment Opportunity Commission (EEOC) prohibits discrimination in hiring. The following topics should be avoided when interviewing a job applicant to assure the applicant's rights are not violated.

RACE	**BIRTHPLACE**
SEX	**NATIONAL ORIGIN** **(may ask for proof that the applicant has authorization to work in the United States)**
COLOR	**MARITAL/FAMILY STATUS** **(do not ask if the applicant has children)**
DISABILITY **(may ask if the applicant has anything that may prevent him or her from fulfilling the job requirements)**	**AGE** **(may ask for proof that applicant is over 18 years of age if appearance justifies it and necessary for position)**
RELIGION	**IF THE APPLICANT HAS OR HAS HAD EEOC MATTERS**

- Managing payroll and benefits including following workers' compensation cases of office employees
- Setting policies involving personnel issues such as an employee grievance process
- Maintaining staff records such as performance evaluations, trainings, and employee health
- Assuring compliance with federal, state, and local income taxes and other regulations related to personnel
- Mediating appropriate issues between staff members

Once again, depending on the size of the organization, all of these responsibilities may fall on the practice manager. Larger organizations have a separate department with its own director, manager, supervisor, or coordinator. This person generally reports to the practice manager. Some offices contract out many HR services such as payroll.

HEALTH AND SAFETY

Regulations from the Occupational Safety and Health Act (OSHA) and state and local authorities regarding a safe work environment must be followed. The practice manager assures compliance by:

- Developing policies and procedures (P&P), which are then incorporated in a safety manual
- Establishing systems to accommodate P&P, for example, establishing a contract with a biohazardous waste company that includes containers, a schedule, and removal
- Educating and training staff in the P&Ps
- Making supplies and equipment available such as personal protective equipment
- Monitoring observance of the P&P

Health and safety also incorporate emergency preparedness plans with directions for office evacuation and posted information. Risk management and quality improvement are also the role of the practice manager and are discussed in Chapter 4, Law and Ethics.

THE PHYSICAL FACILITY

The physical facility or plant is the building or buildings, offices, parking structures, furniture, and mechanical systems (elevators, electrical, heating, cooling, plumbing, etc.) that make up the medical practice. To promote an efficient workplace the practice manager facilitates the following.

- Utilization of space
- Payment of mortgage or rental, utilities, etc.
- Selection and purchase or lease of capital equipment such as copy machines and telephone systems
- Establishment of contracts and oversight of janitorial, biohazardous waste disposal, and other services
- Required maintenance of elevators and heating, air conditioning, and other equipment; pavement of parking lot; replacement of light bulbs
- Replacement of worn furniture, carpeting, etc.
- Compliance with Americans with Disabilities Act (ADA) requirements
- Availability of adequate supplies and materials
- Emergency repairs such as clogged drains
- Security
- Landscape maintenance
- Plans for future needs

These elements interface with other legal, business, and health and safety responsibilities. The practice manager must have the capability of "wearing many hats," which requires the ability to prioritize and perform more than one task at a time. This referred to as multitasking or being multifocal.

TERMS

Practice Management Review

The following list reviews the terms discussed in this chapter and other important terms that you may see on the exam.

agenda the list of meeting topics and the order in which they will be addressed

autocratic management style the manager makes all the decisions (directive); appropriate when rapid decisions must be made; an autocratic manager may make decisions but allows staff some autonomy in carrying out the work (permissive)

budget the predicted expenses and revenues to operate over a given period of time

chain of command demonstrates how each rank is accountable to those directly superior and how the authority passes from one link in the chain to the next, or from the top to the bottom; reporting hierarchy

democratic (participatory or teamwork) management style staff takes part in the decision making;

democratic managers may monitor staff closely (directive) or not (permissive); should not be used when there is not enough time to get appropriate employee input; this style helps employees grow and develop

in-service education and training conducted in the facility

itinerary the schedule of travel and events, with arrival and departure times and other specifics such as contact numbers

midlevel providers examine, diagnose, and provide some treatments that must be signed off by a supervisor; generally, physician assistants and nurse practitioners

minutes the meeting record; contains the date and time, who was present and absent, what was discussed, and who is responsible for any actions

open door policy a practice giving staff the freedom to come talk any time the manager's office door is opened

organizational chart a model showing the supervisory structure and reporting relationships between different functions and positions; who is responsible for whom and what

REVIEW QUESTIONS

All questions are relevant for the CMA (AAMA), RMA (AMT), and CMAS (AMT) exam.

1. The model that shows the chain of command is called the:
   A. practice management.
   B. staff assignments.
   C. practice ownership.
   D. organizational chart.
   E. corporate plan.

Answer: **D**

Why: An organizational chart contains the formal supervisory structure and reporting relationships between different functions and positions of the management and staff. This is referred to as the chain of command.

Review: Yes ❑ No ❑

---

2. The hiring and firing role of the practice manager comes under the category of:
   A. health and safety.
   B. communications.
   C. human resources.
   D. quality improvement.

Answer: **C**

Why: Human resources is a common term involving services directly related to the people or staff in the organization. Hiring and firing are directly related to staff. Health and safety, communications, and quality improvement involve patients and other entities outside of the organization.

Review: Yes ❑ No ❑

---

3. If a medical practice has a health and safety violation, the organization involved would be:
   A. CDC.
   B. MSDS.
   C. CMS.
   D. P&P.
   E. OSHA.

Answer: **E**

Why: Workplace health and safety is under the Occupational Safety and Health Administration. The CDC is involved with public health, and the CMS is involved with Medicare and Medicaid health insurance. P&P refers to policies and procedures and is not an organization.

Review: Yes ❑ No ❑

---

4. The topics discussed at a staff meeting are reported in the:
   A. minutes.
   B. agenda.
   C. chain of command.
   D. itinerary.

Answer: **A**

Why: The agenda is the schedule of topics to be addressed at a meeting. The chain of command refers to the reporting structure of the business, and the itinerary refers to travel details.

Review: Yes ❑ No ❑

---

5. Management of the physical plant involves:
   A. leasing the facility.
   B. selecting the EHR system.
   C. complying with OSHA.
   D. managing payroll.
   E. mailing and shipping.

Answer: **A**

Why: The physical plant, also referred to as the physical facility, makes up the building and the systems, equipment, and supplies that are directly involved in the functioning of the building, whether it associated with a medical practice or another business such as an attorney's practice.

Review: Yes ❑ No ❑

6. The topics to be discussed at a staff meeting are included in the:
   A. agenda.
   B. minutes.
   C. chain of command.
   D. itinerary.

Answer: **A**

Why: The minutes are the topics of a meeting that already took place. The chain of command refers to the reporting structure of the business, and the itinerary refers to travel details.

Review: Yes ❑ No ❑

---

7. Through which of the following is the manager most likely to discover a problem?
   A. Policies and procedures
   B. Organizational chart
   C. Risk management
   D. Physical plant
   E. Human resources

Answer: **C**

Why: Risk management is a process to routinely assess, identify, correct, and monitor any potential problems to prevent harm and loss.

Review: Yes ❑ No ❑

---

8. The office manager role includes all of the following EXCEPT:
   A. developing policy and procedure manuals.
   B. verifying licenses and other credentials.
   C. negotiating contracts.
   D. documenting in the medical record.

Answer: **D**

Why: Unless a person is providing direct care, he or she would not be documenting in the medical portion of the patient's record. If the practice manager functions in a different role, such as a medical assistant, this is not part of the manager's role.

Review: Yes ❑ No ❑

---

9. The schedule of travel and events is called the:
   A. minutes.
   B. agenda.
   C. chain of command.
   D. in-service.
   E. itinerary.

Answer: **E**

Why: The minutes are the topics of the meeting that already took place. The chain of command refers to the reporting structure of the business, and the agenda refers to the topics of the upcoming meeting. In-service refers to training activities offered in the organizations.

Review: Yes ❑ No ❑

---

10. The physical plant must comply with:
   A. ADA.
   B. HIPAA.
   C. CMS.
   D. MSDS.

Answer: **A**

Why: The physical plant refers to the building, parking area, hallways, elevators, and so on. All of these structures are expected to meet the specifications of the Americans with Disabilities Act (ADA), which requires adequate access to people with special needs.

Review: Yes ❑ No ❑

---

11. If a manager does not include others in the decision making or how the decision should be implemented, this management style is referred to as:
   A. diplomatic.
   B. autocratic.
   C. democratic.
   D. bureaucratic.
   E. laissez-faire.

Answer: **B**

Why: Rationale needed. Diplomatic is handling situations with tact; democratic is allowing others to participate in decision making; bureaucratic is very structured and "goes by the book"; laissez-faire is an easy going leadership style permitting lots of leeway to employees

Review: Yes ❑ No ❑

12. Training conducted in the workplace is referred to as:
    A. staff meetings.
    B. seminars.
    C. in-service.
    D. supervision.

Answer: **C**

Why: A staff meeting is a get together of all members of the practice to discuss various topics with a planned agenda. A seminar is an educational program attended outside of the office and usually conducted by a professional organization. Supervision is what the person above you on the chain of command does.

Review: Yes ❑ No ❑

---

13. All of the following are common methods used by the practice manager to communicate with staff EXCEPT:
    A. bulletin boards.
    B. e-mails.
    C. communication books.
    D. newsletters.
    E. certified letters.

Answer: **E**

Why: The practice manager would not normally send a staff member a certified letter unless he or she was unable to reach the person using the common methods. Certified mail is used to reach patients with important information that may require documentation that it was received.

Review: Yes ❑ No ❑

---

14. When dealing with supplies, the role of the practice manager would most likely be to:
    A. assure they were ordered.
    B. order the supplies.
    C. put them away.
    D. receive the supplies when they arrive.

Answer: **A**

Why: Ordering, receiving, and putting away supplies are usually the duties of the medical assistant or medical administrative specialist. The manager's role is to assure that the functions are taking place.

Review: Yes ❑ No ❑

---

15. A job description usually contains all of the following elements EXCEPT:
    A. summary of the position.
    B. name of the supervisor.
    C. responsibilities.
    D. qualifications.
    E. organization.

Answer: **B**

Why: The job description usually includes the title of the supervisor, such as director, but does not include the person's actual name. The names of supervisors may change, but the organization's job descriptions are usually in place for a long period of time.

Review: Yes ❑ No ❑

---

16. The major purpose for monitoring a budget is to:
    A. determine who is spending too much money.
    B. ascertain if Medicare is paying on time.
    C. assure the revenue is meeting the expenses.
    D. decide how much money is left for raises.

Answer: **C**

Why: A budget is done to estimate what the annual expenses will be and what the revenues will be. If the revenue does not cover the expenses, adjustments in the budget must be made.

Review: Yes ❑ No ❑

17. An example of a typical job requirement to work in a medical office is:
    A. ability to lift 25 lbs.
    B. proof of citizenship in the United States.
    C. being unmarried.
    D. age between 18 and 40 years.
    E. 20/20 vision.

Answer: **A**

Why: Working in a medical office usually requires lifting, whether it may be in assisting a patient or dealing with supplies and equipment. It is not acceptable to require or ask about citizenship (may ask for documentation regarding working in this country legally which may be done on a work visa), marital status, age (unless person looks under 18 years old), and unreasonable physical requirements such as 20/20 vision.

Review: Yes ❑ No ❑

---

18. A question that you would not ask during an interview would be whether the applicant:
    A. is certified in his or her field.
    B. has a college degree.
    C. is able to work on Sundays.
    D. has a religious affiliation.

Answer: **D**

Why: Whether the person has a certification or went to college could very well be a job requirement or preference. If the office is open on Sundays or may hold special events on Sundays, such as immunization clinics prior to the beginning of school, then asking the applicant if he or she is able to work on Sundays is appropriate. It is never appropriate to ask about an applicant's religious affiliation.

Review: Yes ❑ No ❑

---

19. When an employee entered incorrect information into a medical record that resulted in an incorrect payment, the manager would most likely:
    A. have the employee apologize to the patient.
    B. terminate the employee.
    C. provide a verbal warning.
    D. not give the employee a raise.
    E. dock the employee's pay.

Answer: **C**

Why: If it is the employee's first offense, the manager would probably give a verbal warning. If it had happened in the past, the employee may be given a written warning and/or additional training.

Review: Yes ❑ No ❑

---

20. When an employee is under a performance improvement plan, the manager will probably meet with the employee:
    A. at the employee's annual evaluation.
    B. on a predetermined schedule.
    C. when the manager has time.
    D. at staff meetings.

Answer: **B**

Why: Part of the improvement plan should be to schedule regular periods to follow up on the employee's progress. The exception is if the contract states that the next time the behavior occurs the employee is terminated.

Review: Yes ❑ No ❑

---

21. When dealing with HIPAA compliance, the manager would most likely use what type of management style?
    A. Democratic
    B. Bureaucratic
    C. Laissez-faire
    D. Diplomatic

Answer: **B**

Why: HIPAA compliance is extremely important and P&Ps should be followed without exception. This is an example when a bureaucratic style should be used regardless of the manager's principal leadership style.

Review: Yes ❑ No ❑

22. A role of the practice manager related to service vendors is to:
   A. make appointments for them with the physician.
   B. provide patients with the vendors' brochures.
   C. negotiate contracts for their services.
   D. request that they supply lunch for staff meetings.
   E. treat them as if they are staff members.

Answer: **C**

Why: The role of the office manager is to get the best service for the best price. Appointments with the physician are usually made by the person scheduling appointments. Patients who require vendor services may be given contact information not marketing information. Vendors will sometimes provide staff lunch if an in-service is involved, but this is sometimes frowned upon as conflict of interest. While vendors should be treated with respect, they are not on the same day-to-day status as staff members.

Review: Yes ❑ No ❑

---

23. If an incident occurs in the medical office that results in a legal action, the manager is expected to:
   A. keep it a secret.
   B. place the information in the staff newsletter.
   C. maintain records of the occurrence.
   D. go to court.

Answer: **C**

Why: The manager is expected to discuss the incident with the appropriated parties involved and keep it to himself or herself. It should not be discussed in the staff newsletter because a newsletter is not confidential. The manager is not usually the person to go to court if it becomes necessary, but the manager is expected to keep accurate records on the incident and save medical records that may be involved.

Review: Yes ❑ No ❑

---

24. When preparing the budget, the office manager would include all the following EXCEPT:
   A. predicted increased costs of supplies.
   B. estimated tax payments.
   C. rumored increases in Medicare payments
   D. inflation-adjusted equipment purchases.

Answer: **C**

Why: Most of the budget is created on predicted costs based on estimates and inflation. Generally, these estimates are higher than the previous year for payments. Rumored increases in any payments or revenue are not a reasonable approach to budgeting, especially since most insurance plans, including Medicare, continually attempt to negotiate lower payments to physicians.

Review: Yes ❑ No ❑

---

25. A function of managing the physical facility may be to:
   A. purchase pharmaceuticals.
   B. contract for landscaping maintenance.
   C. upgrade the electronic health record system.
   D. replace the electrocardiogram (ECG) machine.
   E. evaluate a new payroll service.

Answer: **B**

Why: Landscaping maintenance is a function of the physical facility. Purchasing pharmaceuticals, upgrading the electronic health record, and replacing the ECG machine are related to direct patient care services. Payroll is a human resources function.

Review: Yes ❑ No ❑

Unit 4

Clinical Practice

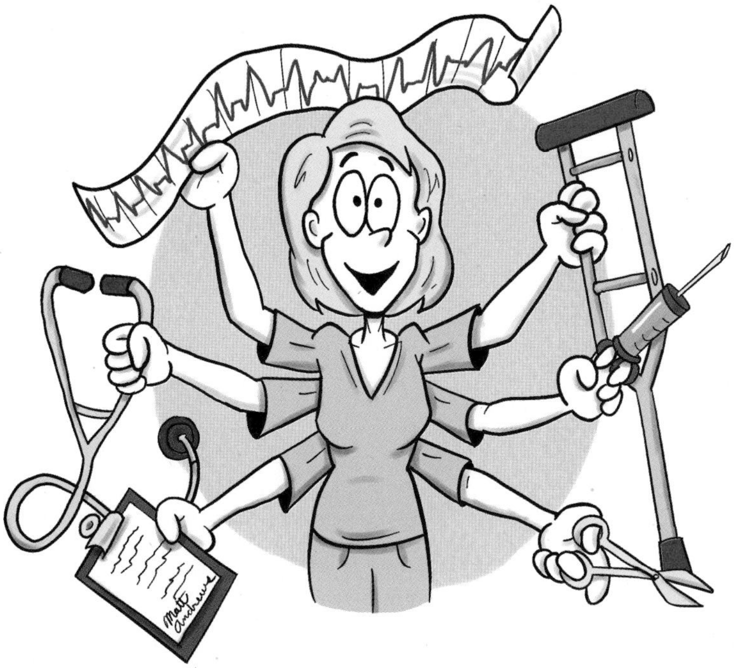

17

Microorganisms and Asepsis

REVIEW TIP

This chapter begins the review of clinical topics. Asepsis is a cornerstone of safe, healthy practices in the medical office and in personal life. To reinforce these principles, look for applications at work and at home as each topic is addressed.

MICROORGANISMS

Microorganisms, or microbes or germs, are living organisms that are too small to see with the naked eye. These organisms surround us and are part of every living process. Some of these microbes cause disease, and others cause disease only under certain circumstances; for example, *Escherichia coli* (*E. coli*), which is found normally in the intestinal tract, may cause sepsis if introduced into the bloodstream.

COMMON PATHOGENS

Common **pathogens** are prevalent microorganisms that cause disease.

- Bloodborne pathogen—any type of pathogen that lives in and is transmitted through blood
  - Bacteria (singular *bacterium*)—one-celled microorganisms; may be found singularly or in chains
    - Types defined by principal shapes
    - Spherical (cocci; singular *coccus*; Latin, meaning "berry")—examples are streptococci, staphylococci, pneumococci
    - Rod (bacilli; singular *bacillus*; Latin, meaning "little staff")—examples are *Bacillus anthracis* (cause of anthrax), *Mycobacterium tuberculosis* (cause of tuberculosis), *Bacillus tetanus* (cause of tetanus)
    - Spiral (spirilla or spirochete; singular *spirillum*; Latin, meaning "spiral"); corkscrew-shaped; an example is *Helicobacter pylori* (one cause of chronic gastritis)
    - Spores—encapsulated (shell or capsule) bacteria in an inactive or resting state; in the medical office, spores are killed only by autoclaving
  - Types defined by air need
    - Aerobic—bacteria that require oxygen for survival
    - Anaerobic—bacteria that live without oxygen
  - Virus—extremely small microbes that pass through most filters; examples of viral diseases include measles, mumps, rubella, herpes, hepatitis B, and influenza
  - Fungus (plural *fungi*)—microbes that grow on other organisms, causing diseases such as tinea (ringworm), candidiasis (thrush), histoplasmosis, or coccidioidomycosis

- Protozoa—simplest form of animal pathogen; parasites; examples of diseases caused by protozoa are malaria, giardiasis, and trichomonas (one cause of vaginitis)

PORTALS OF ENTRY

Portals of entry are the ways microorganisms enter the body.

- Respiratory system—nose, mouth (air)
- Gastrointestinal system—mouth, rectum (food and water)
- Integumentary system—any break in the skin
- Eyes and ears
- Vascular system—through blood supply

CHAIN OF INFECTION

The **chain of infection** illustrates the elements necessary for disease to spread (Fig. 17-1).

1. Reservoir host—initial carrier of the microbe; may be a person, an animal, an insect
2. Means of exit—method of leaving the reservoir host (e.g., sneezing, coughing, feces, blood)
3. Means of transmission—method of moving from the exit of the reservoir host to the entrance of the susceptible host, such as air, contaminated materials called **fomites** (such as food or water), or soiled hands
4. Means of entrance—see "Portals of Entry"

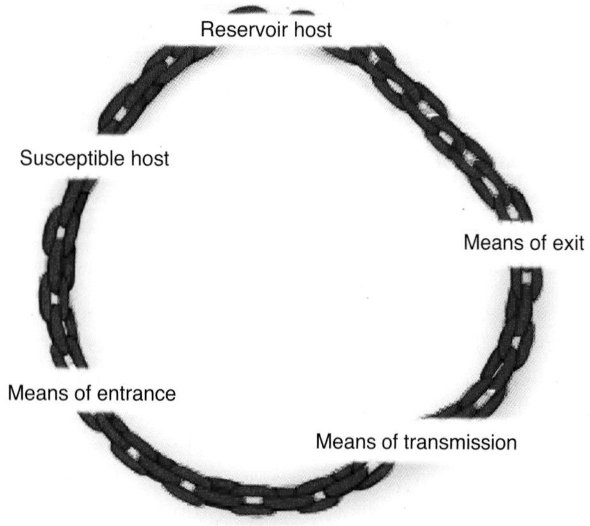

Figure 17-1 Chain of infection.

5. Susceptible host—person with no previous immunity or with weakened immunity resulting from illness, injury, or poor nutrition, or if the pathogen is too virulent (strong) for a normal immune system to resist

LOCALIZED VERSUS GENERALIZED INFECTIONS

- Localized—infection confined to one area of the body (e.g., a pustule)
- Generalized or systemic—infection spread throughout the body (e.g., septicemia)

BIOCHEMICAL AGENTS TO COMBAT PATHOGENS

- Antibiotics—substances ingested, injected, or applied to a living being that have the power to inhibit the growth of or to destroy bacteria
- Chemotherapy—ingestion, injection, or application of chemical agents in treating disease
- Immunizations—biological or chemical agents that create immunity to specific diseases when ingested or injected (see Box 6-7, "Types of Immunity," and Box 6-8, "Common Vaccine-Preventable Diseases" in Chapter 6)

ASEPSIS

Asepsis is the absence or the control of microorganisms. Many of the U.S. Occupational Safety and Health Administration (OSHA) guidelines and mandates address asepsis.

PURPOSES OF ASEPSIS

- Protect patient/public
- Protect health care worker
- Prevent infectious disease from starting
- Stop infectious disease from spreading

TYPES OF ASEPSIS

- Medical asepsis (clean technique)—techniques and procedures to reduce number of microorganisms in an environment and decrease opportunities for further spread
- Surgical asepsis (sterile technique)—techniques and procedures to eliminate *all* microorganisms in an environment

COMMON METHODS OF ASEPSIS

■ Medical handwashing

1. Remove jewelry (wedding and engagement rings usually remain)
2. Use hand- or foot-controlled faucet
3. Wash hands and wrists for 2 to 3 minutes
4. Use brush and cuticle stick on nails
5. Hold hands in downward position while rinsing
6. Dry hands with paper or clean cloth towel
7. Turn off hand faucets with paper or clean cloth towel
8. Lotion may be applied

■ Surgical handwashing

1. Remove all jewelry
2. Use foot- or knee-controlled faucet
3. Wash hands, wrists, and forearms for 10 minutes with brush (first surgical scrub of day)
4. Use cuticle stick on nails
5. Hold hands in upward position while rinsing
6. Dry with sterile towel
7. Do not apply lotion
8. Keep hands upright and do not touch anything until sterile gloves are applied

■ Antiseptics—bacteriostatic chemical cleaning agents used on skin to remove and to inhibit the growth of bacteria; these agents do not destroy all pathogens

■ Disinfectants—bacteriostatic chemical agents used to clean and to decrease the pathogens on inanimate objects (e.g., surgical instruments, countertops); these agents do not destroy all pathogens

■ Sterilization—process of destroying all living organisms

- Gas—used for wheelchairs, beds, and other large equipment; very toxic
- Dry heat—used for instruments that corrode easily; requires at least 1 hour at 320°F
- Chemical (cold sterilization)—used for heat-sensitive equipment such as fiberoptic endoscopes; equipment is soaked in closed containers with strong agents (e.g., glutaraldehyde); specific time recommendations are determined by the manufacturer of the chemical agent
- Steam heat (autoclave)—the most common method of sterilization used in the medical office; the steam is under pressure to achieve higher temperatures
  - Water temperature must be 212°F
  - Steam temperature must be 250°F to 254°F
  - Time required is between 20 and 40 minutes, depending on how tightly items are wrapped (the looser the wrap, the shorter the time required)
  - Sterilization bags or pouches, disposable paper wraps, or surgical towels are used for autoclaving surgical instruments, including those that will be placed on sterile fields; usually, double wrapping is required when using disposable paper wraps or surgical towels
  - Packages must be dry before removing them from the autoclave
  - Procedure:

1. Place cleaned and dried instruments in center of wrap (hinged instruments in open position) with sterilization indicator tape
2. Position opened wrap on a flat surface in a diamond shape with a point toward you
3. Fold the corner closest to you over the instrument
4. Fold the first side corner toward the center, completely covering the instrument; fold extra material back to form a tab; repeat with the second side corner
5. Fold the last corner toward the center and around the packet, ensuring the instrument is completely covered
6. Fasten the packet with sterilization-sensitive tape

■ Standard or universal precautions

- Treat all blood and bodily fluids as contaminated
- Protect the patient from you (especially when patient's immune system is compromised)
- Protect yourself from the patient

■ Personal protective equipment (PPE)

- Gloves (nonsterile used for majority of patient procedures; sterile used only for procedures requiring sterile aseptic technique, e.g., surgery)
- Goggles or eye shields
- Masks
- Gowns
- Aprons

■ Other safety materials and actions

- Safety plan and policies and procedures
- Material Safety Data Sheets (MSDS) and labels for all hazardous agents
- Employee training
- Sharps (needles, scalpels, glass vials, etc.) containers
- Other biohazard receptacles for non-sharp material contaminated with body fluids
- Eyewash stations
- Showers

TERMS

Microorganisms and Asepsis Review

The following list reviews the terms discussed in this chapter and other important terms that you may see on the exam.

antibiotic a substance ingested, injected, or applied to a living being that has the power to inhibit the growth of or to destroy bacteria

antiseptic a chemical cleaning agent used on the skin to remove or to inhibit the growth of bacteria

asepsis the absence of or the control of microorganisms

bacteria (singular *bacterium*) one-celled microorganisms; may be found singularly or in chains

bacteriocide an agent or a process that kills bacteria

bacteriology the study of bacteria

bacteriostasis the process of inhibiting or controlling bacterial growth

bloodborne pathogen any type of disease-causing organism that lives in and is transmitted through blood

chain of infection elements necessary for disease to spread: reservoir, host, portal of exit, means of transmission, portal of entry, susceptible host

disinfectant a bacteriostatic chemical agent used to clean and to decrease the number of pathogens on inanimate objects (such as surgical instruments, countertops); does not sterilize

fomite contaminated food or drink and contaminated objects such as soiled hands; provide avenue for indirect transmission of microbes

health care–acquired infection (HAI) infection a patient acquires when in a health care facility, typically a hospital setting; also known as nosocomial infection

medical asepsis (clean technique) techniques and procedures that reduce the number of microorganisms in an environment and decrease opportunities for further spread

microorganisms microbes or germs; living organisms that are too small to see with the naked eye

mycology the study of fungi

OSHA (Occupational Safety and Health Administration) a federal agency that develops and monitors guidelines and mandates that address health and safety in the workplace

parasite an organism that lives at the expense of another organism

parasitology study of worms, protozoa, and other parasites

pathogens microorganisms that cause disease

portals of entry routes by which microorganisms enter the body

spores encapsulated bacteria in an inactive or resting state

sterilization process of destroying all living organisms

surgical asepsis (sterile technique) techniques and procedures intended to eliminate all microorganisms in an environment

virology study of virus

REVIEW QUESTIONS

All questions are relevant for the CMA (AAMA) and RMA (AMT) exams. Questions 1 through 17 are relevant for the CMAS (AMT) exam.

1. The specific name used for any type of pathogen that lives in and is transmitted through blood is:
   A. anaerobic bacteria.
   B. parasitic amoeba.
   C. bloodborne pathogen.
   D. aerobic pathogen.

Answer: **C**

Why: A bloodborne pathogen is a microorganism that lives in and is transmitted through blood.

Review: Yes ❑ No ❑

---

2. The chain of infection requires the microorganism to find a means of exit from the host. These means of exit include the following EXCEPT:
   A. sneezing.
   B. ingestion.
   C. coughing.
   D. blood.
   E. feces.

Answer: **B**

Why: Ingestion is the process of taking food or water into the body. This is a means by which a microorganism can enter the body but is not a means of exit.

Review: Yes ❑ No ❑

---

3. An example of a viral disease is:
   A. ringworm.
   B. candidiasis.
   C. malaria.
   D. measles.

Answer: **D**

Why: Ringworm and candidiasis are examples of conditions caused by fungus. Malaria is caused by protozoal parasites.

Review: Yes ❑ No ❑

---

4. A bacteria that lives without oxygen is:
   A. aerobic.
   B. aseptic.
   C. anemic.
   D. anoxic.
   E. anaerobic.

Answer: **E**

Why: An anaerobe is a microorganism that can live and grow in the absence of oxygen. The term **anaerobic** describes this type of bacteria. Aerobic means requiring oxygen for life and growth. Anoxic is a term used to describe the absence of oxygen in arterial blood. Anemic describes a condition in which the number of red blood cells or hemoglobin of the blood is below the normal level. Aseptic describes the absence or control of microorganisms.

Review: Yes ❑ No ❑

---

5. The major reason for using proper aseptic procedures is to:
   A. follow office policies.
   B. destroy all bacteria on surfaces.
   C. control the patient's immune system.
   D. protect patients and health care workers.

Answer: **D**

Why: Aseptic technique is practiced to protect patients, the public, and health care workers from the transmission of disease-causing microorganisms. Asepsis is a condition in which living pathogenic organisms are absent: the environment is sterile.

Review: Yes ❑ No ❑

6. The process that destroys all living organisms is:
   A. handwashing.
   B. sanitizing.
   C. autoclaving.
   D. cleansing.
   E. disinfecting.

Answer: **C**

Why: Autoclaving is the only process listed that ensures that all bacteria are destroyed and the items autoclaved are sterile.

Review: Yes ❑ No ❑

---

7. Personal protective equipment includes the following EXCEPT:
   A. needles.
   B. gowns.
   C. gloves.
   D. masks.

Answer: **A**

Why: Personal protective equipment (PPE) includes any device or garment that protects the individual from contact with blood and body fluid that may contain bloodborne pathogens.

Review: Yes ❑ No ❑

---

8. Ringworm is an example of a:
   A. bacteria.
   B. fungus.
   C. protozoa.
   D. virus.
   E. parasite.

Answer: **B**

Why: Fungus is a simple parasitic plant. Ringworm is a type of fungal skin disease that forms a red, ringlike lesion on the skin.

Review: Yes ❑ No ❑

---

9. The organization that develops and monitors guidelines and mandates health and safety practices in the workplace is:
   A. AMA.
   B. CDC.
   C. FDA.
   D. OSHA.

Answer: **D**

Why: The Occupational Safety and Health Administration (OSHA) is a federal agency that has developed policies for the workplace that include guidelines for health care workers to prevent the transmission of bloodborne pathogens.

Review: Yes ❑ No ❑

---

10. A chemical agent used to clean countertops to decrease the number of disease-causing organisms is a(n):
    A. antibiotic.
    B. disinfectant.
    C. antiseptic.
    D. sterile solution.
    E. germicidal soap.

Answer: **B**

Why: A disinfectant is used to clean surfaces to free them of pathogenic organisms. Antibiotics, antiseptics, and germicidal soaps are used on or in the body, not on inanimate objects. A sterile solution is any product that is free of microorganisms.

Review: Yes ❑ No ❑

---

11. Characteristics of a susceptible host include the following EXCEPT:
    A. lack of hygiene.
    B. poor nutrition.
    C. intact immune system.
    D. chronic illness.
    E. injury to the body.

Answer: **C**

Why: A susceptible host is a person who is more vulnerable to a disease or disorder. Chronic illness, injury to the body, poor nutrition, and a lack of good hygiene contribute to the environment for microorganisms to cause infection or disease. A person with an intact immune system is more likely to be able to resist infections caused by pathogens.

Review: Yes ❑ No ❑

12. One difference between a localized and a generalized infection is that a:
    A. localized infection is contained within a specific area.
    B. generalized infection has spread to one specific area of the body.
    C. localized infection is the same as a systemic infection.
    D. generalized infection is caused by nonspecific microorganisms.

Answer: **A**

Why: A localized infection is confined to one area or part of the body, whereas a generalized infection has spread to many areas of the body or may be systemic.

Review: Yes ❑ No ❑

---

13. The most important guideline stated in the universal precautions is to:
    A. always wear gloves even if there is no risk for contact with bloodborne pathogens.
    B. treat all blood and bodily fluids as contaminated.
    C. label specimens from patients who are suspected of having a bloodborne pathogen such as HIV.
    D. conserve supplies by reusing gloves but changing them when visibly soiled with blood.

Answer: **B**

Why: All patients' blood and bodily fluids are considered contaminated, even if they are not. This practice will ensure you always use universal precautions with all patients, not just those suspected of having a bloodborne pathogen. It is not necessary to use gloves when performing procedures that will not put you at risk for contact with blood or body fluids. This includes most noninvasive procedures. Never reuse gloves on different patients.

Review: Yes ❑ No ❑

---

14. When a patient acquires an infection while in a medical facility, it is referred to as a:
    A. bacterial infection.
    B. causative infection.
    C. health care–acquired infection.
    D. pathogenic infection.

Answer: **C**

Why: A health care–acquired infection is an infection separate from the patient's original condition that is acquired while the patient is being treated in a hospital or health care facility.

Review: Yes ❑ No ❑

---

15. The chain of infection does not include:
    A. susceptible host.
    B. means of transmission.
    C. reservoir.
    D. asepsis.

Answer: **D**

Why: Asepsis is the absence or the control of microorganisms. The use of aseptic technique inhibits the spread of disease.

Review: Yes ❑ No ❑

---

16. Which of the following is a chemical cleaning agent used on the skin to remove bacteria?
    A. Disinfectant
    B. Antiseptic
    C. Immunization
    D. Cold sterilization solution
    E. Sterile water

Answer: **B**

Why: A disinfectant is a chemical agent used to clean inanimate objects. An immunization is a biological or chemical agent that creates immunity to specific diseases. Immunizations are ingested or injected. Cold sterilization solution is used to soak instruments before autoclaving. Sterile water is not a chemical cleaning agent.

Review: Yes ❑ No ❑

17. Hepatitis B and rubella are examples of diseases caused by:
    A. yeasts.
    B. fungi.
    C. bacteria.
    D. protozoa.
    E. viruses.

Answer: **E**

Why: Viruses are the smallest form of microorganisms and are not susceptible to antibiotics. They are difficult to treat.

Review: Yes ❑ No ❑

---

18. Steps to follow for proper autoclaving include:
    A. keeping hinged instruments in an open position.
    B. wrapping instruments while they are wet.
    C. wearing sterile gloves to wrap autoclave packs for processing.
    D. storing autoclaved packs while they are damp.

Answer: **A**

Why: Instruments should be dry before they are wrapped for autoclaving. It is not necessary to wear sterile gloves to process wraps for autoclaving. After autoclaving, packs need to be dry before being placed in storage.

Review: Yes ❑ No ❑

---

19. Which of the following are bacteria normally found in the intestinal tract but that cause infection if introduced into the urinary tract or bloodstream?
    A. *Clostridium tetani*
    B. *Bacillus anthracis*
    C. *Escherichia coli*
    D. *Treponema pallidum*
    E. Coccidioidomycosis

Answer: **C**

Why: Escherichia coli is abbreviated to *E. coli*. It is a bacterium found in the intestinal tract and usually causes no problem except when it invades other body systems. *Clostridium tetani* causes tetanus, *Bacillus anthracis* causes anthrax, and *Treponema pallidum* causes syphilis.

Review: Yes ❑ No ❑

---

20. The process that kills spore-producing bacteria is:
    A. handwashing.
    B. chemical soaking.
    C. disinfecting.
    D. autoclaving.

Answer: **D**

Why: Autoclaving is the same as sterilizing. It is the use of steam under pressure. The autoclave is used at an average temperature of 250°F for an average time of 30 minutes. This process is used to ensure that spores will be killed.

Review: Yes ❑ No ❑

---

21. Which of the following is not part of proper surgical handwashing technique?
    A. Remove jewelry.
    B. Dry hands with sterile towel.
    C. Hold hands in a downward position while rinsing.
    D. Use foot- or knee-controlled faucet.
    E. Use a cuticle stick on nails.

Answer: **C**

Why: When performing a surgical handwash, hands should be held upward while rinsing so the water does not carry bacteria from the unscrubbed portion of the upper arm to the scrubbed portion of the arms and hands.

Review: Yes ❑ No ❑

---

22. The unique characteristic of spore-forming bacteria is that they:
    A. are easily destroyed with the use of chemical cleaners.
    B. are only found in cocci shapes or formation.
    C. account for most of the known viruses.
    D. are able to form a resistant capsule around themselves.

Answer: **D**

Why: Spore-forming bacteria are able to form a capsule or shell around themselves that is resistant to most means of asepsis, such as heat or chemicals. Autoclaving or sterilizing is the only method known to kill spores.

Review: Yes ❑ No ❑

23. Objects that provide an avenue for indirect transmission of microbes are called:
    A. spores.
    B. pathogens.
    C. PPE.
    D. fomites.

Answer: **D**

Why: Spores are bacteria that are able to form a capsule or shell around them that is resistant to most means of asepsis, such as heat or chemicals. Pathogens include any disease causing microorganisms. PPE is personal protective equipment used for protection during procedures where there is a chance of contact with pathogens.

Review: Yes ❑ No ❑

---

24. A type of protozoa that causes vaginitis is:
    A. *Candida*.
    B. staphylococci.
    C. *Trichomonas*.
    D. tinea.

Answer: **C**

Why: Candida is an example of yeast, tinea is ringworm, and staphylococci are bacteria. *Trichomonas* are protozoa, single-celled parasites.

Review: Yes ❑ No ❑

---

25. The temperature setting and timing for proper autoclaving is:
    A. 175°F for 10 minutes.
    B. 212°F for 15 minutes.
    C. 250°F for 30 minutes.
    D. 275°F for 45 minutes.
    E. 300°F for 30 minutes.

Answer: **C**

Why: Most autoclave loads are processed at 250°F for 30 minutes. The timing or temperature may vary slightly because of the tightness of the wrap.

Review: Yes ❑ No ❑

---

26. Which of the following is an example of spherical or round bacteria?
    A. Staphylococci
    B. Tetanus
    C. *E. coli*
    D. *Shigella*

Answer: **A**

Why: Round or spherical-shaped bacteria are called *cocci*. Under the microscope, staphylococci appear as clusters or groups of round bacteria. Tetanus bacteria, *E. coli*, and *Shigella* are rod shaped.

Review: Yes ❑ No ❑

18

Patient Exams

REVIEW TIP

The national exams often require you to identify instruments and equipment from a picture. Practice recognizing various instruments and their medical uses. Also, study the body positions described in this chapter, since they usually are incorporated in the exams.

The medical assistant, from the moment of contact, observes the patient for baseline behaviors, changes, and signs and symptoms. This first observation begins the patient exam, and observations continue throughout the patient visit. Specific medical record forms are used to record the information. The medical assistant should note the data from previous visits as a comparison to the newly obtained information. Appropriate asepsis should be followed throughout procedures (refer to Chapter 17).

PATIENT INTERVIEW

The interview process discussed in this chapter incorporates the knowledge, techniques, and skills from previous chapters—including medical terminology, anatomy and physiology, communication, law and ethics, patient education, medical records, and microorganisms and asepsis. Professionalism and confidentiality are expected standards.

- Chief complaint—a summary of the **patient's words** explaining why he or she is seeking health care; best determined by asking an open-ended question such as "What brings you here today?"
- Symptoms—subjective descriptions of altered health indicators (e.g., nausea, headache); complaints that cannot be seen or measured
- Medical-related histories—accounts of past health status or practices and exposures that affect health status
  - Family history—medical history of the patient's close biological relatives (e.g., grandparents, parents, siblings)
  - Patient medical history—the patient's past health status; usually conducted by a review of body systems
  - Social and environmental history—the patient's past and current personal habits and exposures that influence health
  - Screen for abuse and domestic violence—a history-type questionnaire recommended by many professional organizations and mandated in some jurisdictions to assist in determining the presence of abuse in the patient's life

COMMON ASSESSMENT MEASUREMENTS

Obtaining assessment measurements is also known as **anthropometry**. Anthropometry comprises signs, functions, and capacities that can be objectively determined by the senses (e.g., sight, hearing, smell, touch) or by specific equipment and tests. Medical asepsis is maintained in preparing, performing, and following all common assessment functions.

VITAL SIGNS

Vital signs are measurements of body temperature, pulse rate, respirations (TPR), and blood pressure (BP).

- Body temperature—measured by a thermometer using one of two scales, degrees Fahrenheit (F) or degrees Celsius (C), also referred to as centigrade; the normal range for infants, children, and adults is the same, but infants and small children are more sensitive to external temperature changes
  - Common anatomic locations to obtain temperature
    - Oral (temperature taken in the mouth) adult norm is 98.6°F or 37°C
    - Rectal (temperature taken in the rectum) norm is 1 degree higher than oral; adult norm is 99.6°F or 37.5°C
    - Axillary (temperature taken in the armpit) norm is 1 degree lower than oral; adult norm is 97.6°F or 36.4°C
    - Aural, otic, or tympanic (temperature taken in the ear) norm is the same as oral; adult norm is 98.6°F or 37°C
  - Thermometer—instrument used to measure temperature
    - Mercury—a glass thermometer with a mercury column. No longer used due to mercury danger
    - Electronic—a thermometer with a power source used for all sites (special type is used for the ear); displays the temperature digitally; converts from °F to °C or vice versa by flipping a small switch; stylus is covered by a disposable sheath
    - Tympanic—electronic thermometer resembling an otoscope that is used in the ear
    - Disposable—one-time-use plastic thermometer strips, dots, or probes used on the skin or orally; considered least reliable
- Pulse—"beat" caused by expansion and relaxation of the artery wall, expressed in beats per minute; the adult norm is 60 to 100 beats per minute (bpm) in a regular rhythm, usually the same rate and rhythm as the heart; the infant norm is 100 to 160 bpm; and the norm of children to age 10 is 70 to 120 bpm
  - Anatomic sites—the pulse may be taken using any artery lying over bone; the most common follow in the order of frequency of use
    - Radial—pulse located on the thumb side of the wrist; most common site used for adults
    - Brachial—pulse located medially on both arms anterior to the elbow; most common site used for children
    - Apical—pulse located at the fifth intercostal space midclavicular; common site used for infants; requires a stethoscope
    - Dorsalis pedis—pulse located medially on the top of both feet, often used to assess circulation to the extremities
    - Carotid—pulse located on both sides of the neck, lateral to the trachea
    - Femoral—pulse located bilaterally in groin
    - Popliteal—pulse located posterior to both knees, also used to assess circulation to the extremities
    - Temporal—pulse located bilaterally over temporal bone
  - Methods to obtain pulse
    - Manual—light compression of the artery with index and middle finger; count beats for 30 or 60 seconds, multiplying beats by 2 if 30-second count is used
    - Doppler—ultrasonic device used to locate, audibly transmit, and sometimes record pulse
    - Electronic sphygmomanometer—device used to measure pulse and blood pressure simultaneously using a blood pressure cuff
- Respiration—measurement of the number of respiratory cycles per minute, usually done by observation; a respiratory cycle consists of inspiration and expiration; the adult norm is 12 to 20 respiratory cycles per minute in a regular rhythm; the younger the infant or child, the more rapid the normal respiratory rate; 0- to 1-year norm is 20 to 40; 2- to 6-year norm is 20 to 30
- BP—measurement of the force of blood on the artery walls during contraction (systole) and relaxation (diastole) of the heart; recorded as a fraction with systole as the numerator and diastole as the denominator; the adult norm is 120/80; BPs are not commonly taken in children younger than 4 years; the most accurate position for taking a blood pressure is placing the arm at the level of the heart

- Korotkoff sounds—sounds heard through the stethoscope during the measurement of blood pressure; there are five phases:
  1. Phase I—faint tapping sounds heard as the cuff deflates (systole)
  2. Phase II—soft swishing sounds
  3. Phase III—rhythmic, sharp, distinct tapping sounds
  4. Phase IV—soft tapping sounds that become faint
  5. Phase V—disappearance of sound (diastole)
- Pulse pressure—the difference between the systolic and diastolic pressures; the adult norm is 40; the difference should be approximately one third of systole
- Orthostatic pressure—blood pressure taken in all three positions (supine, sitting, and standing) at least 1 to 2 minutes apart
- Sphygmomanometer—the instrument used to measure BP; composed of a cuff for the arm, thigh, wrist, or finger, and a measurement device; the correct size and cuff fit influence the accuracy of the readings
  - Mercury sphygmomanometer—no longer in use because of mercury danger
  - Aneroid sphygmomanometer—a blood pressure cuff with a numeric gauge to measure readings; stethoscope required
  - Electronic sphygmomanometer—blood pressure cuff with an electronic device to measure blood pressure and pulse readings; no stethoscope required
- Stethoscope—the instrument's diaphragm or bell is placed at the artery to be used to hear the sounds that compose the BP

OTHER MEASUREMENTS

Height

Height or length is commonly measured by a rod attached to a weight scale or fixed bar on a wall; a measuring tape is used for measuring the length of neonates and also the head circumference. Measurements are recorded in feet (ft) and inches (in), or centimeters (cm); conversion is 2.5 cm per inch.

Weight

Weight is commonly measured in the medical office using a balance beam or an electronic scale. Measurements are recorded in pounds (lb) or kilograms (kg); conversion is 2.2 lb per kg.

Comparisons of Height and Weight

Using the height and weight in formulas and charts provides the practitioner with an approximation of the patient's size related to normal standards. These methods are used to determine the patient's health risk for various diseases and conditions.

- **Body mass index**—a health risk assessment tool for adults and children to estimate the percentage of body fat by using a formula based on the individual's height and weight; calculations are found online.
  - Normal range = 18.5 to 24.9
  - Underweight = <18.5
  - Overweight = 25 to 29.9
  - Obese = 30 and above
- **Pediatric growth chart**—supplied by the Centers for Disease Control and Prevention (CDC); the form is specific to the current age and sex of the child and contains the height, weight, and head circumference; the individual's measurements are compared by percentile to an established reference group (Fig. 18-1)

Vision

Visual acuity is the measurement of how well a person can see at specified distances; the **Snellen chart method** is used with various letters of the alphabet for adults; the E chart is commonly used for preschoolers. The right eye and the left eye are measured individually, and then both eyes are measured together. The adult norm is 20/20: the numerator indicates the distance the chart is placed from the patient, usually 20 feet; the denominator indicates the distance at which people with normal acuity could read the last line read by the patient—for example, 20/30 vision indicates that the patient sees at 20 feet what someone with normal vision sees at 30 feet (Fig. 18-2 and Fig. 18-3).

- **Ishihara color vision test**—used to determine color vision deficiencies (color blindness); consists of a series of pages or plates with imbedded numbers of various colors; depending on the degree of the deficiency, the person would not see the number or would see it in a different color
- **Tonometer**—an instrument used to measure the intraocular pressure of the eye to diagnose glaucoma; the procedure is called tonometry
- **Ophthalmoscopy (funduscopy) exam**—an examination of the interior eye with an instrument that reflects light through the pupil to determine the health of the interior of the eye; the abbreviation **PERRLA** is used to document the normal finding of "pupils equal round and reactive to light and accommodation"

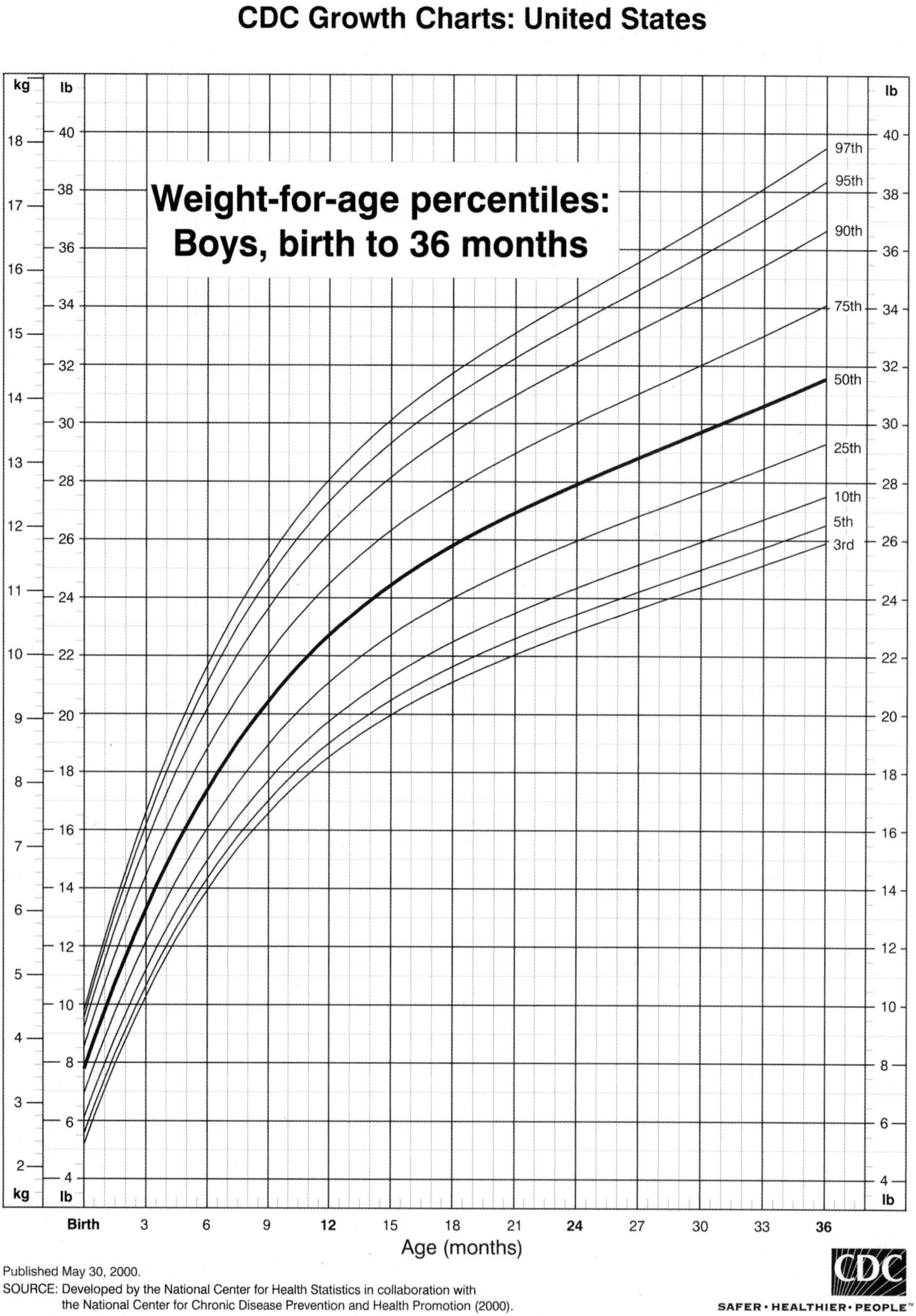

Figure 18-1 Centers for Disease Control and Prevention (CDC) growth chart for U.S. males, birth to 36 months of age (from the CDC).

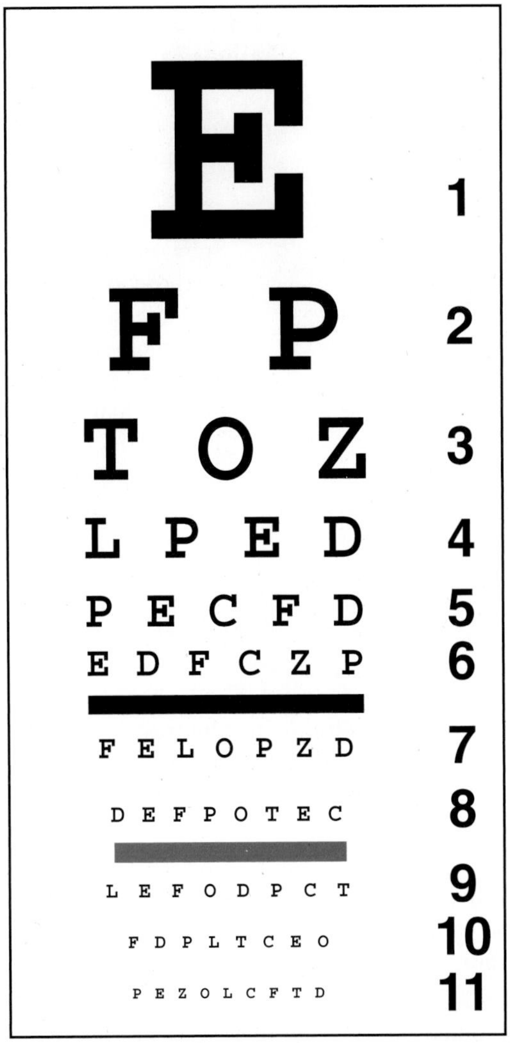

Figure 18-2 Snellen eye chart for those who know the alphabet (from Wikipedia).

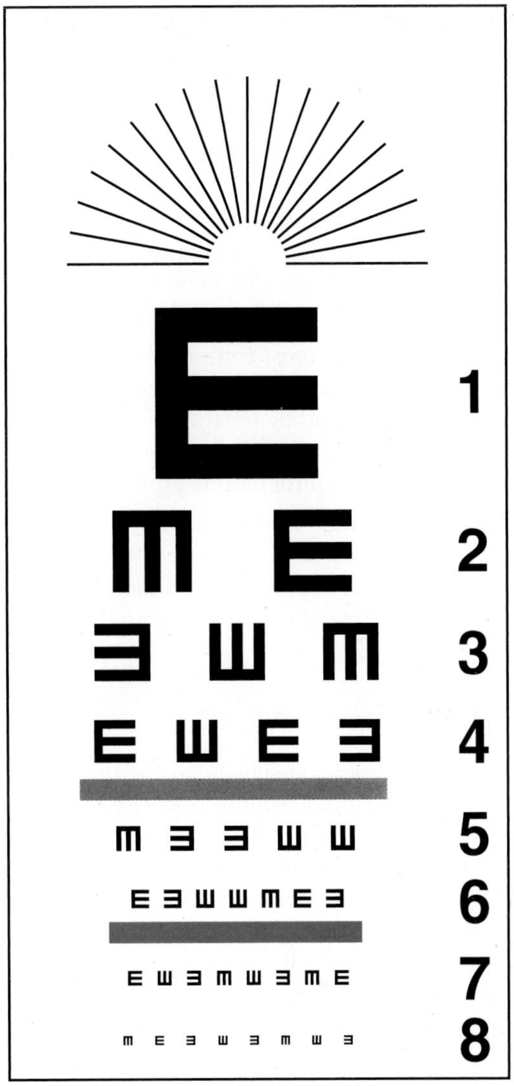

Figure 18-3 Snellen "E" eye chart for preschoolers (from Wikipedia).

All measurements of hearing should be preceded by a visual exam of the auditory canal and eardrum using an otoscope. Hearing measurements may be gross or highly defined.

- Startle—gross measurement used with neonates; a loud noise such as a clap will be initiated; the expected result is that the infant will react with a jerk or a cry
- Whisper—gross measurement; the health care provider will whisper to the patient and the patient repeats what is said; each ear is done separately
- Tuning fork—gross measurement; instrument is activated by striking it with a hand and is then placed on top of the patient's head, beside each ear, and on each side of the patient's mastoid bone; determines hearing and conduction
- Audiometry—a hearing test using an audiometer with earphones that measures the patient's response to tones; it is recorded in decibels (db) and frequencies
- Impedance audiometry—a hearing test using an audiometer and an ear probe that measures tympanic membrane and ossicle mobility
- Tympanometry—a test that uses a tympanometer (air pressure) to measure tympanic membrane mobility

Common Respiratory Tests

Part of the physical exam is to determine how well the lungs are functioning. The practitioner performs an initial evaluation by listening for normal breath sounds with a stethoscope. Other common respiratory tests are performed by the medical assistant.

- **Pulse oximetry**—a test using a pulse oximeter on the patient's digit to measure the percentage of oxygen (O_2) in the blood; this is a common test done with vital signs when visiting the medical office
- **Pulmonary function test (PFT)**—used to diagnose and measure the severity of lung problems by evaluating how well the lungs work: the amount of air the lungs can hold and how quickly the lungs move air in and out; measurements also include the efficiency of oxygenating the blood and removing carbon dioxide
  - **Spirometry**—the most common lung function test; measures how much and how quickly air is moved in and out of the lungs by breathing into a mouthpiece attached to a recording device (spirometer); a graph with the results (spirogram) is produced
  - **Peak flow meter**—a handheld device used to measure the peak expiratory flow rate (PEFR) to monitor asthmatics; the ranges are established by the practitioner; height may be used as a factor.

Box 18-1

Common Supplies and Tools for Routine Patient Exam

4 × 4 gauze (nonsterile)	Slide and fixative or Thin Prep–type container and applicator (pelvic exam)
Exam gloves (nonsterile)	Sphygmomanometer
Laryngeal mirror	Stethoscope
Lubricant (pelvic and rectal exams)	Tape measure
Nasal speculum	Thermometer
Ophthalmoscope	Tissues
Otoscope	Tongue depressor
Penlight	Tuning fork
Percussion hammer	Vaginal speculum (pelvic exam)

PHYSICAL EXAM PREPARATION

The type of examination scheduled for the health care provider to perform determines how the medical assistant prepares the patient and the supplies and tools used. Ensure privacy is maintained, requesting that the patient undress to facilitate access to the body areas that will be examined; provide gowns and draping accordingly. Consideration for the patient's comfort includes room temperature, lighting, sound, and physical position while waiting and during the exam.

- Common supplies and instruments—the medical assistant is responsible for ensuring all supplies and equipment are readily available for the physical exam; Box 18-1 lists common supplies and tools for a routine patient exam; Figure 18-4 illustrates some of those tools
- Patient positions (Fig. 18-5)
  - Supine—patient lies on back with arms to the sides; commonly used for abdominal exams
  - Dorsal recumbent—patient lies on back with knees bent and feet flat on the exam table; commonly used to check progress of labor
  - Lithotomy—patient lies on back with buttocks on edge of exam table, legs elevated and resting in stirrups; commonly used for pelvic exams
  - Sims'—patient lies on left side with left leg slightly flexed and left arm behind body as comfortable; right leg is flexed toward chest and right arm is over the chest; commonly used for rectal exams
  - Prone—patient lies on stomach; commonly used for exam of posterior and administration of intramuscular injections on adults
  - Knee-chest position—patient rests on knees with chest and arms on table and arms flexed over the head; commonly used for rectal and sigmoidoscopic exams
  - Fowler's—patient lies face up on table with upper body elevated to a 45° to 90° angle; commonly used for patients short of breath and for head and neck exams
  - Semi-Fowler's—the Fowler's position at a 45° angle is sometimes referred to as semi-Fowler's
- Examination techniques
  - Observation—visual review of the body, inspecting for symmetry, abnormalities, and skin color and conditions
  - Palpation—use of fingertips and hands to feel for sizes and positions of specific organs, masses, and other abnormalities; texture and firmness; skin temperature and moisture; and flexibility of joints
  - Percussion—process of determining density of specific internal structures by the sound (e.g., dull, hollow) produced by external tapping, usually with fingers or with a percussion hammer for testing neurologic reflexes
  - Auscultation—use of an instrument, usually a stethoscope, to listen to internal body sounds for abnormalities
  - Manipulation—passive movement of body joints to determine the extent of movement
  - Mensuration—measurement of height or length and weight

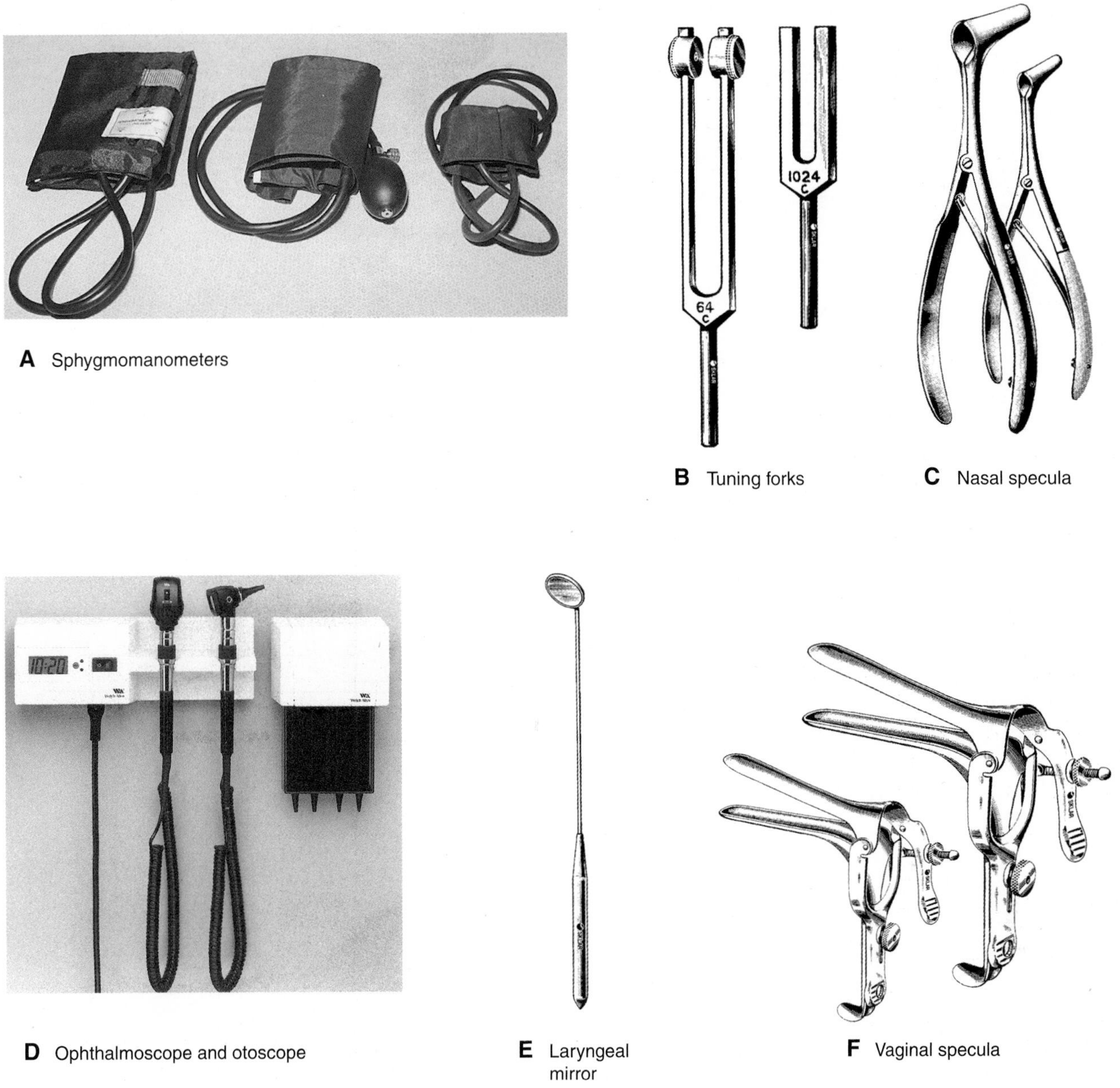

Figure 18-4 Select tools for routine physical exam (Sklar Instruments, West Chester, PA).

TERMS

Patient Exams Review

The following list reviews the terms discussed in this chapter and other important terms that you may see on the exam.

anthropometry obtaining assessment measurements; comprises signs, functions, and capacities that can be objectively determined by the senses (e.g., sight, hearing, smell) or by specific equipment or tests

audiometry a hearing test using an audiometer with earphones that measures the patient's response to tones; it is recorded in decibels (db) and frequencies

auscultation use of an instrument, usually a stethoscope, to listen to internal body sounds for abnormalities

body mass index (BMI) a health risk assessment tool for adults and children to estimate the percentage of body fat by using a formula based on the individual's height and weight

chief complaint a summary of the patient's words explaining why he or she is seeking health care

Doppler an ultrasonic device used to locate, audibly transmit, and sometimes record pulses

impedance audiometry a hearing test using an audiometer and an ear probe that measures tympanic membrane and ossicle mobility

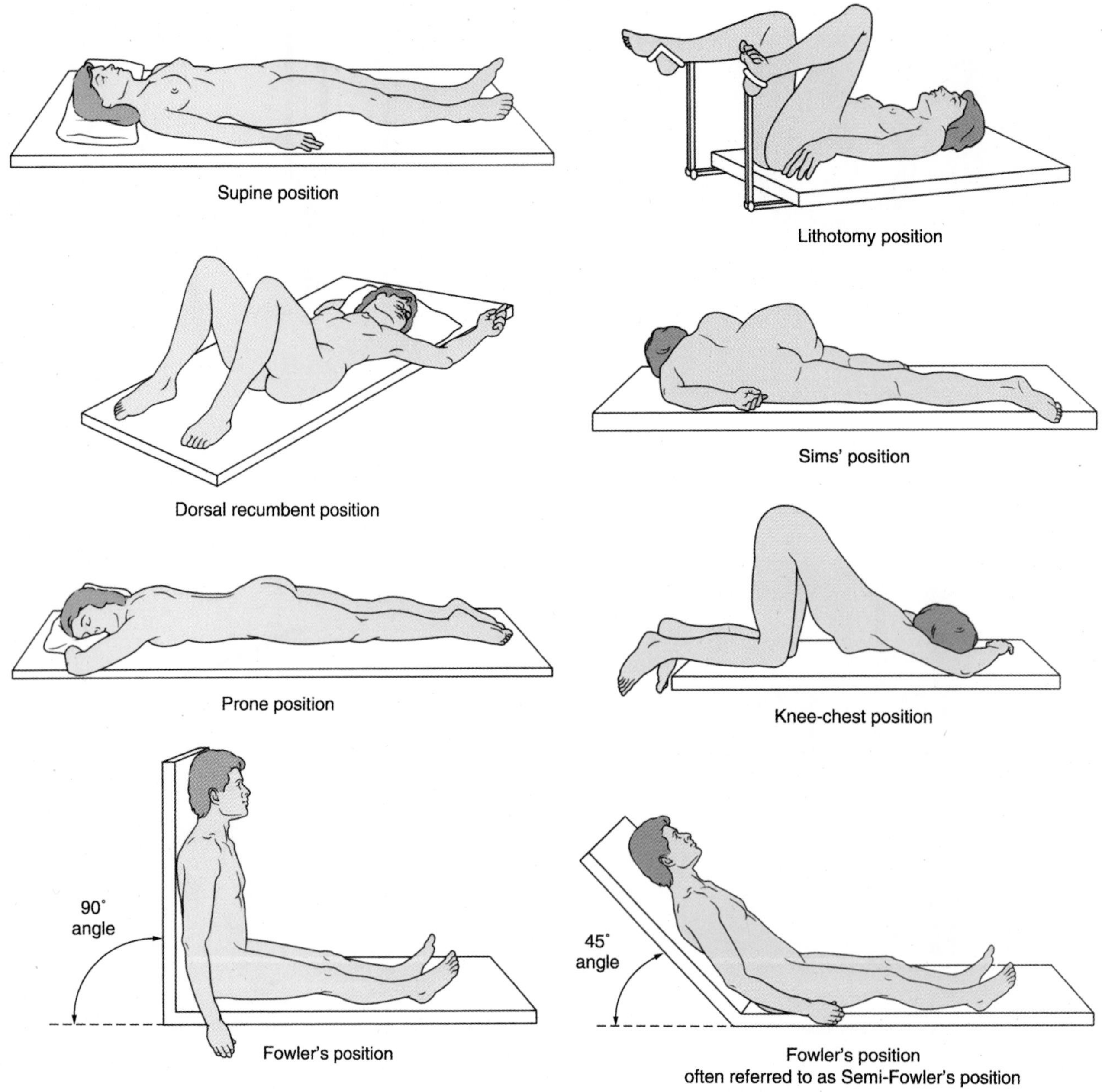

Figure 18-5 Patient positions for exams and procedures. (Reprinted with permission from Hosley JB, Jones SA, Molle-Matthews EA. Lippincott's Textbook for Medical Assistants. Philadelphia: Lippincott-Raven Publishers, 1997.)

Ishihara color vision test used to determine color vision deficiencies (color blindness); consists of a series of pages or plates with imbedded numbers of various colors; depending on the degree of the deficiency, the person would not see the number or would see it in a different color

Korotkoff sounds sounds heard through the stethoscope during the measurement of blood pressure; there are five phases

manipulation passive movement of body joints to determine the extent of movement

mensuration measurement of height or length and weight

observation visual review of the body, inspecting for symmetry, abnormalities, and skin color and conditions

ophthalmoscope (funduscope) an instrument that reflects light throughout the pupil to determine the health of the interior of the eye

orthostatic pressure comparative blood pressures taken in the supine, sitting, and standing positions

otoscope an instrument to examine the auditory canal and eardrum

palpation use of fingertips and hands to feel for sizes and positions of specific organs, masses, or other abnormalities; texture and firmness; skin temperature and moisture; and flexibility of joints

peak flow meter a handheld device used to measure the peak expiratory flow rate (PEFR) to monitor asthmatics

percussion process of determining density of specific internal structures by the sound produced by external tapping, usually with fingers or with a percussion hammer for testing neurologic reflexes

PERRLA pupils equal, round, reactive to light and accommodation; abbreviation used to describe the normal pupil of the eye

pulmonary function test (PFT) used to diagnose and measure the severity of lung problems by evaluating how well the lungs work: the amount of air the lungs can hold and how quickly the lungs move air in and out; measurements also include the efficiency of oxygenating the blood and removing carbon dioxide

pulse oximetry a test using a pulse oximeter to measure the percentage of oxygen in the blood

Snellen chart poster with letters in rows of graduated sizes used to measure how well a person can see at specified distances

sphygmomanometer instrument used to measure blood pressure; the instrument is composed of a cuff for the arm, thigh, wrist, or finger and a measurement device

spirometry the most common lung function test; measures how much and how quickly air is moved in and out of the lungs by breathing into a mouthpiece attached to a recording device (spirometer); a graph with the results (spirogram) is produced

symptoms subjective descriptions of altered health indicators (e.g., nausea, headache); complaints that cannot be seen or measured

tonometry a test using an instrument (tonometer) to measure the intraocular pressure of the eye to diagnose glaucoma

tuning fork used for gross measurement for hearing and sound conduction; the instrument is activated by striking it with the hand and is then placed on top of a patient's head, beside each ear, and on each side of the patient's mastoid bone

tympanometry a test that uses a tympanometer, which uses air pressure to measure tympanic membrane mobility

vital signs measurements of body temperature, pulse rate, respirations (TPR) and blood pressure (BP)

REVIEW QUESTIONS

All questions are relevant for the CMA (AAMA), RMA (AMT), and CMAS (AMT) exams.

1. The main reason why an ill patient is seeking medical care is referred to as the:
   A. assessment.
   B. symptoms.
   C. chief complaint.
   D. observation.

Answer: **C**

Why: When a patient seeks medical care, the medical assistant should summarize the patient's words explaining why the patient has come to see the doctor. The abbreviation of "chief complaint" is CC. Assessment means to evaluate or measure. Symptoms are subjective health indicators such as nausea and headache. Observation is a visual inspection of the body.

Review: Yes ❑ No ❑

---

2. What is the normal adult pulse range in beats per minute?
   A. 50–120
   B. 60–100
   C. 70–130
   D. 80–140
   E. 90–140

Answer: **B**

Why: The normal adult pulse should be between 60 and 100 beats per minute and should have a regular rhythm.

Review: Yes ❑ No ❑

---

3. The pulse point located behind the knee is the:
   A. femoral.
   B. dorsalis pedis.
   C. temporal.
   D. popliteal.

Answer: **D**

Why: The popliteal pulse, located behind the knee, is used to assess circulation to the extremities. The temporal pulse is located on the side of the head above the eye, the dorsalis pedis on the top of the foot, and the femoral in the groin.

Review: Yes ❑ No ❑

---

4. The instrument used to measure the blood pressure is a(n):
   A. pulse oximeter.
   B. Doppler.
   C. sphygmomanometer.
   D. tympanometer.
   E. audiometer.

Answer: **C**

Why: The medical terminology root *sphygm* means "pulse," and *meter* means "an instrument for measuring." A pulse oximeter measures the amount of oxygen in the blood. A Doppler is an ultrasonic device used to locate and audibly transmit a pulse. A tympanometer uses air pressure to measure tympanic membrane mobility. An audiometer measures the patient's hearing based on his or her response to tones.

Review: Yes ❑ No ❑

---

5. The instrument used in the physical exam to determine hearing and conduction is a:
   A. reflex hammer.
   B. stethoscope.
   C. tuning fork.
   D. speculum.

Answer: **C**

Why: A tuning fork is a metal device that vibrates and produces a humming sound. It is used to determine whether a patient can hear. After striking the tuning fork, it is placed on the patient's head or mastoid bone to examine conductive and sensorineural hearing loss.

Review: Yes ❑ No ❑

6. The formula used to change pounds to kilograms is:
   A. 22 lb = 1 kg
   B. 2.2 kg = 1 lb
   C. 100 lb = 1 kg
   D. 1 lb = 100 kg
   E. 2.2 lb = 1 kg

Answer: **E**

Why: Remember, it takes approximately twice the number of pounds to equal a kilogram.

Review: Yes ❑ No ❑

---

7. The examination technique used to listen to internal body sounds is:
   A. palpation.
   B. percussion.
   C. mensuration.
   D. auscultation.

Answer: **D**

Why: Auscultation is performed with the use of a stethoscope. The physician can listen to the sounds made as air moves in and out of the lungs. Bowel sounds are also heard when the stethoscope is placed over the abdomen.

Review: Yes ❑ No ❑

---

8. Which of the following items is not considered necessary for a routine patient exam?
   A. Ophthalmoscope
   B. Percussion hammer
   C. Sterile gloves
   D. Tongue depressor
   E. Otoscope

Answer: **C**

Why: Nonsterile exam gloves are used during a routine patient exam. Sterile gloves are only used when performing a procedure that requires sterile aseptic technique.

Review: Yes ❑ No ❑

---

9. A Snellen chart is used to:
   A. record a child's growth.
   B. measure a patient's vision.
   C. determine normal values in spirometry.
   D. monitor vital signs.

Answer: **B**

Why: The Snellen chart is a poster with rows of letters in graduated sizes and is used to measure vision at specific distances. A person with 20/20 vision can see the letters at 20 feet away from the chart the same as a person with normal vision can at 20 feet.

Review: Yes ❑ No ❑

---

10. The average adult respiration rate is:
   A. 20 to 24 per minute.
   B. 10 to 12 per minute.
   C. 12 to 20 per minute.
   D. 25 to 30 per minute.
   E. 30 to 35 per minute.

Answer: **C**

Why: Respiration ranges vary by age. Infants have a respiration rate of at least 20 per minute or greater, children's respiratory rate is 18 to 20 per minute, and the average adult breathes in and out (one respiration) 14 to 20 times a minute.

Review: Yes ❑ No ❑

---

11. The patient exam position used for a patient who is having difficulty breathing is:
   A. dorsal recumbent.
   B. lithotomy.
   C. prone.
   D. Fowler's.

Answer: **D**

Why: In Fowler's position, the patient lies face up on the exam table with the upper body elevated at a 45° to 90° angle.

Review: Yes ❑ No ❑

12. The pulse point located on the thumb side of the wrist is the:
    A. apical.
    B. brachial.
    C. carotid.
    D. radial.
    E. popliteal.

Answer: **D**

Why: The radial pulse is palpated at the wrist on the thumb side over the radial bone—the bone in the lower arm on the lateral side.

Review: Yes ❑ No ❑

---

13. The systolic pressure is described as:
    A. soft tapping sounds that become faint, or phase IV.
    B. faint tapping sounds heard as the cuff deflates, or phase I.
    C. rhythmic, sharp, distinct tapping sounds, or phase III.
    D. a soft swishing sound, or phase II.

Answer: **B**

Why: The Korotkoff sounds are those sounds heard through the stethoscope during the measurement of blood pressure. There are five phases; phase I is the determination of the systolic pressure. This is the sound made when arterial blood starts flowing back through the blood vessels as the cuff is deflated.

Review: Yes ❑ No ❑

---

14. A percussion hammer is used for which kind of examination?
    A. Orthopaedic
    B. Neurologic
    C. Gynecologic
    D. Urologic
    E. Otologic

Answer: **B**

Why: A percussion hammer is used to test neurologic reflexes. Neurologic refers to the nerves. If a patient has diminished reflexes, this may indicate some nerve involvement. Orthopaedic refers to the skeletal and muscular system. Otologic refers to the ear. Gynecologic refers to women, and urologic refers to the urinary system.

Review: Yes ❑ No ❑

---

15. The instrument used to visualize the ear canal and tympanic membrane is the:
    A. otoscope.
    B. audiometer.
    C. nasoscope.
    D. ophthalmoscope.

Answer: **A**

Why: The root *oto* refers to the ear. A scope is an instrument used to examine a body part. Sometimes a scope has a light source attached. An otoscope is a lighted instrument used to look into the ear canal and examine the eardrum (tympanic membrane). An audiometer is used to measure hearing (*audio* means hearing or sound). A nasoscope is an instrument used to examine the nose, and an ophthalmoscope is used to examine the eyes.

Review: Yes ❑ No ❑

---

16. The exam method used to check for conjunctivitis (pinkeye) is:
    A. auscultation.
    B. palpation.
    C. percussion.
    D. inspection.
    E. mensuration.

Answer: **D**

Why: Conjunctivitis, or pinkeye, is an inflammation of the conjunctiva of the eye. The physician visually inspects the eyes for the signs of infection and inflammation.

Review: Yes ❑ No ❑

17. The exam method used when a physician is determining a patient's range of motion is:
    A. auscultation.
    B. palpation.
    C. manipulation.
    D. mensuration.

Answer: **C**

Why: Manipulation is the passive movement of the joints of the body to determine the extent of movement. Mensuration refers to the measurement of height, weight, and length. Auscultation is the act of listening to internal body sounds, usually using a stethoscope. Palpation is using the fingertips and hands to feel for sizes and positions of specific organs, masses, and abnormalities.

Review: Yes ❑ No ❑

---

18. An oral temperature registers 99.4°F, which equates to a(n):
    A. rectal reading of 101.4°F.
    B. axillary reading of 98.4°F.
    C. otic reading of 100.4°F.
    D. rectal reading of 99.4°F.
    E. axillary reading of 99.4°F.

Answer: **B**

Why: The temperature reading taken rectally is 1 degree higher than oral. An axillary temperature, under the arm, is 1 degree lower, and a temperature taken in the ear is the same as an oral temperature.

Review: Yes ❑ No ❑

---

19. If the blood pressure is 130/90, the pulse pressure is:
    A. 40
    B. 60
    C. 90
    D. 130

Answer: **A**

Why: The pulse pressure is the difference between the systolic and diastolic readings. Therefore, 130 minus 90 equals 40.

Review: Yes ❑ No ❑

---

20. What position would be used to examine the back or spine?
    A. Fowler's
    B. Supine
    C. Knee-chest
    D. Dorsal recumbent
    E. Prone

Answer: **E**

Why: In the prone position, the patient is lying face down on the exam table. Supine is face up, and dorsal recumbent is face up with knees bent and feet flat on the table. The knee-chest position requires the patient to kneel on the table and lower the chest to the table. The knee-chest position is used to perform rectal exams.

Review: Yes ❑ No ❑

---

21. Which of the following pulse sites requires a stethoscope to take the pulse?
    A. Brachial
    B. Carotid
    C. Apical
    D. Femoral

Answer: **C**

Why: The apical pulse is located at the fifth intercostal space midclavicular. A stethoscope is placed on the chest at this location to listen to the pulse.

Review: Yes ❑ No ❑

---

22. When performing a physical exam, the abbreviation PERRLA is used to describe what part(s) of the body?
    A. Abdomen
    B. Nose and sinuses
    C. Ears
    D. Eyes
    E. Heart

Answer: **D**

Why: PERRLA means pupils equal, round, and reactive to light and accommodation. This abbreviation is used to describe normal pupils in the eye.

Review: Yes ❑ No ❑

23. Which of the following instruments and supplies is not included for a pelvic exam?
    A. Lubricant
    B. Cytology slide
    C. Sterile gloves
    D. Vaginal speculum

Answer: **C**

Why: It is not necessary to include sterile gloves with a pelvic exam tray setup; only regular nonsterile exam gloves are used.

Review: Yes ❑ No ❑

---

24. When measuring the blood pressure, the medical assistant will normally place the stethoscope over which artery?
    A. Apical
    B. Brachial
    C. Carotid
    D. Radial
    E. Aorta

Answer: **B**

Why: The term **brachial** means "relating to the arm." The brachial artery is located on the inner aspect of the anterior of the arm, and the pulse is felt at the elbow region.

Review: Yes ❑ No ❑

---

25. Blood pressure readings taken 1 to 2 minutes apart in the supine, sitting, and then standing position, are the:
    A. pulse pressure.
    B. metastatic pressure.
    C. orthostatic pressure.
    D. orthopaedic pressure.

Answer: **C**

Why: The term **orthostatic** refers to "erect posture or position." A patient's blood pressure can fluctuate when changing positions from lying down to standing up.

Review: Yes ❑ No ❑

19

Minor Surgical Procedures

REVIEW TIP

Chapter 17, "Microorganisms and Asepsis," has direct application to surgical procedures–be sure you understand those concepts before reviewing this chapter. Minor surgery is another area of the national exams that contains questions requiring identification, care, and usage of surgical instruments.

Most states define and regulate types of surgery that are considered appropriate for the medical office. Medical malpractice insurance carriers also play a role. Refer to Chapter 4, "Law and Ethics," for issues concerning licensure, scope of practice, patient rights, informed consent, malpractice, and confidentiality. As in all areas of medical assisting, patient education is an important component (see Chapter 8).

General anesthesia is not usually administered for surgery in the medical office and is not covered in this book.

PREPARATION

Surgical asepsis must be maintained throughout the preparation and performance of surgical procedures.

- Sterile field—a pathogen-free area containing sterile instruments, solutions, sponges, and other items that will come in direct contact with another sterile item or the surgical field; this includes the hands and anterior neck to waist of the surgical team
  - Ensure sterile indicators and dates on instruments and solutions are intact and current before opening and placing on a sterile field
  - Examine sterile items for signs of break in packaging or presence of moisture (discard item if either is noted)
  - Open the sterile package(s)
    - Open the top flap first; open away from you to avoid reaching over sterile field
    - Open the right and left flaps to the sides
    - Open the last flap toward you
  - Allow only sterile items to come into contact with other sterile items
  - Keep all sterile items and hands above the waists of the surgical team
  - Maintain a border of 1 inch between nonsterile and sterile areas
  - Do not turn your back to a sterile field or leave it unattended
  - Do not lean or reach over sterile field
  - Do not pass contaminated or nonsterile items over a sterile field
  - Pour liquids such as sterile saline or an antiseptic into a sterile waterproof container on the sterile field
  - Do not touch the container with the nonsterile bottle

- Do not drip or spill liquid on the sterile field
- Do not talk, cough, or sneeze over a sterile field

■ Surgical handwashing (scrub)—remove all jewelry; use foot- or knee-controlled faucet; wash hands, wrists, and forearms for 10 minutes (first surgical scrub of day); hold hands in upward position while rinsing; use brush and cuticle stick on nails; do not apply lotion; dry with sterile towel; apply sterile gloves

■ Personal protective equipment (PPE) for surgery
- Gloves—sterile
- Goggles or eye shields—nonsterile
- Masks—nonsterile
- Gowns—sterile
- Aprons—sterile if worn over surgical gown

■ Surgical site preparation
- Hair removal—shave or cut hair at surgical site only with physician order (usually in procedure file); use only disposable blades; sterile instruments should be covered during hair removal; all loose hair should be removed before application of antiseptic
- Skin cleansing—using an antiseptic cleansing solution (check for patient allergies) such as Betadine® or Hibiclens®, cleanse the surgical site using a circular motion from the point of the incision outward; use a clean sponge to repeat
- "Painting" and draping—after performing the previous steps, a sterile member of the surgical team will use a sterile sponge stick and sterile sponges to apply, or "paint," an antiseptic solution on the surgical site, using circular motions beginning with the incision site and working outward (one sponge per layer of antiseptic); fenestrated drapes (a drape with a hole or opening) or sterile towels, held in place by sterile towel clips, are applied, as well as any other drapes (sterile coverings) required by the size of the sterile field
- When local anesthetic is required on a sterile field, the physician will hold the sterile syringe with sterile gloved hands; the medical assistant shows the physician the label on the vial and holds the vial upside down for the physician to draw out the required amount of medication

INSTRUMENTATION

All instruments or parts of instruments that enter the sterile field must be sterile. Chapter 17 covered the two common procedures for sterilization: autoclaving and cold or chemical sterilization. Safety (e.g., the use of sharps containers and other biohazard receptacles) was also addressed in Chapter 17.

COMMON INSTRUMENTS (FIG. 19-1)

■ Curette—sharp or smooth spoon-shaped instrument used to scrape tissue or other substances from a body orifice or organ; the most common types are ear and uterine

■ Dilator—solid instrument used to stretch or widen the opening to an anatomic structure

■ Forceps—a two-handled instrument used to grasp, move, or crimp tissue; may be with or without "teeth"
- Splinter forceps—fine-pointed, tweezer-like forceps without teeth used to remove splinters and other foreign objects
- Thumb forceps—smooth (without teeth) forceps; the general-use forceps
- Adson forceps—tweezer-like forceps, with or without teeth, with a smaller tip for smaller areas
- Bayonet forceps—tweezer-like forceps shaped like a bayonet used for packing in areas (e.g., the nostrils)
- Ring (sponge) forceps—long, two-handled forceps with open ovals on the ends to grasp tissue, hold sponges, or transfer sterile instruments
- Hemostat—sometimes referred to as a forceps; straight or curved instrument used to compress or crimp capillaries and other blood vessels to stop bleeding; also referred to as a *clamp* or a *crile*; types are
  - Kelly hemostat—a medium-size hemostat; may be curved or straight
  - Mosquito hemostat—a small hemostat used for pediatric, plastic, or microsurgery; may be curved or straight

■ Needle holder—a two-handled instrument that clasps a suture needle, allowing the physician to push and pull the needle with suture material through various anatomic structures

■ Probe—a straight instrument with ends of various shapes, used primarily to explore ducts, canals, and other anatomic structures

■ Retractors—instruments of various shapes used to hold back tissue and organs to facilitate exposure to the operative site

■ Scalpels—knives of various blade shapes and sizes, used to make surgical incisions; the blade is always disposable; the knife handle may or may not be disposable

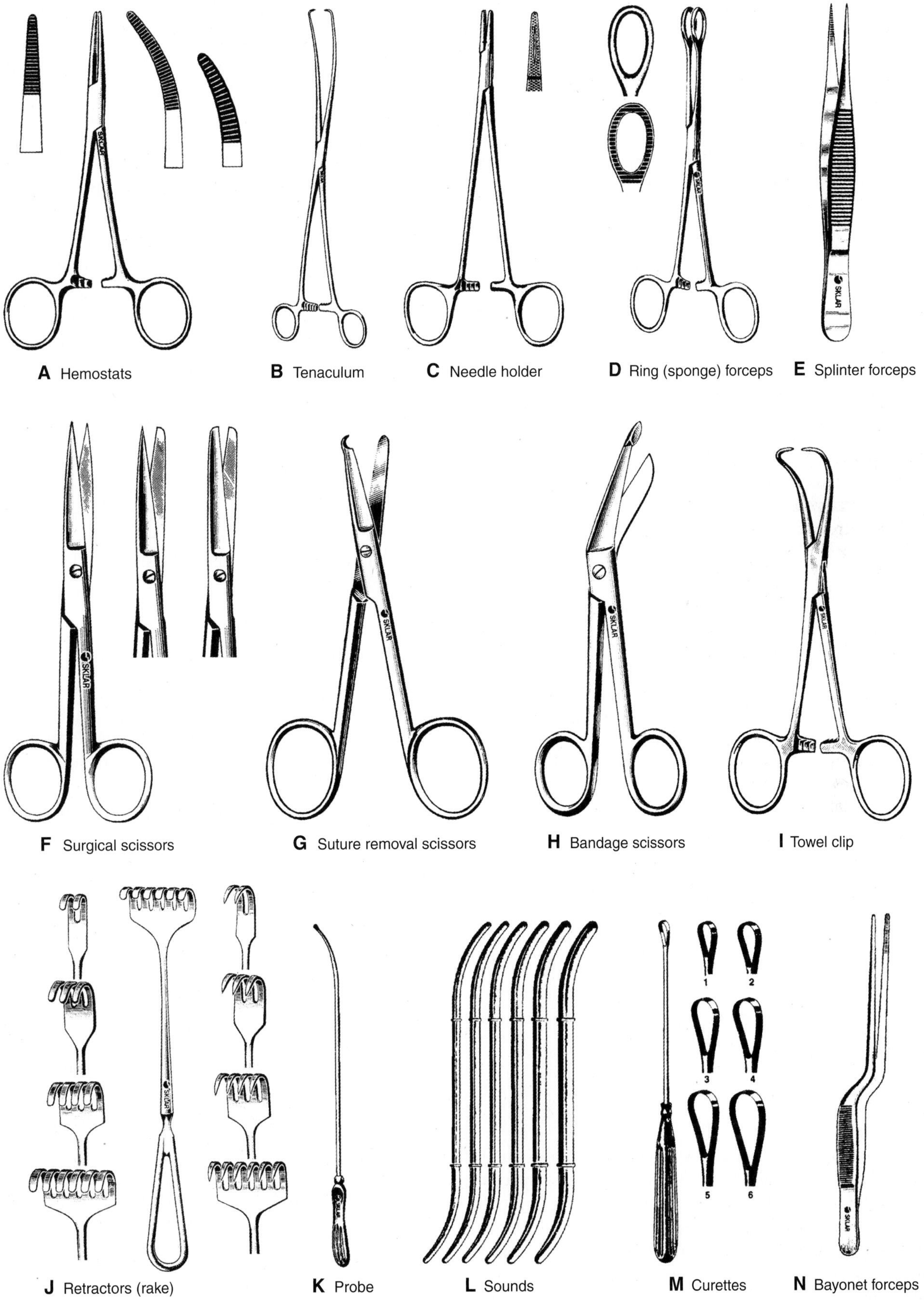

Figure 19-1 Common surgical instruments (Sklar Instruments, West Chester, PA).

- Scissors—two-bladed instrument used to cut tissue and materials during surgical procedures
  - Surgical/operating scissors—scissors used during surgery to cut and dissect tissue; may be curved or straight, blunt or sharp (e.g., Mayo scissors)
  - Suture scissors—scissors used to cut suture material; straight-bladed suture scissors are used in suturing; suture scissors with a hook on the end of one side are used to remove sutures
  - Bandage scissors—angled scissors with a blunt knobbed end to insert under dressings to remove them without injuring tissue
- Sound—a straight or curved instrument used to explore body cavities for measurement of depth and presence of masses or foreign bodies
- Tenaculum—a long, two-handled instrument with pointed ends used to grasp tissue during surgery; a cervical tenaculum is commonly used in well-woman exams
- Towel clamps (clips)—small instruments of various shapes used to keep sterile towels used as drapes in place during surgery

Other Common Instrumentation With Power Sources

- Electrosurgery—a method of dissection and cauterization using an electric current directed to a specific anatomic area to cut, destroy, or coagulate; the power source is initiated and controlled through a boxlike unit that transmits to a hand piece with sterile removable tips that come in direct contact with the surgical site; the patient must be grounded and safety precautions enforced
- Cryosurgery—a method of destroying tissue by freezing (cryogenics) using liquid nitrogen applied from a tank with a gauge and removable hand pieces (e.g., for removal of cervical lesions), or other cryomaterials requiring simple spray canisters (e.g., for removal of skin lesions)
- Laser surgery—a method using high concentrations of electromagnetic radiation in narrow beams for surgical and diagnostic applications (e.g., coagulation of retinal hemorrhage); uses vary and are dependent on the color spectrum; common terms associated with laser surgery are *argon*, *continuous wave*, *pulsed wave*, *excimer*, *krypton*, *KTP*, *YAG*, and *Q-switched*; goggles should be worn and special training provided before assisting in laser surgery

COMMON SURGICAL TRAY INSTRUMENTS

Each office maintains a file of all instruments, supplies, and equipment needed for each surgical procedure. The following are select surgical trays and their instruments.

- General minor surgery tray used for procedures such as removal of lesions—towel clips (four), scalpel and blade, curved and straight hemostats (two each), surgical scissors, thumb forceps, forceps with teeth, suture scissors, needle holder (retractors and other instruments may be added as needed), specified type of surgical sponge; sutures and sizes may be on the file card or requested by the physician during the procedure
- Suture tray—towel clips (four), curved hemostat, forceps with teeth, thumb forceps, suture scissors, needle holder, sterile 4 × 4 gauze; sutures identified by the physician and added to the setup
- Suture or staple removal tray—suture scissors or staple remover, thumb forceps, sterile 4 × 4 gauze

ENDOSCOPE

An **endoscope** is a special instrument used to examine the interior of canals and hollow viscus; the specific design and name is dependent on the organ (e.g., gastroscope, bronchoscope). The instrument usually contains fiberoptic technology that allows lighting, video transmission, and other technologic procedures; biopsies and select surgical procedures may be performed through the endoscope, eliminating or minimizing a surgical incision.

CLOSURE MATERIALS

The type of material used for closure is dependent on several factors. Is the closure on an internal anatomic structure or on the skin? What are the depth, thickness, and length of the closure site? What are the healing capacity factors of the patient (e.g., nutritional status, diabetes, recent history of steroid administration, smoking)?

- Suture—derived from Latin, meaning "a sewing"; threadlike materials (ligature) and needle used to close a wound; the needle and ligature used in the medical office are usually mechanically attached (swaged) by the manufacturer
- Ligature
  - Absorbable—material that dissolves in the body (e.g., catgut); used for internal suturing
  - Nonabsorbable—material that does not dissolve (e.g., silk, nylon and other synthetics, wires); generally for external use, although some wires may be used internally; most nonabsorbable sutures are removed after healing takes place
  - Size—determined by the thickness of the diameter; the range is approximately from 7, the largest, to 11-0, the smallest (Box 19-1)
- Needle
  - Cutting—needle with sharp, flat edge used on tough tissue (e.g., skin)

Box 19-1

Range of Common Suture Material Sizes

Larger to smaller

7	6	5	4	3	2	1	0	1-0	2-0	3-0	4-0	5-0	6-0	7-0	8-0	9-0	10-0	11-0

Large ←——→ Small

- Noncutting—needle with sharp, smooth, rounded edge used on finer tissue, such as peritoneum
- Curved—the shape of the needle; may have cutting or noncutting edge; needle holder used
- Straight (Keith)—the shape of the needle; may have cutting or noncutting edge; no needle holder required
- Size—determined by the size of the ligature to be used; physician will ask for ligature size on a cutting or noncutting, curved or straight needle

■ Staples—metal clips used to approximate skin edges during healing or occlude internal structures; materials vary per use (e.g., stainless steel used on skin, silver used for neurosurgery); external staples must be removed with a staple remover

■ Steri-Strips—adhesive strips of material used in minor lacerations or as a follow-up to sutures to hold wound edges together during healing

■ Glue—bonding material used externally to approximate skin edges or internally to affix structures; often used in neurologic or orthopaedic surgeries

WOUNDS

Wounds are traumas to body tissues caused by physical means. The trauma may be unintentional, such as a fall, or intentional, such as surgery. The type of wound determines the treatment and the potential for healing. Surgical wounds are considered clean wounds because they are initiated under sterile conditions. Dirty wounds are those sustained under contaminated conditions (e.g., a knife wound while preparing a meal).

■ Abrasion—outer layers of skin scraped off, resulting in a small amount of sanguineous or serosanguineous drainage, such as a "skinned" knee

■ Contusion—bleeding below unbroken skin caused by blunt trauma; a bruise

■ Incision—a smooth cut as in surgery or as made with a razor; the amount of bleeding depends on the location and depth

■ Laceration—a jagged traumatic cut resulting in irregular wound edges

■ Puncture—a hole in the skin made by a sharp pointed object

■ Healing—physiologic process of wound closure; there are two predominant types

- First intention (primary)—wound edges are approximated and healing process occurs in all layers (e.g., incision, laceration)
- Secondary intention (granulation)—wound edges do not approximate and healing begins at wound bottom, forming granular projections on the wound surface (e.g., a wound from a drain)

■ Dressings—defined as sterile coverings placed over a wound but often used synonymously with bandaging; types of dressing include gauze, occlusives (e.g., Vaseline gauze), nonstick (e.g., Telfa), nonopaque (e.g., BioDerm), and commercial gauze impregnated with medication (e.g., NuGauze); dressings should be applied using sterile technique

■ Bandages—sterile or nonsterile materials that splint or protect injured tissue (e.g., Kerlix, Ace bandages, triangular slings, tube gauze [frequently used on digits]), maintain pressure over an area (such as abdominal pads, Coban), and hold sterile dressings in place (e.g., Montgomery straps, rolled gauze)

TERMS

Minor Surgical Procedures Review

The following list reviews the terms discussed in this chapter and other important terms that you may see on the exam.

abrasion outer layers of skin scraped off, resulting in a small amount of sanguineous or serosanguineous drainage, such as a "skinned" knee

contusion bleeding below unbroken skin caused by blunt trauma; a bruise

cryosurgery a method of destroying tissue by freezing (cryogenics) using liquid nitrogen applied from a tank with a gauge and removable hand pieces, or other cryomaterials requiring simple spray canisters

curettes sharp or smooth spoon-shaped instruments used to scrape tissue or other substances from a body orifice or organ; most common are ear and uterine

dilators solid instruments used to stretch or widen the opening to an anatomic structure (e.g., uterine, urethral sounds)

electrosurgery a method of dissection or cauterization using an electric current directed to a specific anatomic area to cut, destroy, or coagulate

endoscope special instrument used to examine the interior of canals and hollow viscus; design and name is dependent on the organ; it usually contains fiberoptic technology allowing lighting, video transmission, and other technologic procedures

forceps a two-handled instrument used to grasp, move, or crimp tissue

hemostat sometimes referred to as a *forceps*; straight or curved instrument used to compress capillaries and other blood vessels to stop bleeding; also referred to as a *clamp* or a *crile*

incision a smooth cut as in surgery or as made with a razor

laceration a jagged traumatic cut resulting in irregular wound edges

laser surgery a method using high concentrations of electromagnetic radiation in narrow beams for surgical and diagnostic applications

needle holder a two-handled instrument that clasps a needle, allowing the physician to push and pull the needle with suture material through various anatomic structures

probe a straight instrument with ends of various shapes; used primarily to explore patency of ducts, canals, and other anatomic structures

puncture a hole in the skin made by a sharp pointed object

retractors instruments of various shapes used to hold back tissue and organs to facilitate exposure to the operative site

scalpels knives with various blade shapes and sizes, used to make surgical incisions

sound a straight or curved instrument used to explore body cavities for measurement of depth and presence of masses or foreign bodies

suture scissors scissors used to cut suture material; straight-bladed suture scissors are used to suture; suture scissors with a hook on the end of one side are used to remove sutures

tenaculum a long, two-handled instrument with pointed ends used to grasp tissue during surgery; a cervical tenaculum is commonly used in well-woman exams

towel clamps (clips) small instruments of various shapes used to keep sterile towels used as drapes in place during surgery

REVIEW QUESTIONS

All questions are relevant for the CMA (AAMA) and RMA (AMT) exams.

1. An instrument used to grasp tissue is a:
   A. probe.
   B. curette.
   C. dilator.
   D. forceps.

Answer: **D**

Why: There are many types of forceps, such as splinter forceps, thumb forceps, Adson forceps, and sponge forceps. These are used to grasp tissue or supplies.

Review: Yes ❑ No ❑

---

2. The instrument used to remove stitches is:
   A. operating scissors.
   B. Kelly hemostat.
   C. suture scissors.
   D. Mayo scissors.
   E. needle holder.

Answer: **C**

Why: Sutures and stitches are the same. Suture scissors have a hook on the end of one of the blades. This hook is slipped under the stitch/suture, and the stitch is cut for removal.

Review: Yes ❑ No ❑

---

3. A procedure that uses liquid nitrogen to freeze and destroy tissue is:
   A. electrosurgery.
   B. laser surgery.
   C. endoscopic surgery.
   D. cryosurgery.

Answer: **D**

Why: The root *cryo* means "cold." Liquid nitrogen produces a freezing effect that destroys tissue. This method is frequently used to destroy cervical lesions.

Review: Yes ❑ No ❑

---

4. Which of the following statements is true regarding the sizing of suture, or ligature?
   A. 2-0 suture is finer than 6-0 suture.
   B. 3 suture is thicker than 6 suture.
   C. 4-0 suture is finer than 2-0 suture.
   D. 5-0 suture is finer than 6-0 suture.
   E. 4 suture is finer than 2 suture.

Answer: **C**

Why: Suture is available in different sizes or gauges. When the size ends in a zero, suture sizes become smaller as the number gets larger. A 2-0 suture is thicker than a 10-0 suture. The opposite is true when the suture size is a whole number. The higher the whole number, the larger or thicker the suture. For example, size 7 suture is thicker than size 2.

Review: Yes ❑ No ❑

---

5. Which of the following sutures does not require removal from the body?
   A. Catgut
   B. Silk
   C. Nylon
   D. Cotton

Answer: **A**

Why: Catgut suture is an absorbable suture made from the intestines of sheep or cattle. It is readily broken down by the body and usually does not require removal.

Review: Yes ❑ No ❑

---

6. The type of wound caused by scraping off the outer layers of skin is a(n):
   A. incision.
   B. abrasion.
   C. contusion.
   D. laceration.
   E. bruise.

Answer: **B**

Why: An example of an abrasion is a skinned knee, in which the top layers of skin are scraped off.

Review: Yes ❑ No ❑

7. Which of the following instruments is used to scrape foreign substance from an ear?
   A. Dilator
   B. Hemostat
   C. Retractor
   D. Curette

Answer: **D**

Why: A curette is a sharp or smooth, spoon-shaped instrument used to scrape tissue or other substances from a body orifice or organ. A dilator is a solid instrument used to stretch or widen the opening to an anatomic structure. A hemostat is used to compress or crimp capillaries and other blood vessels to stop bleeding. A retractor is used to hold and separate tissue.

Review: Yes ❑ No ❑

---

8. The type of bandage material that is not intended to apply pressure but to hold a dressing in place on the forearm is:
   A. elastic bandage.
   B. rolled gauze.
   C. triangular bandage.
   D. tubular gauze.
   E. 4 × 4 gauze.

Answer: **B**

Why: Rolled gauze is available in different widths from 1 inch to 6 inches and in various lengths. It is used to wrap around a body part such as an arm or a leg. Elastic bandage is made from a stretchy material and is used to apply pressure. Triangular bandages are used to make a sling for the arm. Tubular gauze is used to bandage toes and fingers. Gauze squares are used to cover wounds and are available in 1-inch to 4-inch squares.

Review: Yes ❑ No ❑

---

9. A type of wound caused by a blunt trauma to the body that results in bleeding below unbroken skin is a(n):
   A. puncture.
   B. laceration.
   C. contusion.
   D. abrasion.

Answer: **C**

Why: A contusion causes a bruise. A bruise forms from bleeding beneath the skin. The skin is not broken, but the injury is visible through the surface of the skin.

Review: Yes ❑ No ❑

---

10. Items that are placed on the sterile field of a biopsy surgical tray setup include the following EXCEPT:
   A. scalpel.
   B. needle holder.
   C. bandage scissors.
   D. hemostat.
   E. curette.

Answer: **C**

Why: Bandage scissors are used to cut through and remove bandages and have a blunt end so they do not injure the patient during use. They are not included on the tray for a biopsy.

Review: Yes ❑ No ❑

---

11. The type of material preferred to bandage a digit is:
   A. 4 × 4 gauze.
   B. tube gauze.
   C. Ace bandage.
   D. 2 × 2 gauze.

Answer: **B**

Why: Tube gauze is gauze manufactured into a tube shape. It stretches and conforms to body parts such as fingers and toes (digits).

Review: Yes ❑ No ❑

12. Which of the following statements is true regarding the sterile tray setup?
    A. All bandage materials are added to the sterile tray for easy access after the procedure.
    B. You should pour solutions into the basin on the sterile tray holding the bottle label down so you can see the liquid in the container.
    C. Surgical handwashing is not required.
    D. You should reach over the sterile field, not around it, to access something on the other side of the tray.
    E. A 1-inch border around the sterile field is considered contaminated.

Answer: **E**

Why: Bandage materials are not placed on the sterile field. Only those items that are sterile are on the tray. For example, adhesive and surgical tape are not sterile. When pouring solutions from a bottle, pour the liquid from the container with the label face up, so that if liquid drips down the bottle, the label will not be destroyed or damaged. Before setting up a sterile tray, it is essential to perform a surgical handwash. You should never reach over a sterile tray.

Review: Yes ❑ No ❑

---

13. A fenestrated sterile drape:
    A. is used to cover the sterile tray after it is set up to protect it from becoming contaminated.
    B. has an opening in the middle and is placed over the area of the patient where a surgical incision will be made.
    C. is a type of bandaging material used to cover a large area of the body.
    D. is a sterile drape impregnated with an anesthetic medication.

Answer: **B**

Why: The word *fenestra* is a Latin term for "window" or "opening." This sterile drape is approximately 18 × 24 inches and has a 2-inch square opening in the middle. The drape is placed over the patient, with the opening over the area where the surgical procedure will be performed.

Review: Yes ❑ No ❑

---

14. To ensure package sterility, the medical assistant should:
    A. use a torn sterile package only if the tear is small.
    B. use sterile packages up to 30 days after the expiration date to conserve the need to re-autoclave.
    C. use only dry, undamaged sterile packages.
    D. only transport sterile packages with sterile gloves.
    E. perform a surgical handwash before wrapping packs for sterilization.

Answer: **C**

Why: You should not use a sterile package if it is wet or damp or has become damaged. Packs sterilized in-house expire 30 days from the preparation date. The outside of the sterile package is not considered sterile, only the contents within the pack. Therefore, sterile gloves are not required to transport the pack. It is not necessary to perform a surgical handwash before wrapping packs.

Review: Yes ❑ No ❑

---

15. Electrosurgery is used to:
    A. retract tissues.
    B. dilate openings in the body.
    C. dissect and coagulate tissue.
    D. freeze tissue.

Answer: **C**

Why: Electrosurgery is a method of cauterization using an electric current to dissect or coagulate tissue. Surgical instruments are used to retract or to hold back structures of the body during surgery. Dilation is the process of making an opening larger. Cryosurgery is the method used to freeze tissue.

Review: Yes ❑ No ❑

16. The first step performed to set up a sterile field is to:
    A. open the sterile package.
    B. pour solutions that will be used during the procedure.
    C. wash your hands.
    D. don sterile gloves.
    E. prepare the local anesthetic in a syringe and place it on the sterile field.

Answer: **C**

Why: Handwashing is performed before any procedure. When setting up a sterile field, a surgical handwashing is performed for 10 minutes.

Review: Yes ❑ No ❑

---

17. After a surgical procedure, the guidelines for discarding materials include:
    A. placing all sharps in a biohazard sharps container.
    B. placing only visibly soiled materials in a biohazard sharps container.
    C. discarding all paper materials in the trash can.
    D. pouring unused solutions back into their proper containers.

Answer: **A**

Why: All items that are disposable and considered sharp are discarded in the biohazard sharps container. This includes suture materials with needles attached, syringes and needles, and scalpel blades. All other materials soiled with body fluids should be placed in a biohazard container, but not in one specifically designed for sharps. Red trash bags are most commonly used for these items.

Review: Yes ❑ No ❑

---

18. An instrument used to explore anatomic structures is a:
    A. hemostat.
    B. curette.
    C. forceps.
    D. dilator.
    E. probe.

Answer: **E**

Why: A probe is a straight instrument with various shaped ends that are usually blunt, used primarily to explore the patency of ducts, canals, and other anatomic structures.

Review: Yes ❑ No ❑

---

19. Instruments used to hold back tissue and organs are:
    A. thumb forceps.
    B. Kelly forceps.
    C. retractors.
    D. curettes.

Answer: **C**

Why: Retractors may be plain or toothed and may be sharp or blunt. They are designed to be either held by an assistant or screwed open to be self-retaining.

Review: Yes ❑ No ❑

---

20. A common antiseptic solution used to prep the surgical site is:
    A. Betadine®.
    B. alcohol.
    C. hydrogen peroxide.
    D. formaldehyde.
    E. sterile saline.

Answer: **A**

Why: Formaldehyde is not intended for use on the skin. Alcohol is used for surface cleansing of the skin for minor invasive procedures and to wipe items such as stethoscopes. Hydrogen peroxide does not have the antiseptic qualities necessary for prepping the skin before surgery. Sterile saline is a salt solution that is free from all microorganisms.

Review: Yes ❑ No ❑

21. A jagged traumatic cut resulting in irregular wound edges is a(n):
A. contusion.
B. laceration.
C. incision.
D. abrasion.

Answer: **B**

Why: A contusion does not break the skin but bleeding occurs beneath the skin, resulting in a visible bruise. An incision is a smooth cut, as made with a razor or a scalpel. An abrasion is a wound caused from scraping away the top layers of skin.

Review: Yes ❑ No ❑

---

22. An instrument used to examine the interior of canals or of hollow organs is a(n):
A. retractor.
B. catheter.
C. dilator.
D. curette.
E. endoscope.

Answer: **E**

Why: An endoscope is an illuminated optic instrument used for visualizing the interior of a body cavity or of an organ. Scopes include a gastroscope, which is used to examine the stomach; a bronchoscope, which is used to examine the bronchi of the lungs; and a sigmoidoscope, which is used to examine the sigmoid colon.

Review: Yes ❑ No ❑

---

23. The procedure for delivering local anesthetic to the sterile field is to:
A. fill the syringe with the proper amount of solution before the procedure and place it on the sterile field.
B. place the vial of solution on the sterile field so the physician can have access to it.
C. remove the syringe from the sterile field, fill the syringe with the amount of solution required, and return the syringe to the sterile field for the physician to use.
D. while the physician holds the syringe with sterile gloved hands, the medical assistant holds the vial of solution for the physician, and the physician draws out the required amount of solution.

Answer: **D**

Why: The vial of medication is not sterile and should not be placed on the sterile field. Using sterile technique, a syringe is placed on the sterile field. The physician holds the syringe and directs the needle into the rubber stopper of the vial and withdraws the required amount of solution. The medical assistant must remember to wipe the top of the vial with alcohol before offering the vial to the physician. Also, it is usually required that the medical assistant either show the physician the vial label or read the label out loud before using the solution to ensure the solution is the correct one.

Review: Yes ❑ No ❑

---

24. The bandage material preferred when pressure is required over the injured area is:
A. 4 × 4 gauze.
B. elastic bandage.
C. roller gauze.
D. triangular bandage.
E. Telfa pad.

Answer: **B**

Why: The elastic (Ace) bandage is form-fitting and used as a pressure bandage. It is important to check the patient's extremities for proper blood return into toes and fingers. If the bandage is too tight, it can restrict blood flow to the body part.

Review: Yes ❑ No ❑

---

25. A wrapped, autoclaved, sterile package is opened on the Mayo stand by opening the top flap of the wrapper:
A. toward the right side of the table.
B. toward the left side of the table.
C. away from you.
D. toward you.

Answer: **C**

Why: The top flap is opened away from you so that as the other flaps are opened you will not have to reach over the sterile contents of the package. After the top flap is open, the right and left flaps are opened to the sides. The last flap, closest to you, is opened by lifting it toward you.

Review: Yes ❑ No ❑

20

The Electrocardiogram

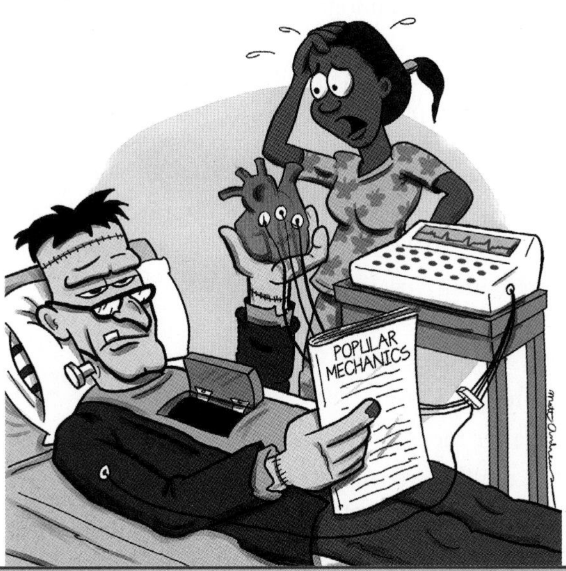

REVIEW TIP

Refer to Chapter 6, "Anatomy and Physiology," and review the cardiovascular system, including the functions, components, cardiac cycle, and cardiac conduction. Exam questions may involve identifying a cardiac rhythm or PQRST waves from a picture of an electrocardiogram strip or identifying cardiac leads.

The **electrocardiogram (ECG or EKG)** is the graphic representation of the electrical activity that passes through the heart. It is monitored at the skin surface with sensors called **electrodes** that produce specific **leads** or views of the heart, which is a three-dimensional organ. The ECG is a painless and noninvasive tool used to collect baseline information (e.g., during a routine physical exam) and to diagnose and monitor various heart diseases such as myocardial infarctions and other ischemia, heart blocks and other conduction defects, benign and life-threatening arrhythmias, and the effects of cardiac drugs.

OVERVIEW

The electrical activity of the heart begins at the cellular level. It then follows the conductive pathway bringing about the cardiac cycle, which results in the heart pumping blood throughout the body (see Chapter 6, Figs. 6-19 and 6-20).

- Cardiac polarity—electrical status of cardiac muscle cells; an attempt to maintain electronegativity (ability to attract electrons) inside these cells to ensure an appropriate distribution of ions (e.g., potassium, sodium, chloride, calcium)
  - Polarization—resting cardiac muscle cells
  - Depolarization—charged and contracting cardiac muscle cells
  - Repolarization—recovering cardiac muscle cells; returning to equilibrium
- Cardiac cycle—the pumping of the heart in a rhythmic cycle of contraction and relaxation (the sound

through a stethoscope is often described as "lub dub")

- Normally 60 to 100 cycles or beats per minute (normal adult heart rate)
- Phases of atrial and ventricle contractions (systole) and relaxation (diastole)
  - Atrial systole—contraction of atria, forcing blood into ventricles through tricuspid and mitral valves
  - Ventricle diastole—relaxation of ventricles, allowing them to fill with blood from atria
  - Ventricle systole—contraction of the ventricles, forcing blood through the aortic and pulmonic valves to the aorta and pulmonary artery
  - Atrial diastole—relaxation of atria, allowing them to fill with blood from the vena cava and pulmonary veins

■ ECG complex—a full cardiac electrical cycle (one heartbeat) represented by PQRST waves (and sometimes U wave) working together as a complex (Fig. 20-1)

- P wave—an upward curve representing atrial contraction; used to measure the atrial rate
- Q wave—a downward deflection after the P wave
- R wave—a large upward spike after the Q wave
- S wave—a downward deflection after the R wave
- T wave—an upward curve after the S wave, representing the repolarization and resting of the ventricles
- U wave—a small upward curve sometimes following the T wave, representing slow repolarization or return to resting
- QRS complex—the QRS waves representing contraction of the ventricles
- PR interval—the P wave and the line connecting it to the QRS complex, representing the time the electrical impulse travels from the sinoatrial (SA) node to the atrioventricular (AV) node

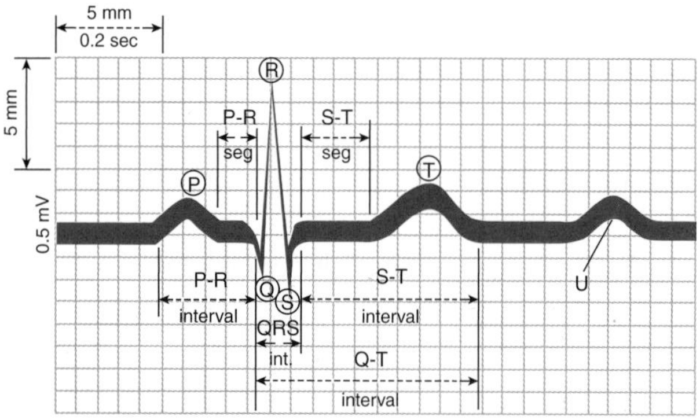

Figure 20-1 Normal cardiac electrical cycle. (Reprinted with permission from Pillitteri A. Maternal and Child Nursing. 4th Ed. Philadelphia: Lippincott Williams & Wilkins, 2003.)

- QT interval—the QRST waves representing a full cardiac electrical cycle
- ST segment—a slight upward line connecting the QRS waves to the T wave and representing the time between contraction of the ventricles and relaxation or recovery

■ Types of ECGs

- Single-lead ECG—information recorded from one view of the heart; a lead is a specific view of the heart, which is a three-dimensional organ; usually, lead II is selected
- 12-lead (multichannel) ECG—information recorded from 10 electrodes, representing 12 views of the heart from 12 different angles
- Telemetry—single-lead or 12-lead ECGs transmitted via radio, electronic, or telephone waves to another site for monitoring or interpretation
- Interpretive ECG—a computerized ECG machine that is programmed to analyze data and produce a printed interpretation with the graph

ELECTRODES, PLACEMENT, AND LEADS

The terms "electrodes" and "leads" are sometimes used synonymously. *This is not correct.* An **electrode** is the sensor attached to the ECG machine that adheres to the skin. A **lead** is the view of the heart produced by a standard combination of electrode placements. The 12-lead ECG is produced using 10 electrodes (Fig. 20-2). The correct placement of these electrodes influences the quality and accuracy of the rhythm strip. The right leg (RL) is the grounding electrode and not used as part of any lead. Electrodes should never be placed over a bony prominence or clothing.

PLACEMENT OF ELECTRODES (10 SENSORS)

■ Chest electrodes (6)

- V1—fourth intercostal space at right margin of sternum
- V2—fourth intercostal space at left margin of sternum
- V3—midway between V2 and V4
- V4—fifth intercostal space at left midclavicular line
- V5—placed midway between V4 and V6
- V6—fifth intercostal space at the left midaxillary line

■ Limb electrodes (4)

- RA—right arm
- LA—left arm
- RL—right leg (ground)
- LL—left leg

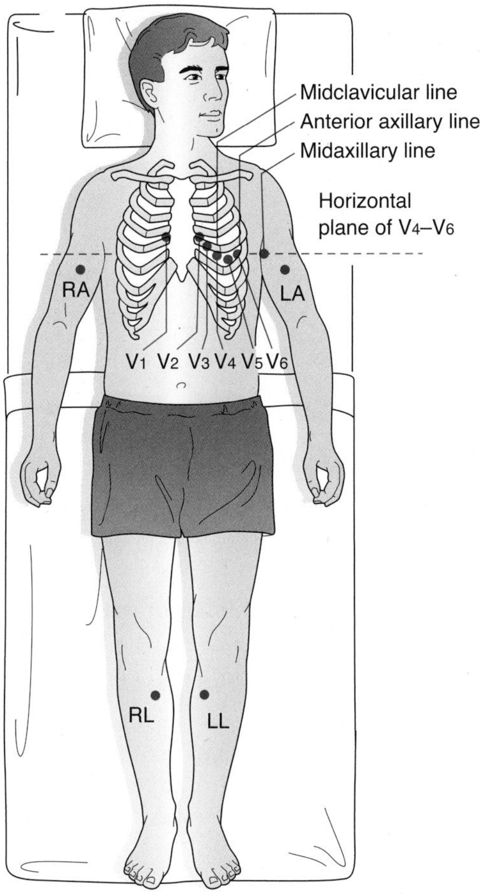

Figure 20-2 Twelve-lead electrocardiogram electrode placement. (Reprinted with permission from Hosley JB, Molle-Matthews E. Lippincott's Pocket Guide to Medical Assisting. Philadelphia: Lippincott Williams & Wilkins, 1999.)

ECG LEADS (12 VIEWS OF THE HEART)

- Limb leads (6)
  - Bipolar limb leads—record cardiac electrical activity between two electrodes
    - Lead I—heart view between LA and RA electrodes
    - Lead II—heart view between LL and RA electrodes
    - Lead III—heart view between LL and LA electrodes
    - Lead I, lead II, and lead III with RL (ground) form **Einthoven triangle** (Fig. 20-3)
  - Unipolar (augmented voltage) limb leads
    - aVR (RA electrode)
    - aVL (LA electrode)
    - aVF (LL electrode)
- Chest (precordial) leads (6)—all chest leads are unipolar and equate to the six chest electrodes
  - V1
  - V2
  - V3
  - V4
  - V5
  - V6

The national certification examinations frequently ask questions about identification of ECG leads.

ECG PAPER

ECG paper is standardized paper designed for ECG machines. It has a combination of small and large blocks to measure the cardiac electrical activity demonstrated on the graph.

- Horizontal line—time
- Vertical line—voltage or amplitude
- Small block—1 mm × 1 mm, representing 0.1 millivolt (mV) on the vertical axis and **representing 0.04 second on the horizontal axis**
- Large block—5 mm × 5 mm, representing 0.5 mV on the vertical axis and **representing 0.20 second on the horizontal axis;** five large horizontal blocks represent1 second
- Vertical slashes above the graph—mark 3-second intervals (15 large blocks); used to calculate heart rate
- Paper speed—25 mm/sec is the usual speed for adults; 50 mm/sec is usual speed for children
- Calibration—10-mm (two large blocks) vertical mark is the normal standard; it is sometimes referred to as the *standardization mark*; the calibration is changed to

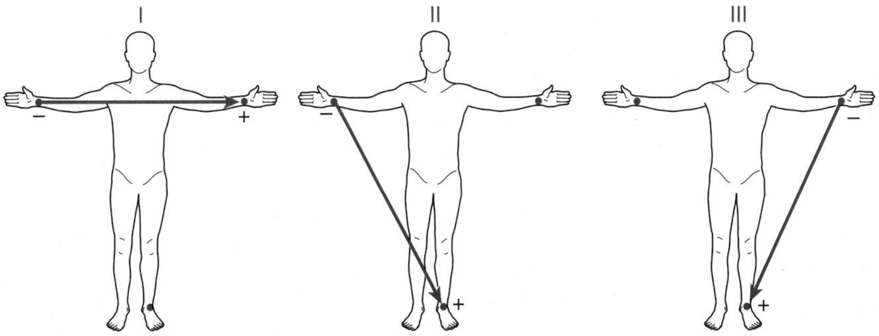

Figure 20-3 Einthoven triangle representing views of the heart in leads I, II, and III.

Box 20-1

ECG Lead Marking Codes

Limb leads: Bipolar (Dot = •)	Limb leads: Unipolar (Dash = —)	Chest leads (Dash = — / Dot = •)
Lead I •	aVR —	V1 — •
Lead II • •	aVL — —	V2 — • •
Lead III • • •	aVF — — —	V3 — • • •
		V4 — • • • •
		V5 — • • • • •
		V6 — • • • • • •

5 mm (one-half standard) in situations where the R wave is too large and the ECG machine amplitude must be decreased to allow the tracing to fit on the paper

- Marking codes—symbols of dots and dashes representing the leads on an ECG tracing (Box 20-1); most model machines identify the leads by placing I, II, III, aVR, aVL, aVF, V1, V2, V3, V4, V5, or V6 in the portion of the graph representing that lead

STYLUS

A **stylus** is a heated penlike instrument of the ECG machine that receives impulses via electrodes and moves on ECG paper, recording the electrical activity of the heart.

NORMAL SINUS RHYTHM (NSR)

Normal sinus rhythm (NSR) is a standard cardiac cycle that begins in the SA node. The role of the medical assistant is not to interpret an ECG. The expectation is that the medical assistant can differentiate normal sinus rhythm from abnormal cardiac rhythms and notify the physician of irregularities. The physician may order a rhythm strip, a long tracing of lead II, as opposed to a complete ECG. The purpose is to evaluate a longer interval of complexes that may be compared to a previous ECG. Criteria for NSR are as follows (Box 20-2):

- Regular rhythm—same number of spaces between all R waves
- Heart rate—normal adult heart rate is 60 to 100 beats per minute
  - Calculation method 1—count number of large blocks between two R waves and divide into 300 (e.g., five large blocks between two R waves = 300/5 = 60 beats per minute)
  - Calculation method 2—count number of R waves between 6-second marks (30 large blocks) and multiply by 10 (e.g., 6 R waves in 6 seconds = 6 × 10 = 60 beats per minute)
- P waves—P waves present before each QRS complex
- Normal PR interval—0.12 to 0.20 second (three to five small blocks)
- Normal-shaped QRS complex—0.06- to 0.10-second duration (1.5 to 2.5 small blocks)

CARDIAC ARRHYTHMIAS

Cardiac **arrhythmias** or dysrhythmias are irregular heart activities resulting in loss of a regular rhythm. If all the criteria for normal sinus rhythm, as stated previously, are not met, the beat is considered abnormal. Figure 20-4 illustrates a normal sinus rhythm and some examples of arrhythmias.

Box 20-2

Template for Identifying Normal Sinus Rhythm

Rhythm	Rate	P wave present	Normal PR interval (0.12–0.20 sec)	Normal-shaped QRS interval (0.06–0.10 sec)

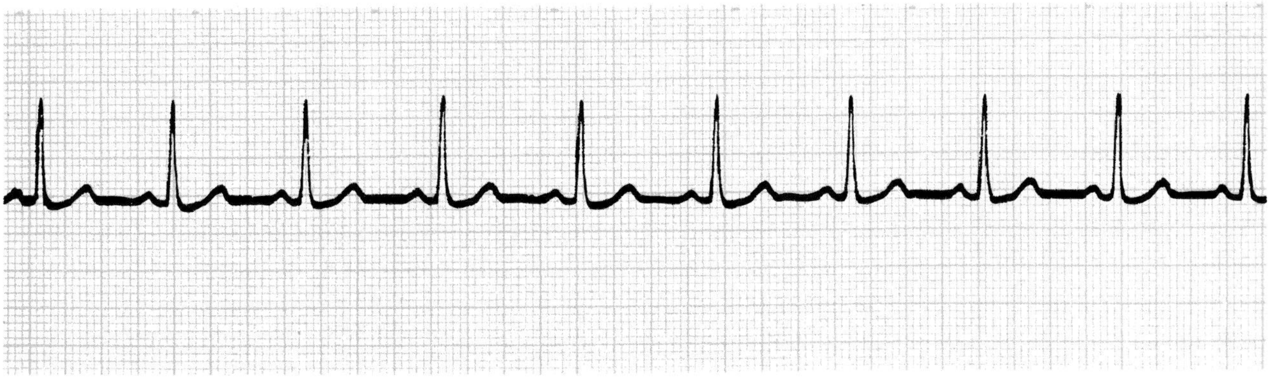

A Normal sinus rhythm

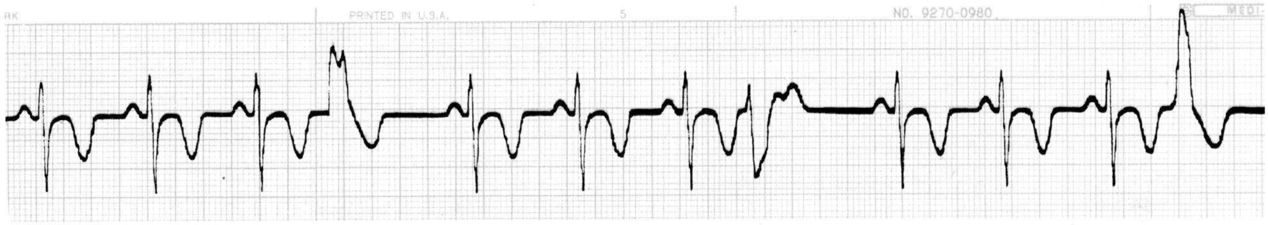

B Premature ventricular contractions (PVCs)

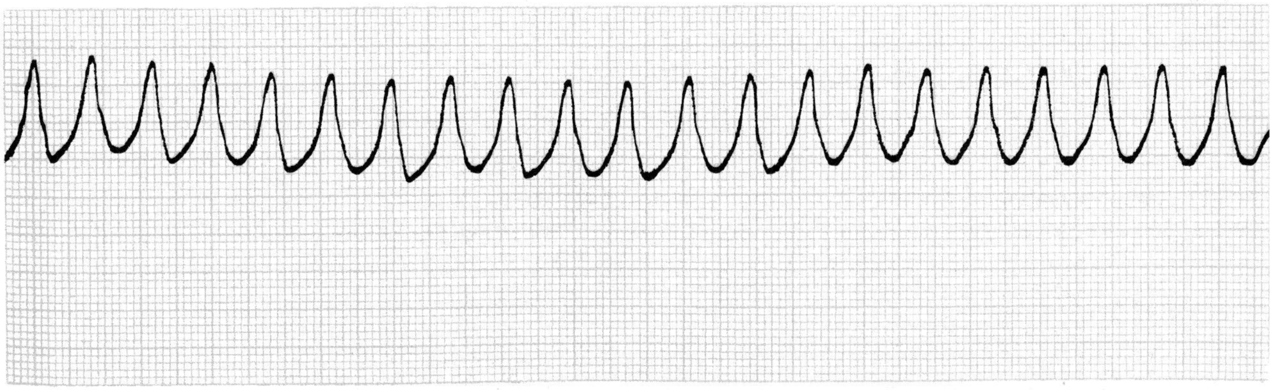

C Ventricle tachycardia

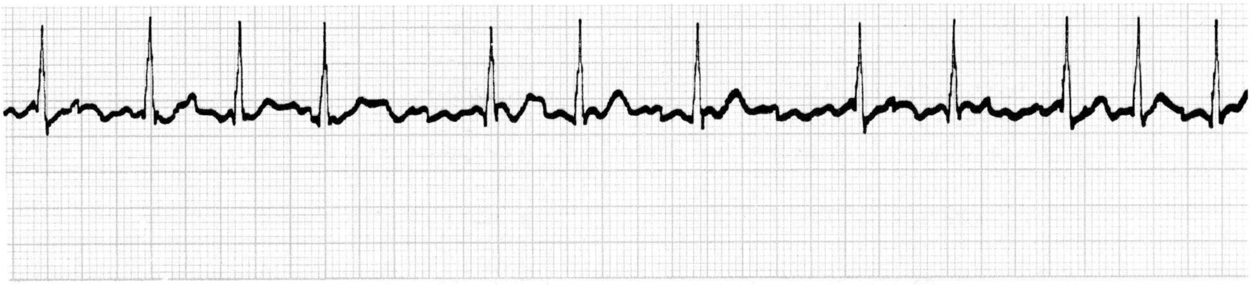

D Atrial fibrillation

Figure 20-4 Select electrocardiogram strips. (Reprinted with permission from Smeltzer SC, Bare BG. Textbook of Medical-Surgical Nursing. 9th Ed. Philadelphia: Lippincott Williams & Wilkins, 2000.)

- Bradycardia—a heart rate slower than 60 beats per minute
- Tachycardia—a heart rate faster than 100 beats per minute
- Asystole—absence of a heart rate, no complexes; flat line; cardiac arrest
- Ectopic beat—a beat originating outside the SA node, the pacemaker of the heart
- Bigeminy—every other beat is ectopic and/or premature
- Ventricular arrhythmias—irregularities in the ventricular activity
  - Premature ventricular contraction (PVC)—a contraction of the ventricles occurring early; may be life threatening, depending on the ratio of PVCs to normal ventricular contractions; report to physician
  - Ventricular tachycardia—ventricular rate of more than 100 to 150 beats per minute, a wide QRS complex; considered a life-threatening arrhythmia and should be reported to the physician immediately
  - Ventricular flutter—ventricular rate of 150 to 300 beats per minute; considered a life-threatening arrhythmia and should be reported to the physician immediately
  - Ventricular fibrillation—uncoordinated, ineffective ventricular contractions, "quivering of the heart"; displayed on the ECG as coarse or fine trembles with no identifiable waves or complexes; considered a life-threatening arrhythmia and should be reported to the physician immediately
- Atrial arrhythmias—irregularities in the atrial activity
  - Premature atrial contraction (PAC)—a contraction of the atria occurring early
  - Atrial tachycardia—also called AT; atrial rate of 150 to 250 beats per minute; P waves are often unidentifiable or hidden in previous T wave
  - Paroxysmal atrial tachycardia (PAT)—atrial tachycardia that starts, and often stops, suddenly
  - Atrial flutter—atrial rate of 250 to 350 beats per minute; "saw tooth" pattern on ECG; the ventricular rate is dependent on the number of nonconducted beats
  - Atrial fibrillation—atrial rate of 350 to 500 beats per minute; P waves not distinct because of rapid rate; R to R waves are usually irregular; often with a rapid ventricular rate

Use Box 20-2 and Figure 20-4 to practice identifying normal sinus rhythm versus an arrhythmia.

ARTIFACTS

Artifacts are interruptions or disturbances in the ECG strip resulting from activity outside the heart. Figure 20-5 demonstrates examples of some of the following artifacts.

- Somatic tremors or movement—involuntary or voluntary muscle or other movement by the patient
- Alternating current (AC) interference—caused by other sources of electricity in the room, such as other equipment including some cell phones, crossed wires, improper grounding
- Wandering baseline—movement of the stylus from the center of the ECG paper in a "roaming" or "wandering" manner; causes may be electrodes that are too loose or too tight, corroded or dirty electrodes, oil or lotion on the patient's skin
- Interrupted baseline—a break between complexes, usually resulting from a wire becoming disconnected from an electrode or a broken wire
- Heat or pressure—imprint on the ECG paper caused by a hot or sluggish stylus

OTHER COMMON CARDIAC TESTS

- Holter monitor—a portable ECG device worn by a patient for 24 hours; monitors heart activity during normal activities of daily living and requires a patient to keep a diary of activities to help physician with diagnosis; electrodes are placed in the following locations:
  - Fourth intercostal space, right sternal margin
  - Right clavicle, lateral to sternal notch
  - Left clavicle, lateral to sternal notch
  - Fifth intercostal space, left axillary line
  - Lower right chest wall
- Stress test—ECG recordings taken while the patient exercises using a treadmill, stationary bicycle, or stair climber; monitors the response of the heart to increased demand
- Echocardiogram—sound waves transmitted through the heart producing a picture on a screen; used to test the heart for structural or functional abnormalities
- Angiogram—an x-ray visualization with contrast material injected into a blood vessel to determine the presence of structural or functional abnormalities
- Cardiac catheterization—insertion of a catheter into a major blood vessel to visualize the heart's activity, to measure pressures, and to identify abnormalities, especially blockages

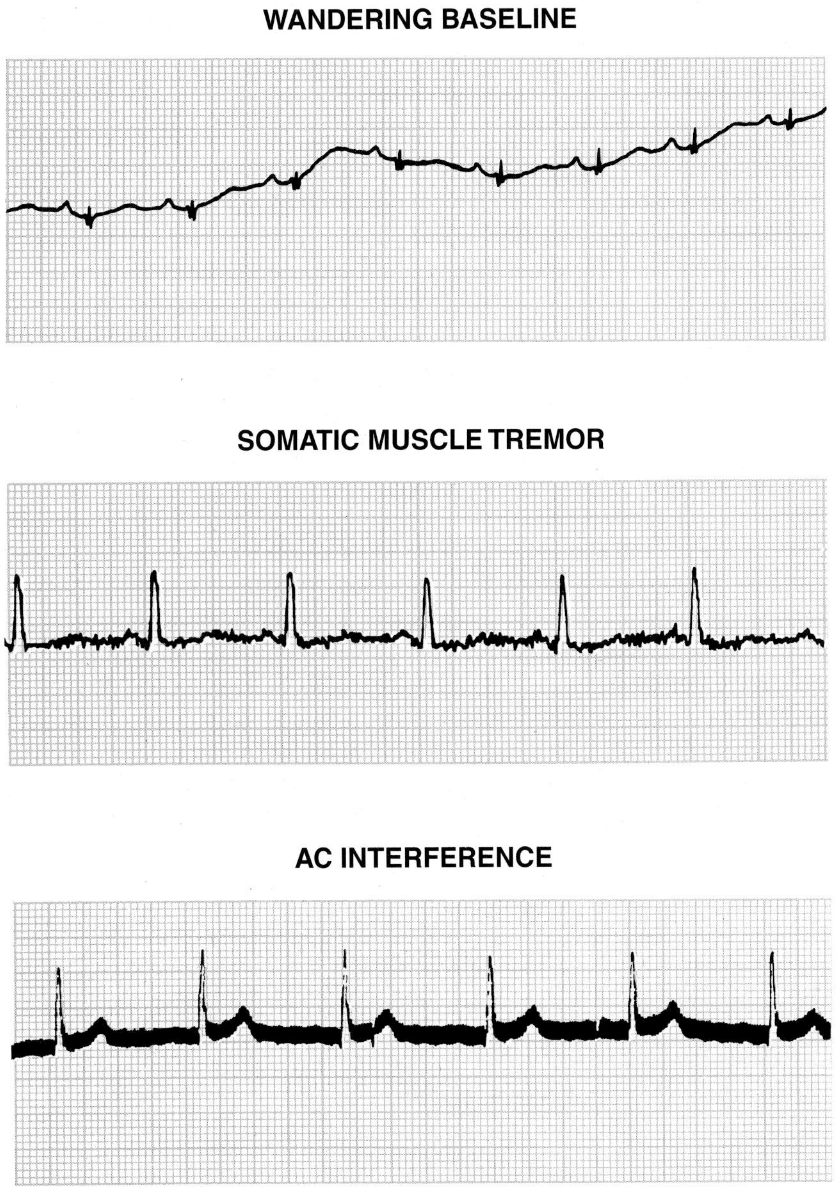

Figure 20-5 Electrocardiogram artifacts. (Reprinted with permission from Hosley JB, Jones SA, Molle-Matthews EA. Lippincott's Textbook for Medical Assistants. Philadelphia: Lippincott-Raven Publishers, 1997.)

TERMS

Electrocardiogram Review

The following list reviews the terms discussed in this chapter and other important terms you may see on the exam.

arrhythmia irregular heart activity resulting in loss of a rhythm

artifacts interruptions or disturbances in the ECG strip resulting from activity outside the heart

asystole absence of a heart rate, no complexes; represented by a flat line; cardiac arrest

atrial fibrillation atrial rate of 350 to 500 beats per minute; P waves not distinct because of rapid rate; R to R waves usually irregular, often with a rapid ventricular rate

atrial flutter atrial rate of 250 to 350 beats per minute; a "saw tooth" pattern on ECG; the ventricular rate is dependent on the number of nonconducted beats

atrial tachycardia (AT) atrial rate of 150 to 250 beats per minute; P waves are often unidentifiable or hidden in previous T wave

bigeminy every other beat is ectopic or premature

bradycardia a heart rate slower than 60 beats per minute

depolarization charged and contracting cardiac muscle cells; systole

ECG complex a full cardiac electrical cycle (one heartbeat) represented by the PQRST (and sometimes U) waves

echocardiogram reflected sound waves used to test the heart for structural or functional abnormalities

ectopic beat a beat originating outside the sinoatrial (SA) node, the pacemaker of the heart

Einthoven triangle the views of the heart from the placement of lead I, lead II, and lead III, which form a triangular shape

electrocardiogram (ECG or EKG) the graphic representation of the heart's electrical activity monitored at the skin surface with sensors called electrodes

electrodes skin sensors used to capture or monitor electrical activity of various organs (e.g., the heart, the brain)

Holter monitor a portable ECG device worn by a patient for 24 hours; heart activity is monitored during normal activities of daily living

lead a standard combination of electrode placements that designates a specific view of the heart

normal sinus rhythm (NSR) a standard cardiac cycle that begins in the SA node

paroxysmal atrial tachycardia (PAT) atrial tachycardia that starts, and often stops, suddenly

polarization resting cardiac muscle cells

premature atrial contraction (PAC) a contraction of the atria occurring early

premature ventricular contraction (PVC) a contraction of the ventricles occurring early; may be life threatening, depending on the ratio of PVCs to normal ventricular contractions

repolarization recovering cardiac muscle cells; diastole; returning to equilibrium

sinoatrial (SA) node pacemaker of the heart

stress test ECG recordings taken while the patient exercises on a treadmill, stationary bicycle, or stair climber

stylus a heated penlike instrument of the ECG machine that receives impulses via electrodes and moves on ECG paper, recording the electrical activity of the heart

tachycardia a heart rate faster than 100 beats per minute

ventricular fibrillation uncoordinated and ineffective ventricular contractions, "quivering of the heart"; displayed on the ECG as coarse or fine trembles with no identifiable waves or complexes; considered a life-threatening arrhythmia

ventricular flutter ventricular rate of 150 to 300 beats per minute; considered a life-threatening arrhythmia

ventricular tachycardia ventricular rate of more than 100 to 150 beats per minute, wide QRS complex; considered a life-threatening arrhythmia

REVIEW QUESTIONS

All questions are relevant for the CMA (AAMA) and RMA (AMT) exams.

1. The measurements of the smallest blocks on standard ECG graph paper are:
   A. 1 mm wide by 5 mm high.
   B. 1 cm high by 1 cm wide.
   C. 5 mm wide by 1 mm high.
   D. 1 mm wide by 1 mm high.

Answer: **D**

Why: The small blocks are 1 mm by 1 mm, and the large blocks are 5 mm by 5 mm.

Review: Yes ❑ No ❑

---

2. Lead I of the ECG tracing is the heart view between the:
   A. right arm (RA) and the left arm (LA).
   B. right arm (RA) and the left leg (LL).
   C. left arm (LA) and the left leg (LL).
   D. right leg (RL) and the left leg (LL).
   E. left arm (LA) and the right leg (RL).

Answer: **A**

Why: Leads I, II, and III are the standard limb leads; they are also known as bipolar leads. Lead I is designated as the first lead, starting at the top of the body with both arms.

Review: Yes ❑ No ❑

---

3. In a standard ECG, lead V3 is located:
   A. at the midaxillary line at the horizontal level of position V4 and position V5.
   B. at the fifth intercostal space and left midclavicular line.
   C. midway between position V2 and position V4.
   D. at the fourth intercostal space at the right margin of the sternum.

Answer: **C**

Why: After the location of V2 and V4 have been determined, V3 is located on an imaginary line midway between V2 and V4.

Review: Yes ❑ No ❑

---

4. Proper preparation of the patient includes the following EXCEPT:
   A. nylon hose should be removed to expose the area of the legs where the sensors will be placed.
   B. place the electrodes or sensors over bony prominences of the arms and legs where the electrical activity is more easily conducted.
   C. position the power cord away from the patient to lessen the chance of artifacts in the ECG tracing.
   D. make the patient comfortable and reassure patient that the procedure is not painful and that there is no transfer of electricity.
   E. place the ground sensor on the right leg.

Answer: **B**

Why: Electrodes or sensors should be placed over fleshy, muscular parts of the upper arms and lower legs. Conduction will be impaired if placed on bony prominences.

Review: Yes ❑ No ❑

---

5. The height of a normal standardization mark on an ECG tracing is:
   A. 5 mm.
   B. 10 mm.
   C. 20 mm.
   D. 25 mm.

Answer: **B**

Why: A normal standardization mark that marks the accuracy of the ECG machine should be 10 mm high. The mark should have a square top. Most ECG machines automatically place a standardization mark at the beginning of the tracing. To manually insert a standardization mark, you need to push the Standard button on the machine.

Review: Yes ❑ No ❑

6. AC interference is an artifact in an ECG tracing that means:
   A. the patient is having a muscle tremor.
   B. there is a loose electrode connection.
   C. there is electrical interference in the room.
   D. the electrodes are too tight on the patient.
   E. the patient may be cold and shivering.

Answer: **C**

Why: There may be electrical machines, computers, or other devices causing interference with the function of the ECG machine. It may be necessary to unplug other appliances or equipment in the room, or the patient may need to be moved to another room to properly complete the ECG.

Review: Yes ❑ No ❑

---

7. The cardiac testing procedure that requires the patient to keep a diary of daily activities is a(n):
   A. cardiac stress test.
   B. echocardiogram.
   C. 12-lead electrocardiogram.
   D. Holter monitor.

Answer: **D**

Why: The Holter monitor is a small, portable ECG device that a patient wears while continuing with daily activities. Usually a 24-hour period is adequate to record and monitor the heart's activity. The patient maintains a written diary or log of activities and events during this time. The physician can determine if there is any correlation between abnormal heart function and the daily activity that took place during that period.

Review: Yes ❑ No ❑

---

8. The ECG grounding lead is the lead attached to the:
   A. right arm.
   B. left arm.
   C. right leg.
   D. chest, midway between V2 and V4.
   E. left leg.

Answer: **C**

Why: The grounding lead helps to reduce alternating current (AC) interference. It keeps the average voltage of the patient the same as the instrument.

Review: Yes ❑ No ❑

---

9. The ECG tracing is printed on graph paper at a standard speed for an adult of:
   A. 25 mm/sec.
   B. 50 mm/sec.
   C. 10 cm/sec.
   D. 20 cm/sec.

Answer: **A**

Why: Each block on the ECG graph paper represents 1 mm. When an ECG tracing is moving at a standard speed, the paper is advancing at 25 millimeters (25 small squares) each second.

Review: Yes ❑ No ❑

---

10. Lead II of the ECG tracing records the electrical activity through the heart from the:
   A. right arm to left arm.
   B. right arm to left leg.
   C. right leg to left leg.
   D. right arm to right leg.
   E. left arm to left leg.

Answer: **B**

Why: The standard limb leads—lead I, lead II, and lead III—form an imaginary triangle when lines connect the reference points. Lead I is the top horizontal line of the triangle, the left side of the triangle is lead II, and the right side of the triangle is lead III.

Review: Yes ❑ No ❑

11. During the electrical heart cycle, **repolarization** refers to the:
   A recovering phase.
   B. discharging phase.
   C. resting phase.
   D. contracting phase.

Answer: **A**

Why: During the heart cycle, cardiac cells are exchanging positive and negative charges within the cell membranes. During repolarization, negative ions are transferred to the inside of the cell, and the positive ions return to the outside. Repolarization is a recovery time for the cells and is a necessary process for another heartbeat to take place.

Review: Yes ❑ No ❑

---

12. The chest lead V1 is located at which intercostal space?
   A. Fourth
   B. Fifth
   C. Between fourth and fifth
   D. Sixth
   E. Third

Answer: **A**

Why: V1 is located at the fourth intercostal space at the right margin of the sternum.

Review: Yes ❑ No ❑

---

13. The image traced on the ECG paper is made by a:
   A. pen filled with an ink cartridge.
   B. needle scratching the image on the paper.
   C. heated stylus tip that melts the coating of the paper.
   D. felt pen.

Answer: **C**

Why: The ECG paper is coated with a finish that is heat sensitive. The stylus is heated and melts away the coating, exposing the dark paper underneath. The tracing can be thick or blurry because of an overheated stylus. The temperature of the stylus needs to be adjusted to ensure a good, clear tracing.

Review: Yes ❑ No ❑

---

14. The purpose of adjusting the normal standard to one-half standard is to:
   A. conserve paper.
   B. enlarge the height of the patient's ECG tracing.
   C. decrease the size of the patient's ECG tracing.
   D. eliminate artifacts in the tracing.
   E. ensure proper lead placement.

Answer: **C**

Why: When the ECG machine setting is changed from the normal 10-mm-high standard mark to one-half standard, 5 mm high, it decreases the size of the patient's ECG tracing. This is necessary when the tracing is so large it goes off the paper. The physician cannot properly measure the complex unless the entire complex is on the paper.

Review: Yes ❑ No ❑

---

15. When a patient has trouble relaxing or cannot remain still for the ECG, the artifact that may occur is:
   A. somatic muscle tremor.
   B. wandering baseline.
   C. AC interference.
   D. electrode interference.

Answer: **A**

Why: A somatic muscle tremor appears as a static line in between the complexes on the ECG paper. To avoid this artifact, make sure the patient is comfortable and not cold. Pillows may be placed under the knees to help the patient relax.

Review: Yes ❑ No ❑

16. The type of cardiac procedure that requires the use of a treadmill is:
    A. echocardiography.
    B. cardiac stress test.
    C. cardiac angiography.
    D. 12-lead ECG.
    E. Holter monitoring.

Answer: **B**

Why: A cardiac stress test is a procedure that measures the body's response to increased demands made on the heart muscle. The patient walks on a treadmill while the ECG tracing is recorded. Some cardiac abnormalities may be exhibited on exertion rather than at rest.

Review: Yes ❑ No ❑

---

17. The medical assistant should gather all the appropriate patient data before the ECG procedure EXCEPT:
    A. patient's height and weight.
    B. date of the patient's first ECG procedure.
    C. patient's current medications.
    D. time and date of the recording.

Answer: **B**

Why: It is not important to know when the patient had his or her first ECG procedure. However, it may be important to know when the patient had his or her last ECG. Some patients have had many electrocardiograms performed. If the patient had a prior ECG with the same physician, the record will be in the patient's file, and the physician can do a comparison.

Review: Yes ❑ No ❑

---

18. The leads aVR, aVL, and aVF are the:
    A. standard leads.
    B. bipolar leads.
    C. limb leads.
    D. chest leads.
    E. augmented voltage leads.

Answer: **E**

Why: Augmented voltage leads provide additional information about the electrical activity of the heart. They use the electrical midpoint of the three limb sensors as the negative pole, and each limb sensor is considered the positive pole. Lead aVR, augmented voltage right, uses a midpoint between the left leg and left arm as the negative pole and the right arm as the positive pole. Lead aVL uses a midpoint between the left leg and right arm as the negative pole and the left arm as the positive pole. Lead aVF uses a midpoint between the right arm and left arm as the negative pole and the left leg as the positive pole.

Review: Yes ❑ No ❑

---

19. The QRS complex of the ECG tracing represents:
    A. atrial depolarization.
    B. atrial repolarization.
    C. ventricular depolarization.
    D. ventricular repolarization.

Answer: **C**

Why: The QRS complex represents the contraction of the ventricles as positive ions enter the cells and negative ions leave them. Depolarization is the electrical activity that causes the heart to contract.

Review: Yes ❑ No ❑

---

20. The ECG marking code that represents lead V1 is:
    A. one dot.
    B. one dash.
    C. two dots.
    D. one dash and one dot.
    E. one dash and two dots.

Answer: **D**

Why: All the chest leads, V1 through V6, are identified as a dash followed by the number of dots that corresponds with the number of the lead.

Review: Yes ❑ No ❑

21. A long strip of QRS complexes of a certain lead used to define certain cardiac arrhythmias is a(n):
    A. monitor strip.
    B. stress strip.
    C. rhythm strip.
    D. artifact strip.

Answer: **C**

Why: A rhythm strip is run to give the physician a tracing longer than the typical lead length. This allows the physician to determine whether the patient has an abnormality that only shows up occasionally and not with each beat.

Review: Yes ❑ No ❑

---

22. If the electrodes are too loose on the patient, what artifact might you find on the ECG tracing?
    A. Wandering baseline
    B. Somatic tremor
    C. AC interference
    D. Electrical interference
    E. Muscle tremor

Answer: **A**

Why: A wandering baseline appears as a tracing that wanders back and forth from the bottom to the top of the paper. The normal baseline should stay within the middle of the paper. Check all electrodes for proper connection. If electrodes are too loose, the baseline may wander on the tracing paper.

Review: Yes ❑ No ❑

---

23. The purpose of setting the ECG paper speed at 50 mm/sec is to:
    A. help record rapid heartbeats.
    B. increase the size of the complex on the paper.
    C. help record slow heartbeats.
    D. decrease the size of the complex on the paper.

Answer: **A**

Why: When a patient has a rapid heartbeat, the faster speed allows the complexes to space farther apart on the paper. It is easier to determine the quality of the complexes when they are not plotted close together. Rapid heartbeats are normal for infants and young children.

Review: Yes ❑ No ❑

---

24. The P wave represents the:
    A. last waveform of the ECG complex.
    B. activity of the ventricles.
    C. resting phase of the heart muscle.
    D. atrial depolarization.
    E. ventricle repolarization.

Answer: **D**

Why: The P wave is the first waveform of the ECG complex and represents the electrical activity that spreads from the SA node through the atria, causing atrial contraction. During this time, the cells are depolarizing.

Review: Yes ❑ No ❑

---

25. What should the medical assistant tell a patient if the patient asks if he or she will feel any discomfort from the ECG procedure?
    A. If you feel any shocks or electrical tingling, please let me know.
    B. Don't worry, we do lots of these exams every day.
    C. The ECG procedure does not hurt and does not send electricity through you.
    D. The electrodes are cold and may feel too tight, but we need to get a good connection.

Answer: **C**

Why: Reassure the patient that the ECG machine does not send out any electricity and that it does not hurt to have the procedure performed. The medical assistant should ask the patient if there is anything that would make him or her more comfortable during the exam, especially if the patient has a problem that could cause discomfort when lying down. Pillows used as support for the arms or legs could help relax the patient.

Review: Yes ❑ No ❑

21
Laboratory Procedures

REVIEW TIP

Review Chapter 17, "Microorganisms and Asepsis," which contains information that is needed for laboratory procedures. Understand the concepts in that chapter before beginning this chapter. Be able to recognize the laboratory norms and other information contained in the tables, boxes, and review terms.

Laboratory procedures, whether for diagnosis or treatment, are an integral part of health care provided in the medical office. The medical assistant plays a major role and is often the one to obtain, prepare, and process the laboratory specimen. The integrity of the specimen and adherence to the processing procedure can determine the correctness of the test results, the accuracy of the patient's diagnosis, and even the efficacy of the treatment.

LABORATORY DIVISIONS

Laboratory procedures are divided into areas or divisions of expertise. The divisions are named according to the types of tissues or organisms to be studied and require different equipment, reagents, and staff training. Although many of the laboratory procedures are not performed in the medical office, the specimens are collected there and general knowledge of divisions is needed.

- Clinical chemistry—analysis that identifies and measures chemical components in blood, urine, spinal fluid, tissue, and other body fluids; common examples include laboratory tests for glucose, cholesterol, calcium, globulin, blood urea nitrogen (BUN), chloride, sodium, potassium, bilirubin, and triglycerides
- Cytology—analysis of cells to determine abnormalities; examples include Pap smears and chromosomal studies
- Hematology—study of blood and blood-forming tissue; analysis of blood to determine abnormalities; examples include tests for hemoglobin, hematocrit, prothrombin time, erythrocyte sedimentation rate, platelet count, and differential white blood cell count (diff) (Table 21-1 lists common blood tests and their normal ranges)
- Histology—microscopic study of cells, tissues, and organs in association with their functions; examples of tests include biopsy and tissue analysis
- Immunology (serology and blood banking)—study of immunity, sensitivity, and induced sensitivity; the presence of antibodies/antigens and pathology; examples include tests for Rh typing, ABO blood typing, Rh antibody titer, rapid plasma reagent (RPR), mononucleosis, human immunodeficiency virus, and pregnancy
- Microbiology—study of microorganisms; in the laboratory, this division usually determines the presence and

Table 21-1 **Common Blood Tests: Normal Ranges**

Test	Adult Normal Range
Bleeding time	2–7 minutes
Blood urea nitrogen (BUN)	10–20 mg/dL
Chloride	98–110 mEq/L
Cholesterol: total	140–200 mg/dL
High-density lipoprotein	30–90 mg/dL
Low-density lipoprotein	30–100 mg/dL
Creatinine	0.6–1.3 mg/dL
Erythrocyte sedimentation rate (ESR, sed rate)	(Results are age- and method-dependent) Male: 0–20 mm/hr Female: 0–30 mm/hr
Glucose (fasting blood sugar, FBS)	70–110 mg/dL
Hematocrit (HCT or "crit")	Male: 39%–49% packed RBCs Female: 35%–45% packed RBCs
Hemoglobin (Hb, Hgb)	Male: 13.2–17.3 g/dL Female: 11.7–16.0 g/dL
Platelets	150–400 × 10^3 cells/µL
Potassium	3.5–5.0 mEq/L
Prostate-specific antigen (PSA)	0–6.5 ng/mL (age-specific ranges)
Red blood cells (RBCs)	Male: 4.3–5.7 × 10^3 cells/µL Female: 3.8–5.1 × 10^3 cells/µL
Rheumatoid factor (RF)	< 30 U/mL
Sodium	135–148 mEq/L
Triglycerides	Male: 40–163 mg/dL Female: 35–128 mg/dL
White blood cells (WBCs)	4.5–11.0 × 10^3 cells/µL

µL = mm^3 (sometimes used to measure WBCs).

identity of microorganisms found in specimens; examples are tests for tuberculosis, meningitis, and diphtheria

- Parasitology—study of human parasites and ova (eggs); examples include tests for hookworm, scabies, pinworms, tapeworms, toxoplasmosis, malaria, and amebiasis
- Urinalysis—physical, chemical, and microscopic analysis of urine; examples include tests for color, clarity, specific gravity (physical), pH, glucose, ketones, nitrites (chemical), red blood cells (RBCs), white blood cells (WBCs), crystals (microscopic), and human chorionic gonadotropin (hCG) for pregnancy; Table 21-2 lists normal ranges for urinalysis

Table 21-2 **Components of Reagent Strip Urinalysis and Normal Results**

Test	Norm
pH	4.5–8
Protein	Negative
Glucose	Negative
Ketone	Negative
Bilirubin	Negative
Blood	Negative
Leukocytes	Negative
Nitrites	Negative
Urobilinogen	2.0 mg/dL
Specific gravity	1.020–1.030
Color	Pale-dark yellow
Clarity	Clear
Odor	Distinct

CLINICAL LABORATORY IMPROVEMENT AMENDMENTS

Enacted in 1988 by Congress, the Clinical Laboratory Improvement Amendments (CLIA) placed all laboratories involved with testing human laboratory specimens under the regulation of the Health Care Finance Administration (now called the Centers for Medicare and Medicaid Services) and the Centers for Disease Control and Prevention (CDC). The standards developed were divided into three areas: personnel, testing, and quality assurance.

The CDC also identifies and publishes a list of CLIA-waived laboratory tests. These are tests generally permitted in a medical office without the stringent standards associated with non–CLIA-waived tests performed in laboratories. The list of waived tests also includes the names of approved commercial products for conducting these tests. The medical assistant may perform the CLIA-waived tests for the following:

- Blood ketone
- High-density lipoprotein cholesterol
- Infectious mononucleosis antibodies (mono)
- Streptococcus, group A (rapid strep)
- Urine hCG by visual color comparison (pregnancy test)
- Blood glucose monitoring devices
- Hemoglobin—copper sulfate, nonautomated

- Hemoglobin by single analyte instruments
- Microhematocrit, spun
- Urine dipstick or tablet analytes
  - Bilirubin
  - Glucose
  - Hemoglobin
  - Ketone
  - Leukocytes
  - Nitrite
  - pH
  - Protein
  - Specific gravity
  - Urobilinogen
- Ovulation test by visual color comparison
- Fecal occult blood
- Erythrocyte sedimentation rate, nonautomated
- *Helicobacter pylori* antibodies

COMMON SPECIMENS COLLECTED IN THE MEDICAL OFFICE

Although only CLIA-waived tests are performed in the medical office, many specimens are collected there and sent to reference laboratories for processing. Correct specimen collection is vital to test results and is often the responsibility of the medical assistant.

- Biopsies—removing tissue from patients for microscopic examination to determine cancer or other abnormalities; may be done surgically or with endoscopes, biopsy punches, or other instruments
- Phlebotomy—incision or needle puncture into a vein to draw blood (see Box 21-1); during insertion, the bevel of the needle should be face up at a 15° to 30° angle
  - Blood components (see Fig. 21-1)
    - Plasma—relatively clear yellow liquid portion of blood; composes 55% of whole blood; upper layer in specimen tube
    - Buffy coat—light grayish liquid portion of blood containing WBCs; composes 1% of whole blood; middle layer in specimen tube
    - Red blood cells (RBCs)—dark red opaque portion of blood containing RBCs; composes 44% of whole blood; bottom layer of specimen tube
    - Serum—liquid portion of blood after clotting factors are removed; composition includes portions of plasma and buffy coat

Box 21-1

Venous Blood Collection Reminders

- Ask the patient about latex and tape allergies.
- The antecubital fossa is the preferred site for blood draw.
- The vein of choice is the median cubital.
- The tourniquet should be placed 3 to 4 inches above the point of puncture.
- The tourniquet should not be left on for more than 1 minute.
- Cleanse the site using a circular pattern beginning at the point of puncture and moving to the outside.
- Allow the antiseptic to dry before inserting safety needle.
- Always anchor the vein.
- Safety needle attached to the tube collection holder (use a butterfly only for difficult draws).
- Release the tourniquet when filling the last tube.
- Gently invert the collection tubes 8 to 10 times to mix tube additives.
- Using a sterile dressing, apply direct pressure to the site.
- Do not tape until bleeding has stopped.

  - Collection tubes—glass and plastic; Box 21-2 lists the order of collection for glass and for plastic tubes
    - Yellow top—used to collect serum for bacteriologic tests; does not contain an additive

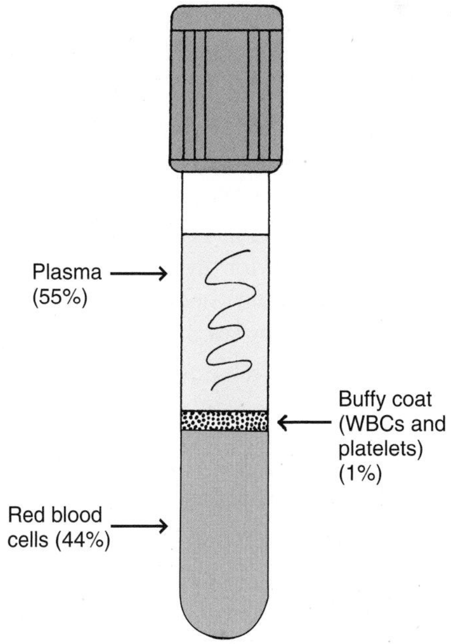

Figure 21-1 Centrifuged blood specimen. (Reprinted with permission from McCall RE, Tankersly CM. Phlebotomy Essentials. 3rd Ed. Philadelphia: Lippincott Williams & Williams, 2003.)

Box 21-2

Order of Draw to Avoid Cross-Contamination of Additives

Order of Draw Using Plastic or Glass Tubes

1. Yellow-top tubes requiring sterility (for blood cultures)
2. Light blue top
3. Red or speckled top
4. Green top
5. Lavender top
6. Gray top

    - Red top—used to collect serum for chemistry and serology; a "clot tube"; does not contain an additive
    - Speckled top (red and black)—used to collect serum for chemistry and serology; different from red top in that it contains a gel that separates serum and RBCs during centrifugation
    - Lavender top—used to collect plasma for hematology testing; contains an anticoagulant
    - Blue top—used to collect plasma for coagulation studies; contains anticoagulant sodium citrate
    - Green top—used to collect plasma for urgent chemistry studies; contains anticoagulant
    - Gray top—used to collect blood for glucose and alcohol testing; contains anticoagulant
  - Capillary puncture—dermal puncture of finger, earlobe, or heel (in infants) to obtain a blood specimen; examples include tests for blood glucose and hemoglobin; also used for mandated neonatal specimen collection
    - Capillary puncture for phenylketonuria (PKU)—capillary specimen from the infant's heel used to detect phenylalanine; required by law in the United States
    - Capillary puncture for thyroid hormones—capillary specimen from infant's heel used to detect hypothyroidism; required by law in the United States
  - Capillary puncture technique
    - Avoid squeezing tip of finger
    - May "milk" hand and finger
    - Discard first drop of blood
    - Avoid scraping collection tube over puncture
    - Avoid air bubbles or spaces in the collection area of the tube
- Cerebral spinal fluid—clear, colorless fluid that covers the spinal cord and brain, obtained for testing by a lumbar puncture performed by a physician or mid-level provider
- Cervical scrapings/brushings—specimens obtained during a pelvic exam; used to test for cancer of the cervix and other diseases
- Sputum—secretions from the respiratory system obtained by deep coughing; used to culture for presence of tuberculosis (*Mycobacterium tuberculosis*) and other disease-causing microorganisms
- Stool—fecal specimen used to test for ova and parasites, pathologic bacteria, and occult blood (e.g., Hemoccult), which may indicate cancer
- Throat swabbing (with sterile cotton applicator)—specimen collected for culture and sensitivity (C&S) to detect disease-causing microorganisms in the throat and to test for the appropriate antibiotic to combat them
- Urethral brushings—specimen collected with a fine brushlike applicator inserted in the urethra; used to test for sexually transmitted infections
- Urine
  - Random sample—urine specimen collected at any time
  - Clean-catch sample—urine specimen collected after cleaning the urinary meatus; the patient then begins to void, stops, collects a portion of urine in the provided container, and finishes voiding in the toilet; referred to as a "midstream" urine; used for tests to determine the presence of bacteria in the urine
  - 24-hour sample—all urine voided in a 24-hour period is collected directly into a specified container; used to determine the presence of substances released only sporadically and to measure the amount of urinary output
  - First voided sample—urine collected in the morning after a night's sleep; used to obtain more concentrated substances for pregnancy testing and microscopic exams
  - Catheterized sample—urine collected by insertion of a sterile tube into the urinary bladder; used to measure the amount of residual urine in the bladder or to obtain a sterile urinary specimen for culturing
  - Postprandial—urine collected after patient has consumed a meal
- Wound swabbings (with sterile applicator)—drainage from wounds; used to culture for pathogens

PREPARATION FOR SPECIMEN EXAMINATION

- Smear—using a swab-type applicator, a small amount of the specimen is applied to a glass slide and allowed to dry

- Wet mount—a drop of normal saline (0.9% sodium chloride) is placed on a slide that has been smeared with the specimen; a cover slide is placed on top, and the specimen is ready for examination with a microscope
- Potassium hydroxide (KOH) mount—primarily used to identify fungal infections; the specimen is prepared as a wet mount, substituting KOH for the saline; the specimen is allowed to sit at room temperature until examination under the microscope
- Stains—a smear of the specimen is prepared; when dry, the slide is heated and a stain material applied; specific bacteria hold certain color stains, allowing identification
  - Purple stain—identifies gram-positive bacteria
  - Red stain—identifies gram-negative bacteria
  - Acid-fast—certain bacteria are not susceptible to color staining; these bacteria are called acid-fast (e.g., *Mycobacterium tuberculosis*)
- Sensitivity—testing to determine a pathogen's susceptibility to specific antibiotics
- Culture—the process of growing pathogens from specimens inoculated into a culture media and maintained at a designated temperature; the purpose is to identify the microorganisms contained in the specimen
  - Common culture media—substances used to promote growth of bacteria by providing a nutrition source; may be a liquid or gel-like state
    - Transport media—usually a tube structure with a substance used to keep the bacteria alive until they can be plated on an appropriate culture media; specific tubes may be used for specific specimens
    - Petri dish—a round plastic dish that contains agar, a gelatin-like culture material made from algae, and has a cover to minimize contamination of the specimen with environmental bacteria the covered petri dish should be placed in the incubator upside down
    - Plating—process of inoculating agar with the specimen swab and sometimes with a sterile inoculating loop

THE MICROSCOPE

The microscope (scope) is an instrument used to magnify very small objects, usually objects not visible to the naked eye. Anton van Leeuwenhoek (17th century) is attributed with being the first to use an instrument with lenses to visualize "germs." Many different types and strengths of microscopes are used in clinical and research laboratories. The most common one found in the medical office is the binocular, or two-eyepiece, scope. It is used to identify microorganisms placed on slides from various body specimens using the processes previously mentioned. The main portions of the microscope are described below and illustrated in Figure 21-2.

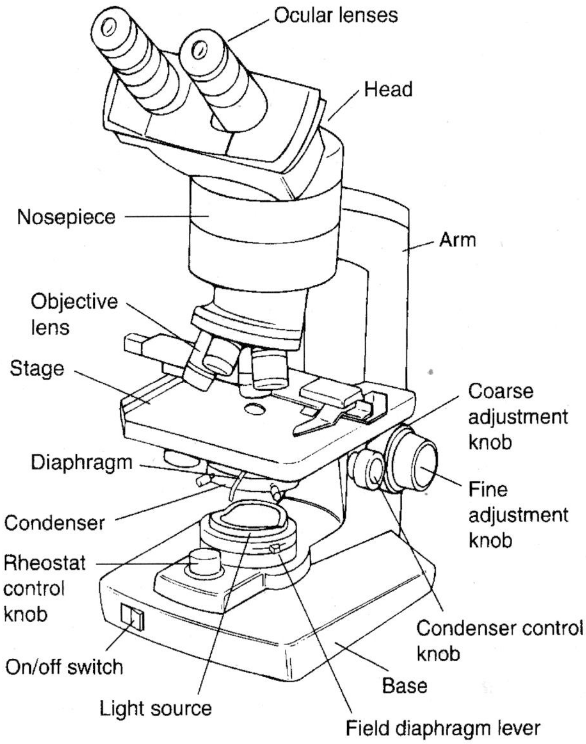

Figure 21-2 Basic parts of the microscope.

- Ocular lens(es)—eyepiece(s)
- Frame—structure that supports the scope
  - Base—bottom portion of the frame that holds entire structure
  - Arm—extension of the frame that holds upper portion of the scope
- Head—portion of the frame below the eyepiece(s)
- Stage—platform that holds the slide during observation
- Condenser—lens beneath the stage that focuses light on the slide; it may be raised or lowered
- Light source—located on base; provides light to the condenser
- Diaphragm—controls the amount of light on the condenser
- Nosepiece—portion below the head that holds the objective lenses
- Objective lenses—lenses below the nosepiece marked with specified magnifications; these are summarized in Table 21-3
  - Low power—magnification 10×; used for initial focus

Table 21-3 **Objective Lens Magnification**

Ocular Lens	Lens Magnification	Total Lens Magnification
Low power	10 × 10×	100×
High-power dry	10 × 40×	400×
Oil immersion	10 × 100×	1000×

- High-power dry—magnification 40×; used to locate and focus on the specimen
- Oil immersion—magnification 100×; used with oil to perform differential count of blood smear

■ Coarse adjustment—outside knob used with low-power objective lens

■ Fine adjustment—inside knob used with both high-power and oil-immersion objective lenses

TERMS

Laboratory Procedures Review

The following list reviews the terms discussed in this chapter and other important terms you may see on the exam.

anticoagulant substance that prevents blood from clotting

biopsy removing tissue from patients for microscopic examination to determine the presence of cancer or other abnormalities; may be done surgically or with endoscopes, biopsy punches, or other instruments

calibration a measurement compared with a standard; a method for testing the accuracy of equipment; a quality assurance procedure

capillary puncture dermal puncture of finger, earlobe, or heel in infants to obtain a blood specimen

centrifuge laboratory instrument that spins at high speeds, separating particles in specimens such as blood and urine

clinical chemistry analysis to identify and to measure chemical components in blood, urine, spinal fluid, tissue, and other body fluids

complete blood count (CBC) panel of blood tests that includes hematocrit, hemoglobin, red blood cells, white blood cells, and differential white blood cells (diff)

control a specimen with known values that serves as a check of test accuracy

crossmatching laboratory testing process to determine compatibility of blood donated by one person with the blood of a potential recipient

culture the process of growing pathogens from specimens inoculated into a culture medium and maintained at a designated temperature; the purpose is to identify the microorganisms contained in the specimen

cytology analysis of cells to determine abnormalities

evacuated tube (ET) a tube, sealed to maintain the vacuum, that is used for obtaining blood specimens; it may have additives, depending on the type of blood specimen to be obtained

fibrinogen a protein in blood plasma that assists clotting

hematocrit percentage of red blood cells in the total blood volume

hematology study of blood and blood-forming tissue; analysis of blood to determine abnormalities

hemoglobin oxygen-carrying portion of red blood cells

histology microscopic study of cells, tissues, and organs in association with their functions

human chorionic gonadotropin (hCG) hormone present in blood and urine during pregnancy; urine or blood tests are used to determine pregnancy by the presence of hCG

immunohematology specialized immunology dealing with blood, the presence of antibodies/antigens, and pathology

immunology study of immunity, sensitivity, and induced sensitivity; the presence of antibodies/antigens and pathology

incubation maintaining a controlled environment to promote growth of microbial or tissue cultures

lancet a sharp, sterile, disposable instrument used to puncture skin for collecting capillary blood

microbiology study of microorganisms; in the laboratory, this division usually determines the presence and the identity of microorganisms found in specimens; examples include tests for tuberculosis, meningitis, and diphtheria

microscope (scope) an instrument used to magnify very small objects usually not visible to the naked eye

parasitology study of human parasites and ova (eggs)

phenylketonuria (PKU) a disease resulting in mental retardation caused by a deficiency in the metabolic process; tested for by using a capillary specimen from an infant's heel, a test required by law in the United States

phlebotomy incision or needle puncture into a vein to draw blood

plasma relatively clear yellow liquid portion of blood; composes 55% of whole blood; upper layer in specimen tube

plating process of inoculating agar with a specimen swab and sometimes a sterile inoculating loop

point of care testing (POCT) laboratory testing performed at the location where the patient is receiving his or her health care (usually the medical office) using small, rapid instruments and methods; these tests are Clinical Laboratory Improvement Amendments (CLIA) waived

qualitative analysis the identification of a type of pathogen by its appearance in the specimen

quantitative analysis the method used to determine the number of bacteria present in a specimen

reagent a substance that, when added to a solution of another substance, participates in a chemical reaction; it may be used to identify or to quantify the presence of another substance

sensitivity testing to determine a pathogen's susceptibility to specific antibiotics

serum liquid portion of the blood that remains after clotting factors are removed

universal donor a person who has O-negative blood, which is theoretically able to be transfused into a person with another blood type in an emergency situation

urinalysis the physical, chemical, and microscopic analysis of urine

urinometer a sealed glass float placed in approximately 15 mL of urine and that measures specific gravity

REVIEW QUESTIONS

All questions are relevant for the CMA (AAMA), RMA (AMT) exam.

1. The process of removing tissue from a patient for microscopic examination is called:
   A. cytology.
   B. microbiology.
   C. biopsy.
   D. histology.

Answer: **C**

Why: The process of removing tissue from the body for examination is called a biopsy. Cytology and histology are both a process of analysis or examination of cells. Microbiology is the study of all microscopic organisms.

Review: Yes ❑ No ❑

---

2. The following blood collection tubes contain an anticoagulant EXCEPT:
   A. blue.
   B. lavender.
   C. gray.
   D. green.
   E. red.

Answer: **E**

Why: A red-stoppered collection tube is used to collect serum for chemistry and serology tests. The tube does not contain any additive, enabling the blood to form a clot and the serum to be separated from the clot or clotted cells.

Review: Yes ❑ No ❑

---

3. A urine specimen that is collected at any time of the day is referred to as:
   A. clean catch.
   B. random.
   C. 24-hour.
   D. postprandial.

Answer: **B**

Why: Random means at any time. Clean catch is a method of collection of urine in which the patient cleans the area of the urinary meatus and collects the urine in midstream. A 24-hour urine is a collection of all urine in a 24-hour period. Postprandial means after a meal.

Review: Yes ❑ No ❑

---

4. The clear liquid portion of blood that composes 55% of whole blood is:
   A. serum.
   B. plasma.
   C. hemoglobin.
   D. fibrinogen.
   E. thrombin.

Answer: **B**

Why: Serum is the fluid portion of blood that remains after coagulation. It contains no fibrinogen, a plasma protein essential to the blood clotting process. Hemoglobin is a protein-iron compound found in the blood; it carries oxygen to the cells from the lungs and carries carbon dioxide away from the cells to the lungs. Fibrinogen, a globulin, and thrombin, an enzyme, are products found in the blood that are required for proper clotting.

Review: Yes ❑ No ❑

5. Appropriate locations for collecting capillary blood include the following EXCEPT:
   A. fingertip.
   B. earlobe.
   C. antecubital space.
   D. heel.

Answer: **C**

Why: The antecubital space, in the inner surface of the bend of the elbow, is where the veins are located that are used for phlebotomy. Capillary punctures are not performed here.

Review: Yes ❑ No ❑

---

6. When multiple tubes of blood are to be drawn, which is drawn first?
   A. Tubes with anticoagulant additive
   B. Blood culture tubes or any test requiring a sterile specimen
   C. Tubes with no additive
   D. Tubes containing heparin
   E. Tubes containing sodium citrate

Answer: **B**

Why: Any time a sterile specimen is required, such as blood cultures, special care is taken not to contaminate the specimen—therefore, these specimens are drawn first. After that, tubes containing no additive are drawn and then tubes with additive. This order of draw prevents contamination of tubes with the additives.

Review: Yes ❑ No ❑

---

7. The specimen used to perform a culture test for the presence of tuberculosis is:
   A. sputum.
   B. capillary blood.
   C. venous blood.
   D. swab from throat.

Answer: **A**

Why: Tuberculosis typically infects the lungs. Sputum is the material coughed up from the lungs. A culture of this material will grow the acid-fast bacillus *Mycobacterium tuberculosis.*

Review: Yes ❑ No ❑

---

8. A blood test used to indicate the level of kidney function is:
   A. sedimentation rate.
   B. complete blood count.
   C. blood urea nitrogen.
   D. human chorionic gonadotropin.
   E. hematocrit.

Answer: **C**

Why: Blood urea nitrogen (BUN) is a measurement of the amount of nitrogenous substance present in the blood as urea. Urea is a major end product of protein and amino acid metabolism. The kidneys are responsible for excreting this product. If the levels are elevated, it may indicate kidney failure. A sedimentation rate is used to monitor the course of inflammation in rheumatoid arthritis. A complete blood count (CBC) will provide information about the formed white and red cells in the body, both quantity and quality. Human chorionic gonadotropin is a hormone present in blood or urine during pregnancy. This test is used to determine pregnancy. A hematocrit is a blood test that determines the percentage of packed cells in a volume of blood.

Review: Yes ❑ No ❑

---

9. The solution used to identify fungal infections is:
   A. 0.9% sodium chloride.
   B. sodium citrate.
   C. PSA.
   D. KOH.

Answer: **D**

Why: Potassium hydroxide (KOH) is mixed with skin scrapings and the mixture is placed on a microscope slide for analysis. Sodium chloride 0.9% is the solution used for a wet mount. Sodium citrate is an additive in a blue-top evacuated tube used for coagulation studies. PSA is an abbreviation for prostate-specific antigen, which is used in the detection of cancer of the prostate.

Review: Yes ❑ No ❑

10. A urine test that compares the weight of urine with that of distilled water is:
   A. sedimentation rate.
   B. clarity.
   C. specific gravity.
   D. pH.
   E. ketone analysis.

Answer: **C**

Why: Distilled water is used as a measure of density against other liquids such as urine. Distilled water with a specific gravity of 1.000 is compared with urine, which has particles dissolved in it. The normal specific gravity of urine is 1.005 to 1.030.

Review: Yes ❑ No ❑

---

11. Which of the following is proper technique when performing venipuncture?
   A. The bevel of the needle is face up, and the insertion angle is 15° to 30°.
   B. The bevel of the needle is face down, and the insertion angle is 30°.
   C. The bevel of the needle is face up, and the insertion angle is 45° to 60°.
   D. The placement of the bevel is not critical, but the insertion angle should be at least 45°.

Answer: **A**

Why: The bevel of the needle should always be face up when performing venipuncture. If it is face down during insertion, the bevel may lodge against the back wall of the vein and no blood would be obtained. Insertion should be at a slight angle, no greater than 30°.

Review: Yes ❑ No ❑

---

12. Proper sites for a capillary puncture include the following EXCEPT:
   A. tip of ring finger.
   B. heel of infant.
   C. tip of index finger.
   D. earlobe.
   E. tip of middle finger.

Answer: **C**

Why: The index finger tends to be more calloused and may not provide proper blood flow from a lancet puncture.

Review: Yes ❑ No ❑

---

13. The normal range of urine pH is:
   A. 3.0–5.0
   B. 5.0–8.0
   C. 5.0–10.0
   D. 8.0–10.0

Answer: **B**

Why: On the pH scale, 7.0 represents a neutral reading. Readings lower than 7.0 are acidic and higher than 7.0 are basic. The normal range of urine is from slightly acid to slightly basic.

Review: Yes ❑ No ❑

---

14. Which of the following is a normal adult WBC count?
   A. 1,000 cells/mm^3
   B. 7,000 cells/mm^3
   C. 20,000 cells/mm^3
   D. 50,000 cells/mm^3

Answer: **B**

Why: The normal range for a white blood cell count is $4.5–11.0 \times 10^3$ cells/mm^3. This means there are 4,500 to 11,000 white blood cells in a cubic millimeter. A white blood cell count range is also reported as $4.5–11.0 \times 10^3$ cells/μL.

Review: Yes ❑ No ❑

---

15. A urine pregnancy test measures:
   A. RPR.
   B. VDRL.
   C. hCG.
   D. HDL.

Answer: **C**

Why: hCG is the human chorionic gonadotropin hormone present in blood and urine during pregnancy.

Review: Yes ❑ No ❑

16. Which of the following is an incorrect technique to use when performing phlebotomy?
    A. Check the expiration dates printed on vacuum collection tubes to make sure they are not expired.
    B. Put on sterile gloves to ensure use of universal standard precautions.
    C. Apply the tourniquet snugly, but not too tightly.
    D. After the puncture site is determined and cleansed, do not touch the site.
    E. Release the tourniquet before removing the needle from the patient's vein.

Answer: **B**

Why: It is not required that you wear sterile gloves for routine venipuncture; however, clean gloves must be used with each patient.

Review: Yes ❑ No ❑

---

17. The color of the stopper of the vacuum collection tube used to collect plasma for coagulation studies is:
    A. yellow.
    B. red.
    C. red and black.
    D. blue

Answer: **D**

Why: The yellow-, red-, and red-and-black-top tubes do not contain any anticoagulant additive. Blood collected in these tubes will clot and cannot be used for clotting or coagulation blood tests.

Review: Yes ❑ No ❑

---

18. The term used to describe cloudy urine is:
    A. pale.
    B. straw.
    C. transparent.
    D. amber.
    E. turbid.

Answer: **E**

Why: Pale, straw, and amber are used to describe the color of urine; transparent is the term to describe clear urine. Turbid or cloudy urine indicates the presence of some particles in the urine, such as chemicals, blood cells, bacteria, or mucus.

Review: Yes ❑ No ❑

---

19. Which department of the laboratory performs hemoglobin and hematocrit tests?
    A. Cytology
    B. Bacteriology
    C. Immunology
    D. Hematology

Answer: **D**

Why: Cytology is the department that analyzes cells to determine abnormalities. Immunology is the study of immunity and antibodies/antigens. Bacteriology is the study of bacteria, culture, and sensitivity. Hematology includes the study of the blood for any abnormalities of the blood-forming tissue and the quality of the blood cells.

Review: Yes ❑ No ❑

20. Which of the following is part of proper capillary blood collection technique?
   A. Use the index finger as the preferred site for capillary puncture.
   B. Squeeze the tip of the finger for at least 30 seconds before a puncture of the skin.
   C. Scrape the tip of the collection tube over the tip of the finger to get every drop of blood in the tube.
   D. After performing the skin puncture, use the first drop of blood that comes to the surface of the skin.
   E. When collecting blood, avoid air bubbles in the microhematocrit collection tube.

Answer: **E**

Why: When using a microhematocrit collection tube, the test will be inaccurate if there are air pockets in the tube. Proper technique requires that the index finger not be used but that the ring or middle finger be used instead. You should not scrape the skin during the collection process, because this encourages platelet activation, which can cause the blood to clot and alter the test results. To encourage blood flow, make sure the site chosen is warm. Gently massage from the base to the top of the site but do not squeeze the finger. Squeezing or milking the site will dilute the specimen with tissue fluid. Always wipe away the first drop of blood before starting to collect the specimen. The first drop of blood contains a higher concentration of tissue fluid, which may alter the test results.

Review: Yes ❑ No ❑

---

21. A hematocrit reading of 40 means that:
   A. 40% of the total blood volume consists of RBCs.
   B. 60% of the total blood volume consists of RBCs.
   C. 40% of the total blood volume is plasma.
   D. 60% of the total blood volume is WBCs.

Answer: **A**

Why: A hematocrit is the percentage of red blood cells contained in whole blood. A reading of 40 means that of 100% total blood volume, 40% is red blood cells and 60% is plasma, WBCs, and platelets.

Review: Yes ❑ No ❑

---

22. When whole blood is allowed to clot, the clear portion visible after centrifugation is the:
   A. plasma.
   B. buffy coat.
   C. serum.
   D. hemoglobin.
   E. fibrinogen.

Answer: **C**

Why: Serum is the clear liquid portion of the blood that contains no blood cells, platelets, or fibrinogen. Plasma is the clear portion of blood that still contains clotting agents. The buffy coat is the light grayish liquid portion of blood containing WBCs; it composes 1% of whole blood and is the middle layer in the specimen tube. Hemoglobin is the oxygen-carrying portion of RBCs. The platelets and fibrinogen are clotting agents that form the clot.

Review: Yes ❑ No ❑

---

23. Which of the following would be considered a normal finding for urine?
   A. Protein—positive, 4+
   B. Clarity—cloudy
   C. Color—straw
   D. Specific gravity—1.055

Answer: **C**

Why: The color of normal urine is yellow and is typically described as straw-colored. The protein content in urine should be negative. A positive reading could indicate a kidney disorder. The clarity or characteristic of urine should be clear, not cloudy or turbid. The specific gravity of urine is 1.003 to 1.035. The higher the reading, the more dense the urine is because of dissolved particles in the urine. These could be blood cells, chemicals, or bacteria.

Review: Yes ❑ No ❑

24. Parasitology includes the study of:
    A. worms.
    B. fungi.
    C. cells.
    D. bacteria.
    E. antibodies.

Answer: **A**

Why: Parasitology is the study of human parasites (worms and scabies) and ova (eggs).

Review: Yes ❑ No ❑

---

25. Which of the following represents an error in performing venipuncture?
    A. Using the proper size needle to avoid hemolysis of the specimen
    B. Vigorously shaking the anticoagulated blood specimens to completely mix the anticoagulant with the blood
    C. Labeling the tube with the date, time of draw, patient's name, and your initials
    D. Allowing the venipuncture site to completely dry before insertion of the needle

Answer: **B**

Why: If a blood specimen is vigorously shaken, the blood cells will rupture (hemolyze) and release hemoglobin into the plasma. This can result in erroneous readings. Blood drawn in anticoagulant tubes should be well mixed by gently tilting the tube back and forth several times.

Review: Yes ❑ No ❑

22
Medical Imaging

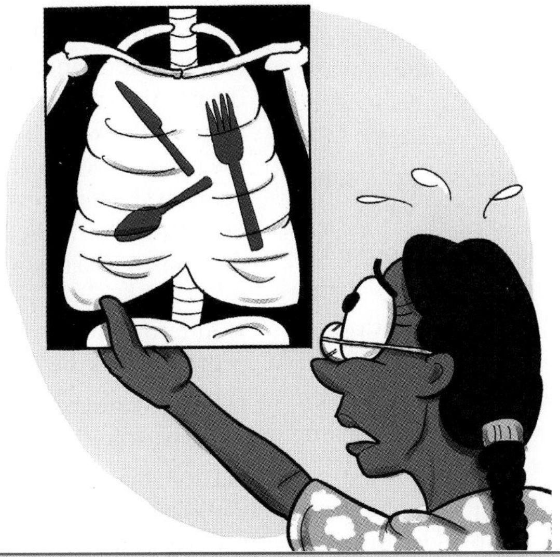

REVIEW TIP

You reached Medical Imaging Chapter 22!
So keep on going–you're almost through.
Stay on the review path–don't go astray
'Cause certification is not far away!

Radiology is the study and use of radioactive substances to visualize an internal structure. The image of the structure is produced on film and called a *radiograph*, *x-ray*, or *roentgenogram* (all synonymous terms). This process was, for many years, the only noninvasive method to penetrate solid objects and obtain "pictures," most commonly of bones and dense organs. The department providing the service was called Radiology. Today, different power sources and technologies are used and different images can be produced. Radiation is also used as a treatment, such as in cancer therapy. Therefore, the Radiology Department has been replaced by the Medical Imaging Department.

Many states require separate certifications to perform any form of medical imaging. The role of the medical assistant and medical administrative specialist, in these states, is not to perform the procedure but to prepare the patient for the test, including providing preparatory education (e.g., fasting, bowel cleansing, ingesting specific substances). Positioning the patient may also be the role of the medical assistant. (*Note:* Endoscopic procedures are generally not performed in the medical imaging department even though they may be considered diagnostic imaging.) Some endoscopic exams are used in tandem with or as a replacement for radiologic exams. For example, the colonoscopy may be done in place of the lower gastrointestinal (GI) series. This eliminates patient exposure to radiation.

COMMON TYPES OF MEDICAL IMAGING

- Radiography—may be used for diagnostic purposes (e.g., to determine a fracture) or therapeutic purposes (e.g., as a treatment for cancer)

- Angiography—radiographic visualization of blood vessels and blood flow by injecting radiopaque material through a subcutaneous catheter
- Arthrography—radiographic visualization of a joint by injection of contrast media
- Barium enema (lower GI series)—rectal administration of barium to radiographically visualize the lower portion of the gastrointestinal system
- Barium swallow (upper GI series)—oral administration of barium to radiographically visualize the upper portion of the gastrointestinal system
- Bone x-ray—flat plates including anteroposterior and lateral; when ordering an x-ray of a bone or bones of a body part that is bilateral, such as a foot, the provider frequently wants an x-ray of the same bone(s) of the opposite side as a comparison.
- Chest x-ray (CXR)—flat plates (x-rays) of the chest; includes anteroposterior (AP) and lateral view
- Cholangiography—radiographic visualization of the bile ducts by injection of contrast media
- Cholecystography—radiographic visualization of the gallbladder structure and function
- Computed tomography (CT)—radiographic visualization of body structures in thin cross sections or layers; much more precise than traditional x-ray
- Intravenous pyelography (IVP)—radiographic visualization of the kidney, ureters, and bladder by injection of contrast media through a vein
- Kidney, ureter, and bladder (KUB)—flat plate (x-ray) of the abdomen
- Mammography—radiographic examination of breasts (usually female) with specialized x-ray equipment
- Myelography—radiographic visualization of the spinal cord and nerve roots by injection of contrast media into the subarachnoid space
- Retrograde pyelography—radiographic visualization of the KUB by administration of contrast media through a urinary catheter

■ Magnetic resonance imaging (MRI)—film visualization of internal structures, including soft tissue, by using a magnetic field in combination with radiation

■ Nuclear medicine—area of medicine using radioisotopes to diagnose and treat specific pathology; used in some cancer therapies

■ Positron emission tomography (PET)—process of producing color images by injecting radioisotopes that combine with particles in the body; used to assess physiology and metabolic activity, not just structures

■ Radiation therapy—using radiation to treat diseases, typically cancer, by shrinking the tumor; may be performed in medical imaging department or outpatient facility

■ Scintigraphy (scintiphotography)—photographic images using a gamma camera to record the distribution of a radioactive agent; used to identify cancer metastasis

■ Ultrasonography (ultrasound)—use of high-frequency ultrasonic waves to produce an image and identify and measure deep body structures and abnormalities

PATIENT POSITIONING FOR RADIOLOGY

The physician usually orders an x-ray based on the view(s) he or she wants, such as "CXR AP and lateral," which means a chest x-ray with anteroposterior and lateral views. The medical assistant and the medical administrative specialist must know the meaning of the positions to properly order the tests and, in some instances, set up the patient to obtain the correct film. Production of a radiograph requires the x-ray beam to go from the machine through the patient's body part(s) to the x-ray plate or cassette that contains the film. Standardized body views or positions are used to perform the x-ray. The views are named for the direction of the beam through the body part (Fig. 22-1).

■ Anteroposterior view (AP)—x-ray beam directed from the front to the back of the body or body part

■ Posteroanterior view (PA)—x-ray beam directed from the back to the front of the body or body part

■ Lateral view (lat)—x-ray beam directed from one side of the body to the other; **view is named after the side closest to the cassette. Caution: This distinction, compared to the AP and PA views, can be confusing.**

- Right lateral view (RL)—x-ray beam **directed from the left side of the body to the right**
- Left lateral view (LL)—x-ray beam **directed from the right side of the body to the left**
- Oblique view—x-ray beam directed at an angle through the body or body part; view is named after body position closest to the cassette, such as the right anterior oblique

RADIATION SAFETY

Radiation is the energy source for producing many of the images described previously. Specific safety measures must be taken to protect the patient, staff, and others in the area of the machine. Some of these measures, such as monitoring the dosimeters and scheduling maintenance, may be the responsibility of the medical assistant or medical administrative specialist.

■ Proper construction of the room(s) in which the machines are housed (e.g., lead-lined walls)

■ Proper care, inspection, and maintenance of machine(s)

■ Personal dosimeter worn by all staff present during x-rays; dosimeters are monitored for absorption of radiation

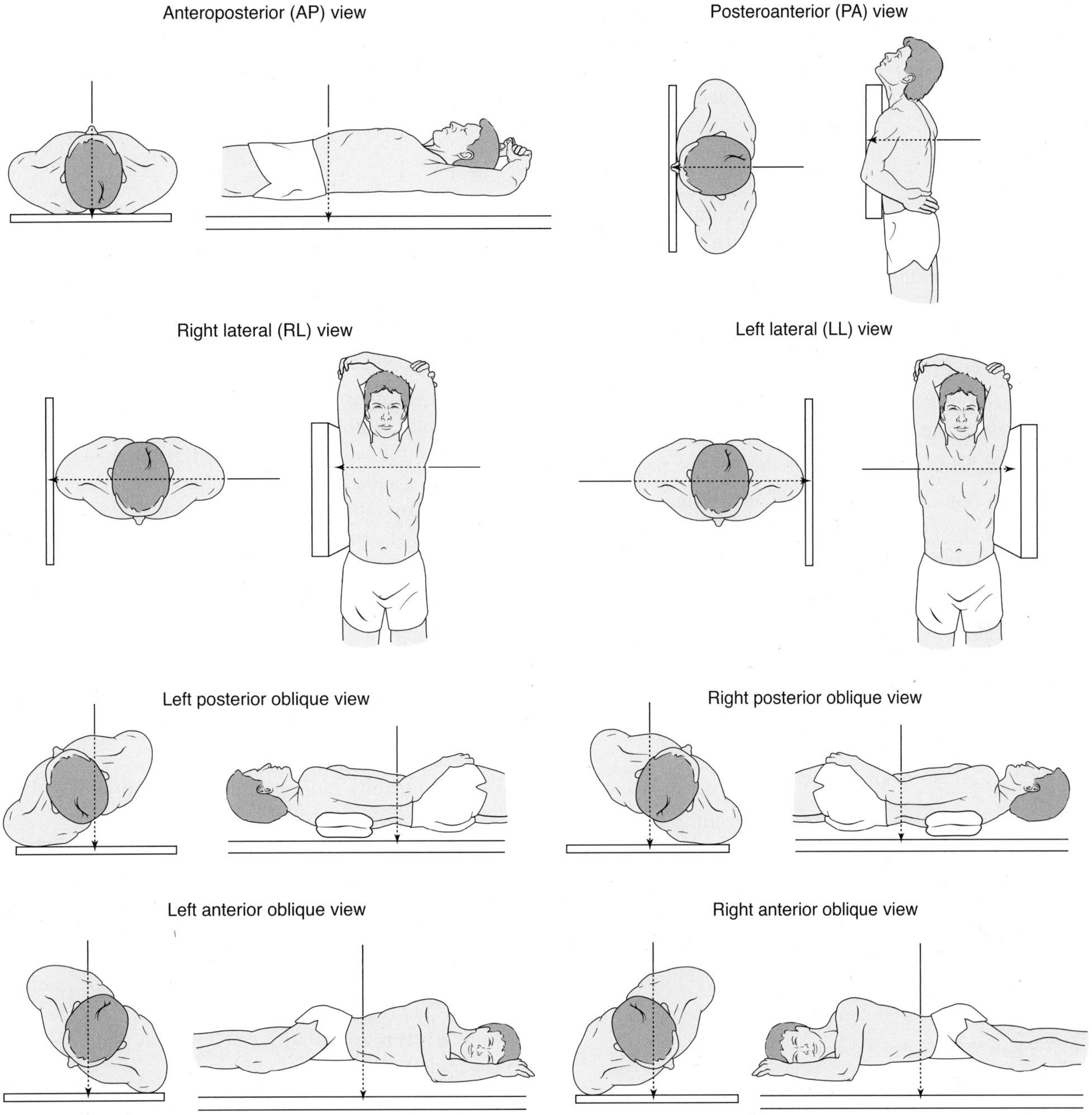

Figure 22-1 Standard positions for specific x-ray views. (Reprinted with permission from Hosley JB, Jones SA, Molle-Matthews EA. Lippincott's Textbook for Medical Assistants. Philadelphia: Lippincott-Raven Publishers, 1997.)

- Lead aprons, gloves, and so on, made available for staff when the staff is not behind protective shield during x-ray procedures
- Female patients should be asked whether they are pregnant; if so, physician should be notified before the x-ray
- Lead shields are used to cover patients' reproductive organs and other organs not involved in exam
- X-ray rooms are properly identified and have a red light displayed outside the room when tests are in progress
- Radioactive materials are disposed of in suitably manufactured and identified containers

COMMON PATIENT PREPARATION

Most medical imaging requires patient preparation. The education required for the patient to prepare for the specific test is generally performed by the medical assistant or certified medical administrative specialist. Regardless of the procedure, *always ask the patient if he or she is allergic to anything* and check the medical record. Be alert for iodine and shellfish allergies if contrast materials are to be used. Some procedures (e.g., angiogram) may be done under emergency conditions, and the usual preparation is waived. Common preparations for scheduled tests follow.

- Angiography
  - Instruct patient to consume nothing by mouth (NPO) for 8 hours before procedure
  - Determine whether the patient is on any blood-thinning medication, including aspirin; report to physician if the patient is on such medication
- Barium enema
  - Instruct the patient to ingest only clear liquids the day before the test
  - Instruct NPO usually 8 hours before the procedure
  - Explain bowel cleansing per facility criteria
  - Instruct the patient to increase fluids after the exam and report if there is no bowel movement within 24 hours after the test
- Barium swallow
  - Instruct patient to have a light evening meal and NPO usually 8 hours before the procedure
  - Instruct the patient to increase fluids after the test; a laxative is usually recommended
- Cholangiogram
  - Instruct patient to have a fat-free evening meal prior to the exam
  - Instruct the patient to take color contrast tablets 2 hours after the evening meal
  - Instruct patient NPO after meal and tablets
  - Bowel cleansing may be ordered per facility criteria
- CT
  - Explain that contrast media will be ingested just prior to procedure
  - Describe whirling sound and motion of machine
- IVP
  - Instruct the patient to ingest only clear liquids the day before the procedure
  - Instruct NPO usually 8 hours before the procedure
  - Explain bowel cleansing per facility criteria
- Mammography
  - Instruct patient not to apply lotion, deodorant, or powder from the neck to the waist
  - Instruct the patient to avoid caffeine 1 week before the test, if this is a facility criterion
- MRI
  - Check for internal metal prostheses or other internal metals (e.g., pacemaker, clips)
  - Instruct patient to not wear metal hair clips or eye makeup for procedure
- Ultrasound
  - Instruct the patient if a full bladder is required for specific ultrasound (e.g., obstetrical ultrasound); provide water
  - Describe the type of transducer and gel to be used

TERMS

Medical Imaging Review

The following list reviews the terms discussed in this chapter and other important terms you may see on the exam.

angiography radiographic visualization of blood vessels and blood flow by injecting radiopaque material through a subcutaneous catheter

arthrography radiographic visualization of a joint by injection of contrast media

barium enema (lower GI series) rectal administration of barium to radiographically visualize the lower portion of the gastrointestinal system

barium swallow (upper GI series) oral administration of barium to radiographically visualize the upper portion of the gastrointestinal system

cholangiography radiographic visualization of the bile ducts using contrast media

cholecystography radiographic visualization of the gallbladder structure and function

computed tomography (CT) radiographic visualization of body structures in thin cross sections or layers

dosimeter badge-like meter worn by radiology personnel to measure the individual's x-ray exposure

intravenous pyelography (IVP) radiographic visualization of the kidney, ureters, and bladder by injection of contrast media through a vein

kidney, ureter, and bladder (KUB) flat plate (x-ray) of the abdomen

magnetic resonance imaging (MRI) film visualization of internal structures, including soft tissue, by using a magnetic field with radiation

mammography radiographic examination of breasts (usually female) with specialized x-ray equipment

myelography radiographic visualization of the spinal cord and nerve roots by injection of contrast media into the subarachnoid space

nuclear medicine area of medicine using radioisotopes to diagnose and treat specific pathology; used in some cancer therapies

oscilloscope screen that displays the visual pattern or picture of an ultrasound

positron emission tomography (PET) process of producing color images by injecting radioisotopes that combine with particles in the body; used to assess physiology and metabolic activity

rad unit of absorbed dose of radiation
radiology the study and use of radioactive substances to visualize an internal structure
radiolucent a substance or structure that x-rays will penetrate
radiopaque substance or structure that is not penetrated by x-rays
retrograde pyelography radiographic visualization of the kidney, ureters, and bladder by administration of contrast media through a urinary catheter
roentgen international unit measuring radiation dose in the air
scintigraphy (scintiphotography) photographic images using a gamma camera to record the distribution of a radioactive agent; used to identify cancer metastasis
ultrasonography (ultrasound) use of high-frequency ultrasonic waves to produce an image and identify and measure deep body structures and abnormalities

REVIEW QUESTIONS

All questions are relevant for the CMA (AAMA), RMA (AMT) and CMAS (AMT) exams.

1. An x-ray study of the urinary system that shows the kidneys, ureters, and bladder following injection of a contrast medium is a(n):
   A. angiogram.
   B. intravenous pyelogram.
   C. cholangiogram.
   D. cholecystogram.

Answer: **B**

Why: An angiogram is a radiographic record of vessels using contrast medium; a cholangiogram is specifically a radiographic record of the bile ducts obtained by cholangiography. A cholecystogram is a radiographic record of gallbladder structure and function.

Review: Yes ❑ No ❑

---

2. The procedure known as diagnostic medical sonography is called:
   A. fluoroscopy.
   B. tomography.
   C. angiography.
   D. CT scan.
   E. ultrasound.

Answer: **E**

Why: Diagnostic medical sonography uses high-frequency sound waves (ultrasound) to create images. Fluoroscopy is the examination of the tissues and deep structures of the body by x-ray using a fluoroscope. Tomography is an x-ray technique that produces a film representing a detailed cross section of tissue. CT scan refers to computed tomography. Angiography is radiographic visualization of blood vessels.

Review: Yes ❑ No ❑

---

3. The exam used to visualize the lower portion of the gastrointestinal system after administration of a radiopaque contrast medium is:
   A. colonoscopy.
   B. intravenous pyelogram.
   C. cholangiogram.
   D. barium enema.

Answer: **D**

Why: A colonoscopy is an exam of the colon with the use of a scope. IVP (intravenous pyelogram) is performed to visualize the kidneys, ureters, and bladder. A cholangiogram is performed to visualize the bile ducts using contrast media.

Review: Yes ❑ No ❑

---

4. The position used in x-ray imaging when the x-ray beam is directed from the front to the back of the body part or body is:
   A. oblique.
   B. anteroposterior.
   C. posteroanterior.
   D. lateral.
   E. anterolateral.

Answer: **B**

Why: The anteroposterior (AP) view describes the position of the x-ray beam as it passes from the front to the back of the body or body part. The oblique view describes the position in which the x-ray beam is directed at an angle through the body or body part. The posteroanterior (PA) view is the opposite of the AP view: the beam passes from the back to the front of the body or body part. The lateral view occurs when the x-ray beam is directed from one side of the body to the other. Anterolateral is not an x-ray imaging position.

Review: Yes ❑ No ❑

5. The term **oblique** used in x-ray imaging means a view of the body or body part from:
   A. a slanting direction.
   B. the side.
   C. the top to bottom.
   D. a perpendicular or horizontal direction.

Answer: **A**

Why: Oblique means any variation from the perpendicular or the horizontal, usually on a slant. The body is slightly tilted, and the x-ray beam enters on an angle.

Review: Yes ❑ No ❑

---

6. The main quality of a contrast medium used in x-ray examinations is that it is:
   A. radiolucent.
   B. radiopaque.
   C. high-frequency sound waves.
   D. high-energy radiation.
   E. nonallergenic.

Answer: **B**

Why: The term **radiopaque** describes a substance through which an x-ray beam will not pass. Bones are relatively radiopaque and show up as white areas on exposed x-ray film. A contrast medium such as barium is also radiopaque and is used to visualize and outline internal structures that would otherwise allow x-rays to pass through and therefore be invisible. Contrast media may contain iodine, which can cause an allergic response in some patients.

Review: Yes ❑ No ❑

---

7. The radiographic examination of the breasts is:
   A. ultrasonography.
   B. mammography.
   C. myelography.
   D. angiography.

Answer: **B**

Why: Mammography is the radiographic examination of the soft tissues of the breast to allow identification of various benign and malignant (cancerous) processes.

Review: Yes ❑ No ❑

---

8. The practice of radiation protection includes wearing a:
   A. transducer.
   B. collimator.
   C. dosimeter.
   D. face mask.
   E. pair of eye goggles.

Answer: **C**

Why: A dosimeter is a device that monitors an individual to see how much radiation he or she has been exposed to over time.

Review: Yes ❑ No ❑

---

9. The radiographic visualization of a joint by injection of contrast media is a(n):
   A. intravenous pyelogram.
   B. angiogram.
   C. cholangiogram.
   D. arthrogram.

Answer: **D**

Why: An arthrogram is used to visualize a joint. The root *arthro* means "joint." IVP (intravenous pyelogram) is an exam of the kidneys, ureters, and bladder after injection of contrast media through the vein. An angiogram is a visualization of blood vessels; a cholangiogram is visualization of bile ducts.

Review: Yes ❑ No ❑

10. It is important to instruct a patient to do this before having an upper GI series performed.
    A. Avoid all medication at least 12 hours before the exam
    B. Use a cleansing enema 2 to 3 hours before the procedure
    C. Have a light or liquid meal early in the evening and then nothing to eat or drink after midnight.
    D. Eat a light meal 2 hours before the exam
    E. Avoid using laxatives

Answer: **C**

Why: Although patients may be asked to avoid some medication, most medication should be taken as scheduled. It is not necessary for a patient to use a cleansing enema before an upper GI series. This exam only visualizes the digestive tract through the duodenum. Patients will be asked to avoid a heavy meal the night before an exam and then not to eat or drink anything for at least 8 hours before the exam. Usually it is recommended that the meal be very light or liquid.

Review: Yes ❑ No ❑

---

11. When positioning a patient for a left lateral view, the patient is positioned so that the:
    A. right side of the body is closest to the film.
    B. left side of the body is closest to the film.
    C. patient is lying down on the x-ray table with the left side closest to the x-ray beam.
    D. patient is lying down on the x-ray table with the right side at a 45° angle to the x-ray cassette.

Answer: **B**

Why: A left lateral view means that the x-ray beam is directed from the right side of the body to the left. This means the body is positioned with the left side closest to the x-ray film.

Review: Yes ❑ No ❑

---

12. Angiography is radiography of the:
    A. kidneys.
    B. heart.
    C. spinal cord.
    D. gallbladder.
    E. blood vessels.

Answer: **E**

Why: Angio is a root word that refers to vessels or, specifically, blood vessels.

Review: Yes ❑ No ❑

---

13. The x-ray examination of the urinary system is a:
    A. GI series.
    B. KUB.
    C. MRI.
    D. CXR.

Answer: **B**

Why: The abbreviation KUB means kidneys, ureters, and bladder. This is a flat-plate x-ray of the abdomen to determine the location and size of the structures. A GI series includes x-rays of the upper and lower gastrointestinal tract. MRI is the abbreviation for magnetic resonance imaging. CXR means chest x-ray.

Review: Yes ❑ No ❑

---

14. A barium enema would be scheduled before an upper GI study because the:
    A. upper GI is completed faster than the barium enema.
    B. barium from the upper GI may take days to clear the patient's system before the barium enema can be performed.
    C. upper GI may show a diagnostic problem sooner than the barium enema.
    D. patient may have an allergy to barium and the reaction will not be as significant when performing the barium enema first.
    E. upper GI series takes longer to perform.

Answer: **B**

Why: Proper scheduling of x-ray exams is a responsibility of the medical assistant. If a barium swallow (upper GI series) is performed first, the patient must wait until all the barium has been eliminated before the preparation for a barium enema can begin. This could take days. The lower GI barium enema requires that only the large intestine be filled with contrast barium. This can be eliminated from the body and not interfere with the upper GI series.

Review: Yes ❑ No ❑

15. If a patient is instructed to be NPO for 8 hours prior to an x-ray exam, it means that the patient should:
A. not eat 8 hours before the exam.
B. ingest only clear liquids before the exam.
C. avoid food but continue to drink fluids as needed.
D. not eat or drink anything 8 hours before the exam.

Answer: **D**

Why: NPO means nothing by mouth (orally). Most x-ray exams require that the patient be NPO for at least 8 hours before the exam. The patient should be instructed that this means liquids also. Occasionally the patient is allowed to take necessary medication.

Review: Yes ❑ No ❑

---

16. When a patient is positioned for a chest x-ray and the patient is facing the x-ray film, this position is known as:
A. posterior oblique.
B. anteroposterior.
C. lateral.
D. decubitus.
E. posteroanterior.

Answer: **E**

Why: Posteroanterior position means that the patient's back or posterior side is closest to the x-ray beam and the anterior or front of the body is facing or closest to the x-ray film.

Review: Yes ❑ No ❑

---

17. The radiographic visualization of the spinal cord by injection of a contrast medium is a(n):
A. intravenous pyelogram.
B. myelogram.
C. cystogram.
D. arteriogram.

Answer: **B**

Why: A myelogram is an x-ray taken after injection of a radiopaque medium into the subarachnoid space to demonstrate any spinal cord or spinal nerve root deformity. An intravenous pyelogram x-rays the kidneys, ureters, and bladder; a cystogram is an x-ray of a sac or bladder; and an arteriogram is an x-ray to visualize the arteries.

Review: Yes ❑ No ❑

---

18. Which of the following is used to produce an MRI?
A. Magnetic field in combination with radiation
B. Injection of radioisotopes
C. High-frequency ultrasonic waves
D. Radioactive chemicals
E. Multiple radioactive iodines

Answer: **A**

Why: MRI means magnetic resonance imaging. It is a form of medical imaging that uses a magnetic field as its source of energy. Radiation is the energy source for producing images on x-ray film.

Review: Yes ❑ No ❑

---

19. Radiation safety principles include the following EXCEPT:
A. placing a dosimeter on the patient.
B. maintaining x-ray machines in a lead-lined room.
C. determining whether a female patient is pregnant.
D. repeating x-rays until the views are absolutely clear.

Answer: **A**

Why: A dosimeter is a device worn by those working in and around the x-ray area, not by the patient. This device measures the amount of accumulated x-rays to which the person is exposed while working in an area where x-rays are taken. A patient is not exposed to additional x-rays, only those required for the exam.

Review: Yes ❑ No ❑

---

20. Before injection of contrast materials, it is important to determine whether the patient has:
A. eaten a fat-free meal the night before the exam.
B. fasted for 8 hours.
C. any allergies.
D. had previous x-rays.
E. ingested any liquids.

Answer: **C**

Why: Patients who are allergic to iodine or shellfish will usually have a serious or life-threatening allergic reaction to the contrast medium.

Review: Yes ❑ No ❑

21. Patient instructions after an exam using barium include the following EXCEPT:
    A. increase intake of water and fluids.
    B. report if no bowel movement within 24 hours of the exam.
    C. remain NPO for 2 hours.
    D. resume a normal diet.

Answer: **C**

Why: There is no need for the patient to remain NPO after the exam. NPO means nothing by mouth.

Review: Yes ❑ No ❑

---

22. The term **radiolucent** means that x-rays:
    A. cannot penetrate the material and it will show as a light or white object on an x-ray film.
    B. will pass through the material and produce a dark image on the x-ray film.
    C. of higher doses are required to produce an image on the x-ray film.
    D. will penetrate the material and will show as a white image on the x-ray film.
    E. will penetrate bony tissue and produce a dark image on the x-ray film.

Answer: **B**

Why: Radiolucent means that x-rays will pass through the materials because they are not dense and do not absorb the radiation; therefore, the materials show dark on the x-ray film. An example is air in the colon. The air will not absorb x-rays and will not show except as a black image on the film.

Review: Yes ❑ No ❑

---

23. The purpose of a cholangiogram is to:
    A. visualize the size of a tumor.
    B. assess the location and size of the kidneys.
    C. view movement of barium through the digestive tract.
    D. visualize the bile ducts.

Answer: **D**

Why: A cholangiogram is a radiographic procedure that uses contrast media to visualize the bile ducts of the gallbladder.

Review: Yes ❑ No ❑

---

24. X-ray films are reviewed and interpreted by a:
    A. radiologic technologist.
    B. registered nurse.
    C. radiologist.
    D. radiographer.
    E. mammographer.

Answer: **C**

Why: A radiologist is a medical doctor who is responsible for interpreting the findings on the x-ray films. A radiologic technologist, also called a radiographer, is a person who is trained to take x-ray films. This person is not licensed or authorized to interpret the films, although most are able to see and identify problem areas on films. A registered nurse is a licensed nurse trained to assess patients' needs and provide clinical care. Nurses are not licensed or trained to perform x-rays. A mammographer is a person trained to perform mammography, that is, imaging of the breasts.

Review: Yes ❑ No ❑

---

25. The abbreviation used to order an x-ray to evaluate the lungs is:
    A. PA.
    B. lat.
    C. CXR.
    D. AP.

Answer: **C**

Why: CXR is the abbreviation for chest x-ray. The x-ray includes an anteroposterior (AP) and lateral view of the chest without use of any contrast medium.

Review: Yes ❑ No ❑

23
Physical Modalities

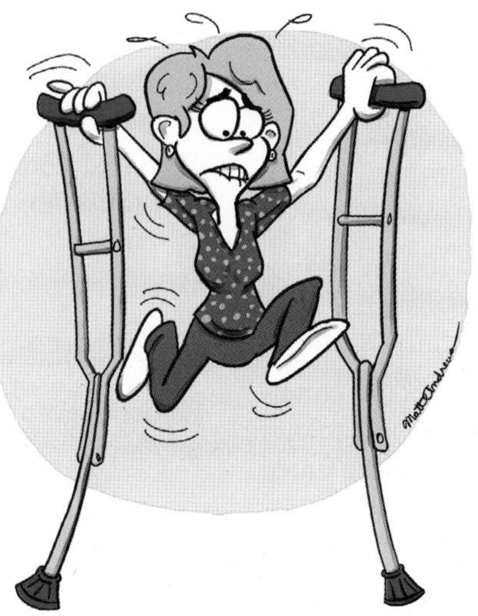

REVIEW TIP

Your medical practice may not provide services for physical modalities or fitting of ambulation devices; however, it is important that the medical assistant recognize improper fitting and use when patients present with crutches, walkers, or canes. Information may be obtained from durable medical equipment vendors or retailers.

Physical modalities are noninvasive therapeutic agents, procedures, and preventive measures used in the following:

- Physical medicine (physiatry)—diagnosis and treatment of disease and disability using physical means, such as diathermy
- Rehabilitative medicine—restores and improves function impaired by disease or injury
- Sports medicine—prevents and treats injuries and impairments that are sports related
- Preventive health—applies techniques and uses devices to prevent injury and impairment (e.g., body mechanics)

MOBILITY TESTING

- Goniometry—measurement of degrees of joint motion using a goniometer
- Range of motion (ROM) test—exam requiring the patient to perform various joint motions to determine the extent of movement (see Chapter 6, Box 6-3, "Joint Movements"); may be active or passive
- Strength tests—exams requiring the patient to perform select muscle or muscle group actions to determine the strength of function
- Activities of daily living (ADL) tests—exams that determine the patient's ability to perform common tasks (e.g., opening doors, brushing hair)

THERAPIES

THERMOTHERAPY

Thermotherapy uses heat to reduce swelling and to decrease pain by dilating blood vessels (vasodilation), increasing circulation to the affected area; it is not used in the initial phase of injury treatment.

- Dry heat—heat without moisture
  - Heating pads—electrically or microwave-heated packs for thermotherapy use; should always be covered with fabric before placing on skin; check cords for safety and frequently monitor temperature to avoid burns
  - Chemical hot packs—heating pads filled with a chemical compound that produce heat when activated (usually by applying pressure); follow same precautions as for heating pads
  - Infrared—heat produced by wavelengths in various lamp-like structures; position a safe distance from skin and monitor frequently to avoid burns
  - Ultraviolet—sunlamps used to treat specific conditions (e.g., psoriasis, newborn jaundice); patient's eyes should be covered and length of exposure timed and monitored to avoid burns
- Moist heat—heat with moisture sources
  - Hot soaks—water or water with antiseptic or other solution is warmed between 100°F and 105°F; affected area requiring treatment is submerged for a specific period
  - Hot compresses—fabric is wet with water or antiseptic or other solutions and placed on affected area; plastic-type wrap may be used to cover compress and conserve heat
- Paraffin—hand or foot is immersed in melted wax with additive such as mineral oil; plastic bags or "mittens" are worn after wax is applied to retain heat; when cool, the wax is peeled off; used for relief of arthritis pain
- Diathermy—deep heat therapy using a mechanical energy source
  - Ultrasound—heat therapy using high-frequency sound waves; a special gel substance is placed on the head of the ultrasound attachment to improve conductivity
  - Microwave—heat therapy using electromagnetic radiation for tissues; should not be used with moisture or on patients with pacemakers

CRYOTHERAPY

Cryotherapy uses cold to prevent swelling and to reduce pain by causing blood vessels to constrict (vasoconstriction); it is used in the initial treatment of an injury.

- Dry cold—cold therapy without moisture
  - Ice pack—waterproof bag filled with ice; air should be removed and bag covered with fabric before placing on skin; monitor to prevent skin damage
  - Chemical ice bag—pack filled with a chemical compound that produces cold when activated (usually by applying pressure); follow same precautions as with ice pack
- Moist cold—cold therapy using moisture
  - Cold soaks—water or water with antiseptic or other solution is cooled with ice and affected area is submerged for a given period
  - Cold compresses—fabric is wet with cold water or antiseptic or other solution and placed on affected area

HYDROTHERAPY

Hydrotherapy uses hot- or cold-water regimens for therapy.

- Whirlpool—a bath or other container in which water is continually circulated to provide massage and heat therapy
- Hot-to-cold plunges—the affected area is alternately plunged between hot and cold baths to contract and dilate vessels

EXERCISES

Exercise is an action to strengthen, develop, or maintain muscle.

- Active exercise—an action to strengthen, develop, or maintain muscle that is performed directly by the patient
  - Isometric exercises—exercises that contract opposing muscles without the muscles shortening
  - Resistance exercise—exercises performed with counter pressure applied to increase the effectiveness and determine improvement
  - Water exercises—exercises performed in water
- Passive exercise—exercises performed on the patient by another person or by a mechanical device
  - Electrical stimulation—electrical device used to stimulate muscles or nerves
  - Passive motion device—a mechanical apparatus placed on a patient to passively exercise the affected area; frequently used on knees after surgery; speed

and flexion may be increased or decreased according to the patient's pain tolerance

- Massage—rubbing, stroking, kneading, and tapping tissue with hands or devices to alleviate pain and improve function

RANGE OF MOTION

Range of motion (ROM) can be passive or active; the patient or caregiver exercises joints by performing standard joint motions such as flexion and rotation to maintain or improve the extent of movement.

OTHER COMMON PHYSICAL THERAPIES

- Manipulation—maneuvers to realign affected area; frequently used on joint dislocations or spinal injuries
- Immobilization—prevention of movement, usually of joint or bone, through the use of splints, casts, and other devices to reduce pain and allow healing to occur
- Traction—application of a slow pulling force; commonly used to realign fractured bones

COMMON ASSISTIVE DEVICES

- Cane—a rod-type device used for minimal standing or walking support as a result of weakness on one side or balance problems; the handle may be candy cane shaped or straight and perpendicular to the rod
  - Types—single-pronged, tripod, or four-pronged (quad); the length may be adjustable or nonadjustable
  - Fit—the patient's elbow should be at a 30° angle when standing to obtain proper cane length
  - Gait—cane is held on patient's strongest side, tip 4 inches to 6 inches lateral to the foot, tip flat on the ground; cane moves forward approximately 12 inches followed by the affected limb, which stops at the cane; the stronger limb moves forward to the cane, and steps are repeated
  - Caution—stronger limb is first going up stairs, weaker limb first going down
- Crutches—assistive walking devices, used singly or as a pair, which transfer weight bearing to upper extremities
  - Common types—standard or axillary crutches usually used for temporary conditions; Lofstrand or forearm crutches usually used for long-term disability
  - Fit—measure with the shoes patient will be wearing; patient standing; normally crutch tips are placed 4 inches to 6 inches lateral to each foot and 2 inches in front of feet; allow 2 to 3 finger widths between the axilla and the axillary support on crutches; adjust crutch height to accommodate; adjust handgrips to 30° of elbow flexion
  - Common gaits—crutches placed on ground 4 inches to 6 inches lateral and 2 inches in front of feet
    - Swing-to gait—patient moves both crutches forward simultaneously, plants them, and lifts body to crutches; repeat steps
    - Swing-through gait—patient moves both crutches forward simultaneously, plants them, and lifts body past crutches; repeat steps
    - Two-point gait—the patient moves one crutch forward and the opposite foot at the same time, followed by the other crutch and other foot
    - Three-point gait (most commonly taught in medical office)—for weight bearing on one leg; patient moves both crutches and affected leg forward simultaneously and follows with unaffected leg; repeat steps
    - Four-point gait—the patient moves right crutch forward, followed by the left crutch, and then the left leg forward parallel to the left crutch, followed by the right leg forward parallel to the right crutch; repeat steps
  - Caution—shoes should be flat and nonskid; avoid throw rugs, wet areas, and other hazards; to avoid axilla nerve damage, support weight using handgrips, not crutch underarm pads
- Gait or transfer belt—a wide woven belt used to assist in lifting or steadying the patient during ambulation or transfer (e.g., car or wheelchair)
  - Placement—buckled over patient's clothes around waist at mid-abdominal area; allow room for two fingers to fit between the waist and the belt
  - Caution—the belt should not be used if patient has no use of lower extremities; check for abdominal, back, or rib conditions and ostomy or feeding devices
- Walker—waist-high assistive walking device with four legs, used when a cane is not enough support; may be folded when not in use
  - Types—standard (fixed) with rubber-tipped legs; or can roll on wheels
  - Fit—client's elbows flexed at 30° angle; hand rests should be approximately at top of patient's femur
  - Gait—patient steps into the walker and grasps handgrips, moves walker forward 6 inches to 12 inches then moves one foot at a time back into walker; repeat steps
  - Caution—walkers should not be used on stairs or narrow passages
- Wheelchair—a mobile chair with adjustable or nonadjustable footrests and brakes, used when a patient cannot ambulate

- Types—nonmechanical or mechanical, standard size or custom fitted to patient
- Caution—always lock brakes when patient is getting into or out of chair; do not allow patient to place arms around your neck

BODY MECHANICS

Body mechanics is defined as the efficient use of the body to prevent injury to the health care provider or patient. The general guidelines follow.

- Keep the back straight
- Keep abdominal muscles tight
- Bend from knees, not back
- Maintain a broad base with one foot slightly forward
- Use the feet, not the body, to pivot
- Carry heavy objects close to your body
- Synchronize lifting, such as "on three—one, two, three"
- Know your limits

TERMS

Physical Modalities Review

The following list reviews the terms discussed in this chapter and other important terms you may see on the exam.

activities of daily living (ADL) common acts performed during a person's normal day

body mechanics the efficient use of the body to prevent injury to the health care provider or patient

cryotherapy (cold) causes blood vessels to constrict, preventing swelling and reducing pain; used in the initial treatment of an injury

diathermy deep heat therapy using a mechanical energy source

ergonomics adaptation of the environment and use of techniques and equipment to prevent injury

hydrotherapy hot- or cold-water regimens used for therapy

isometric exercise a type of exercise that contracts opposing muscles without the muscles shortening

passive exercise exercises performed on the patient by another person or a mechanical device

physical medicine (physiatry) deals with the diagnosis and treatment of disease and disability using physical means, such as diathermy

range of motion (ROM) passive or active; the patient or caregiver exercises joints by performing standard joint motions (e.g., flexion and rotation) to maintain or improve the movement

rehabilitative medicine deals with restoring or improving function impaired by disease or injury

resistance exercise exercises performed with counter pressure applied to increase the effectiveness and to determine improvement

thermotherapy (heat) reduces swelling and decreases pain by improving circulation; it is not used in acute phase of injury

ultrasound heat therapy using high-frequency sound waves; a special gel substance is placed on the head of the ultrasound attachment to improve conductivity

ultraviolet heat lamps to treat specific conditions (e.g., psoriasis, newborn jaundice)

whirlpool bath or other container in which water is continually circulated to provide massage and heat therapy

REVIEW QUESTIONS

All questions are relevant for the CMA (AAMA) and RMA (AMT) exams.

1. Heat applied to a large part of the body will cause:
   A. vasoconstriction.
   B. vasodilation.
   C. decreased blood flow to the body part.
   D. increased blood pressure to the area.

Answer: **B**

Why: Cold application causes the blood vessels to constrict, or become smaller, thus increasing blood pressure in the area and decreasing blood flow to the body part or area. Heat application has the opposite effect on the area.

Review: Yes ❑ No ❑

---

2. Infrared therapy uses heat produced by:
   A. electricity.
   B. water.
   C. chemicals.
   D. sound waves.
   E. wavelengths.

Answer: **E**

Why: Infrared therapy is treatment by exposure to various wavelengths of infrared radiation. Infrared treatment relieves pain and stimulates circulation of blood.

Review: Yes ❑ No ❑

---

3. Cryotherapy is a form of treatment that uses:
   A. sound waves and microwaves.
   B. ice packs and cold packs.
   C. paraffin wax.
   D. hot compresses and hot water.

Answer: **B**

Why: The root *cryo* refers to the use of cold or freezing. Cryotherapy is a form of treatment that utilizes different forms of cold such as chemical ice bags, cold soaks, and ice packs.

Review: Yes ❑ No ❑

---

4. Which of the following is necessary to do when measuring crutches so they fit properly?
   A. The patient should be fitted without shoes on, barefooted.
   B. With the patient standing normally, the crutch tips should be touching the sides of the shoes.
   C. There should be a gap of 2 to 3 finger widths between the underarm and the top of the crutch.
   D. When the hands are resting on the handgrips, the elbows should be straight, not flexed.
   E. The handgrips on the crutches should be at the same height as the patient's waist.

Answer: **C**

Why: There should be some space between the underarm and the top of the crutch to make sure the patient's underarm does not rub on the crutch. Two to three finger widths, or approximately 2 inches is adequate. The patient should have shoes on, and the crutch tips should be placed at least 4 inches to 6 inches from the shoes. The elbows should be flexed slightly when the hands are on the handgrips. The handgrips are positioned slightly above the hip but not at the waist.

Review: Yes ❑ No ❑

---

5. A device used to measure the extent of joint movement is a(n):
   A. diathermy machine.
   B. passive motion machine.
   C. electrical stimulation device.
   D. goniometer.

Answer: **D**

Why: A goniometer is used to perform goniometry, the measurement of degrees of joint motion. Diathermy is the use of shortwaves to heat the body tissues. A passive motion machine is a device that moves a body part without the patient assisting. Electrical stimulation is the use of intermittent electrical stimuli to cause muscles to contract.

Review: Yes ❑ No ❑

6. The realignment of a dislocated finger is an example of which kind of therapy?
   A. Immobilization
   B. Manipulation
   C. Traction
   D. Resistance exercise
   E. Passive exercise

Answer: **B**

Why: Manipulation is the use of the hands in therapy to reduce a dislocation or move a body part into alignment. Immobilization of a body part does not allow movement. An example is placing a splint or cast on the body part. Traction is a method of applying force on a body part to pull or stretch the body part. Resistance exercise is the act of exercising while applying opposite force—for example, using weights while exercising. Passive exercise requires another person to perform the movement for the patient. The patient does not move the body part.

Review: Yes ❑ No ❑

---

7. When the tips of both crutches and one leg are advancing at the same time, it is referred to as a:
   A. three-point gait.
   B. two-point gait.
   C. swing-to gait.
   D. swing-through gait.

Answer: **A**

Why: A three-point gait refers to two crutch tips and one foot touching the ground at the same time.

Review: Yes ❑ No ❑

---

8. The type of exercise used when the patient is unable to move the affected body part without help is:
   A. range of motion.
   B. active exercise.
   C. isometric exercise.
   D. resistant exercise.
   E. passive exercise.

Answer: **E**

Why: In passive exercise, someone or something moves the body part without patient assistance. Passive exercise is frequently used after surgery to increase flexion and extension in joints.

Review: Yes ❑ No ❑

---

9. Kneading and tapping tissue with the hands is a form of:
   A. manipulation.
   B. traction.
   C. range of motion.
   D. massage.

Answer: **D**

Why: Massage is a type of passive treatment used to alleviate pain and improve function of body parts. Massage includes rubbing, stroking, kneading, and tapping tissue with the hands or with devices.

Review: Yes ❑ No ❑

---

10. When instructing a patient on the use of a cane, you should tell him or her to:
    A. use the cane only when using stairs.
    B. use the cane on his or her weaker side.
    C. go up steps with the stronger limb first.
    D. go down steps with the cane first.
    E. adjust the cane low enough so that the arm is straight when walking.

Answer: **C**

Why: Proper technique when using a cane includes using the cane on the stronger side. The cane will provide support on the strong side when moving the weak side. The patient then has a smoother gait and does not have the tendency to limp. When going up steps, the stronger side goes first; going down steps, the weaker limb goes first. When using the cane, the arm is slightly bent.

Review: Yes ❑ No ❑

11. Good body mechanics include the following guidelines except:
    A. when lifting, maintain a narrow base with feet together.
    B. carry heavy objects close to your body.
    C. bend from the knees, not the back.
    D. use feet to pivot, not the body.

Answer: **A**

Why: When lifting, the feet should be slightly apart with one foot forward. This provides a broad base to support the weight of the load.

Review: Yes ❑ No ❑

---

12. The area of medicine that deals with restoring or improving function impaired by disease is:
    A. preventive health.
    B. ergonomics.
    C. rehabilitative medicine.
    D. thermotherapy.
    E. disability management.

Answer: **C**

Why: Rehabilitative medicine deals with restoration of an individual or a part of the body to normal or near normal function after a disabling disease or injury.

Review: Yes ❑ No ❑

---

13. Cold therapy is frequently applied to:
    A. increase blood flow to the affected part.
    B. promote healing by increasing circulation.
    C. increase nerve sensitivity.
    D. decrease swelling.

Answer: **D**

Why: Cold has the effect of decreasing pain by numbing the nerve pathways. Cold therapy decreases circulation (blood flow), thus decreasing swelling.

Review: Yes ❑ No ❑

---

14. The use of a whirlpool is an example of:
    A. diathermy.
    B. cryotherapy.
    C. hydrotherapy.
    D. thermotherapy.
    E. ultrasound therapy.

Answer: **C**

Why: The root word *hydro* means "water." A whirlpool is a tank in which warm water is circulated to provide massage and heat therapy.

Review: Yes ❑ No ❑

---

15. An example of a deep heating agent is:
    A. diathermy.
    B. hydrocollator pack.
    C. infrared lamp.
    D. paraffin bath.

Answer: **A**

Why: Deep heating agents produce heat through energy that will penetrate the tissues as deep as 30 to 50 millimeters. Superficial heating agents affect tissues approximately 10 millimeters beneath the skin's surface. Hydrocollator packs (hot packs), infrared lamps, and paraffin baths are all considered superficial heating agents.

Review: Yes ❑ No ❑

---

16. To evaluate the extent of movement of a patient's knee, the following exam would be performed:
    A. isometric exercise.
    B. range of motion.
    C. manipulation.
    D. gait evaluation.
    E. body mechanics.

Answer: **B**

Why: Range of motion testing is performed to determine the extent of movement of various joints. The patient is evaluated to see how many degrees of flexion and extension the joint will perform. Isometric exercises are exercises that contract opposing muscles without the muscles shortening. Manipulation involves maneuvers to realign affected areas such as joint dislocations or spinal injuries. Gait evaluation is the evaluation of the manner of walking. Body mechanics is defined as the efficient use of the body to prevent injury.

Review: Yes ❑ No ❑

17. The preferred method used in the initial treatment of an injury is:
A. hot compresses.
B. paraffin.
C. hydrotherapy.
D. ice pack.
E. ultrasound.

Answer: **D**

Why: Cold therapy is initially used after an injury to prevent swelling and reduce pain. There is decreased blood flow to the affected part, limiting the initial edema in the area.

Review: Yes ❑ No ❑

---

18. The type of gait in which the patient advances the left foot and right crutch and then the right foot and left crutch is a:
A. swing-through gait.
B. two-point gait.
C. three-point gait.
D. four-point gait.

Answer: **B**

Why: A two-point gait means there are two "points" on the ground at the same time. One crutch and the opposite foot are on the ground at the same time, followed by the other crutch and foot. This is used for a patient who is partially weight bearing and can place some weight on both sides of his or her body.

Review: Yes ❑ No ❑

---

19. Exercises performed by the patient without assistance are:
A. active exercises.
B. passive exercises.
C. range of motion exercises.
D. water exercises.

Answer: **A**

Why: Active exercise refers to those movements the patient is able to perform without assistance. Passive exercise requires another person to move the body part. Range of motion and water exercises both can be performed passively.

Review: Yes ❑ No ❑

---

20. The common acts performed during a person's normal day are referred to as:
A. body mechanics.
B. activities of daily living.
C. ergonomics.
D. isometric exercises.
E. passive exercises.

Answer: **B**

Why: ADL, activities of daily living, are the common tasks that a person performs each day, such as brushing hair and opening doors. Body mechanics refers to the efficient use of the body while performing activities, and ergonomics is the adaptation of the environment and use of techniques and equipment to prevent injury—for example, equipment designed for better posture when sitting in a desk chair. Isometric and passive exercises are used in rehabilitative therapy.

Review: Yes ❑ No ❑

---

21. A therapeutic method used to treat jaundice in newborns is:
A. ultrasound.
B. infrared.
C. diathermy.
D. ultraviolet.

Answer: **D**

Why: Ultraviolet is light beyond the range of human vision. It occurs naturally in sunlight and burns or tans the skin. Ultraviolet lamps are also used to treat psoriasis and other skin conditions.

Review: Yes ❑ No ❑

22. Physiatry deals with:
    A. prevention and treatment of sports injuries.
    B. prevention of injury and impairment.
    C. diagnosis and treatment of disease and disability using physical means.
    D. restoring and improving function through rehabilitation.
    E. diagnosis and treatment of mental disorders.

Answer: **C**

Why: Physiatry, or physical medicine, deals with the diagnosis and treatment of disease and disability using physical means, including such therapies as diathermy.

Review: Yes ❑ No ❑

---

23. Which of the following therapeutic methods uses melted wax?
    A. Chemical hot packs
    B. Paraffin bath
    C. Diathermy
    D. Cryotherapy

Answer: **B**

Why: Paraffin is a type of wax that is melted to create a liquid. The affected body part—usually a hand, a foot, or a joint—is submerged in the wax, or the wax is painted on the body part. The wax hardens, and the heat of the wax penetrates the skin and provides a soothing effect to the painful area. It is frequently used to treat arthritic joint pain and stiffness.

Review: Yes ❑ No ❑

---

24. A method of physical therapy used to realign fractured bones is:
    A. electrical stimulation.
    B. massage.
    C. passive exercise.
    D. infrared heat.
    E. traction.

Answer: **E**

Why: Traction is the application of a slow pulling force on a body part and is commonly used to realign fractured bones.

Review: Yes ❑ No ❑

---

25. The purpose of heat therapy includes the following EXCEPT:
    A. relieve muscle spasm.
    B. decrease bleeding or hemorrhage.
    C. relieve pain.
    D. increase blood flow to the body part.

Answer: **B**

Why: Heat causes an increase in blood flow to an area of the body, causing muscles to relax, and relieves pain. Cold therapy is indicated for decreasing blood flow and to control hemorrhage.

Review: Yes ❑ No ❑

---

24 Nutrition

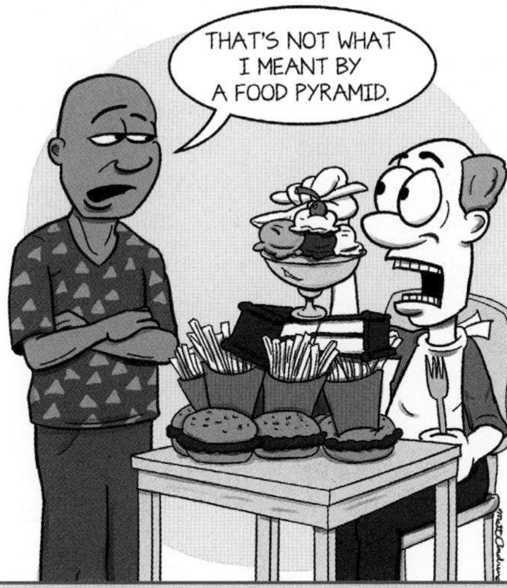
THAT'S NOT WHAT I MEANT BY A FOOD PYRAMID.

REVIEW TIP

Increasing emphasis is placed on nutrition in treating disease and maintaining wellness. The certification exams always include questions on therapeutic diets, as well as vitamins and their functions in the body.

Nutrition is the process of taking food into the body and using it.

STEPS OF NUTRITION

1. Ingestion—taking in of nutrients; eating and drinking
2. Digestion—physical and chemical changing of nutrients in the body to allow absorption
3. Absorption—transferring of digested nutrients from the gastrointestinal system to the blood circulation
4. Metabolism—synthesizing of nutrients from the bloodstream, producing energy

NUTRIENTS

Nutrients are components of food necessary for the body to perform physiologic functions.

ENERGY NUTRIENTS

Energy nutrients produce energy/calories when metabolized. Table 24-1 lists calorie distribution for energy nutrients.

- Carbohydrates—sugars and starches, the body's primary energy source; they produce 4 calories per gram
- Proteins—nutrients with amino acids (building blocks); build and heal body tissue; they produce 4 calories per gram
  - Complete—protein nutrient that contains all nine essential amino acids
  - Incomplete—protein nutrient that does not contain all nine essential amino acids
- Fats (lipids)—greasy material in nutrients; transport fat-soluble vitamins, insulate the body from the cold,

Table 24-1 **Calorie Distribution**

Nutrient	Calories per Gram
Carbohydrate	4
Protein	4
Fat	**9**

and provide fatty acids; they produce 9 calories per gram

- Saturated fats—primarily found in meat, butter, and egg yolks; usually solid at room temperature; increase blood cholesterol
- Unsaturated fats—primarily found in vegetable and olive oils; usually liquid at room temperature; help decrease blood cholesterol
- Cholesterol—found in animal foods and manufactured by the body; not a true fat or lipid but a lipoprotein; necessary for vitamin D and acid bile production
  - High-density lipoprotein, or HDL (good cholesterol)—works to stabilize LDL by transporting select amounts of it to the liver for elimination
  - Low-density lipoprotein, or LDL (bad cholesterol)—waxy material that clogs blood vessels, causing cardiovascular disease
- Triglycerides—component molecule of fat found in fatty foods; a combination of fatty acids and glycerol; high levels clog blood vessels, causing cardiovascular disease

NONENERGY NUTRIENTS

- Fiber—nondigestible but edible portion of plants; necessary for the gastrointestinal elimination function
- Vitamins—organic substances found naturally in foods; needed in small amounts for metabolism and prevention of certain diseases (*Note:* The certification exams ask questions about which vitamins are water-soluble and which are fat-soluble.)
  - Vitamin B_1 (thiamin)—water-soluble vitamin primarily found in whole grains and beans necessary for carbohydrate metabolism
  - Vitamin B_2 (riboflavin)—water-soluble vitamin primarily found in animal products and broccoli; necessary for protein metabolism
  - Vitamin B_6—water-soluble vitamin primarily found in brewer's yeast, whole grains, and nuts; aids in regulation of central nervous system

Table 24-2 **Major Minerals**

Mineral	Major Food Source	Purpose
Calcium (Ca)	Dairy products, salmon	Bone and tooth development, nerve impulse transmission; disorders include osteoporosis and rickets
Chloride (Cl)	Table salt, meats	Acid-base balance; disorders include decreases in mental capacities
Magnesium (Mg)	Green vegetables, whole grains	Enzyme activity, metabolism, heartbeat regulation; deficiencies include metabolic disorders
Phosphorus (P)	Dairy products, meats, fish, nuts	Bone and tooth development, acid-base balance, protein and glucose metabolism; disorders include anemia, abnormal growth, bone loss
Potassium (K)	Oranges, dried fruits	Protein metabolism, acid-base balance correction, nerve impulse transmission, heartbeat regulation; disorders include hyperkalemia and hypokalemia
Sodium (Na)	Table salt, processed food	Fluid balance maintenance; disorders include hypertension

Table 24-3 Trace Minerals

Mineral	Major Food Source	Purpose
Copper (Cu)	Organ meats, whole grains, nuts	Hemoglobin formation, iron absorption, enzyme function
Fluoride (Fl)	Fish, some water supplies	Tooth decay resistance; disorders from overuse include tooth mottling
Iodine (I)	Saltwater fish and crustaceans, iodized table salt	Metabolism regulation, element of thyroid hormone; disorders include goiter
Iron (Fe)	Organ meats, dark green leafy vegetables	Hemoglobin element, oxygen transport; disorders include anemia
Zinc (Zn)	Organ meats, other foods high in protein	Enzyme element, wound healing, growth; disorders include dwarfism

- Vitamin B_{12} (cyanocobalamin)—water-soluble vitamin primarily found in animal products and soybeans; promotes red blood cell (RBC) formation; a deficiency causes pernicious anemia
- Vitamin C (ascorbic acid)—water-soluble vitamin primarily found in citrus fruits and tomatoes; promotes stress resistance, wound healing, and oral health
- Vitamin A—fat-soluble vitamin primarily found in milk and yellow vegetables; promotes good eyesight and protects skin from infection; a deficiency causes night blindness
- Vitamin D—fat-soluble vitamin primarily found in sunlight and dairy products; strengthens bone development; a deficiency causes rickets
- Vitamin E—fat-soluble vitamin primarily found in green leafy vegetables, nuts, and whole grains; protects RBCs; a deficiency causes anemia
- Vitamin K—fat-soluble vitamin primarily found in green leafy vegetables and tomatoes; promotes blood clotting

■ Minerals—elements usually found in the earth's crust, the human body, and some foods; necessary to carry out bodily functions

- Major minerals—essential elements needed by the body in larger amounts: calcium (Ca), chloride (Cl), magnesium (Mg), phosphorus (P), potassium (K), sodium (Na); Table 24-2 lists the major minerals, their sources, and their purposes
- Trace minerals—essential elements needed by the body in very small amounts: copper, fluoride, iodine, iron, zinc; Table 24-3 lists the trace minerals, their sources, and their purposes

DIETARY GUIDELINES

The United States Department of Agriculture (USDA) developed guidelines to assist the general population in making healthy food choices. Prior to 2005, these guidelines were displayed in a food pyramid that divided foods into groups. The group with the most recommended servings per day was on the bottom, and the group with the fewest recommended servings per day was on the top, forming the pyramid shape. The new version was introduced in 2005 when the Dietary Guidelines Advisory Committee met and the latest in 2010. The major change is that the **estimated energy requirement (EER)** is more specific and based on gender, age, height, weight, and activity level. EERs decrease with age, and children have separate recommendations. The food groups in the new pyramid are displayed in a vertical presentation rather than horizontal (Fig. 24-1).

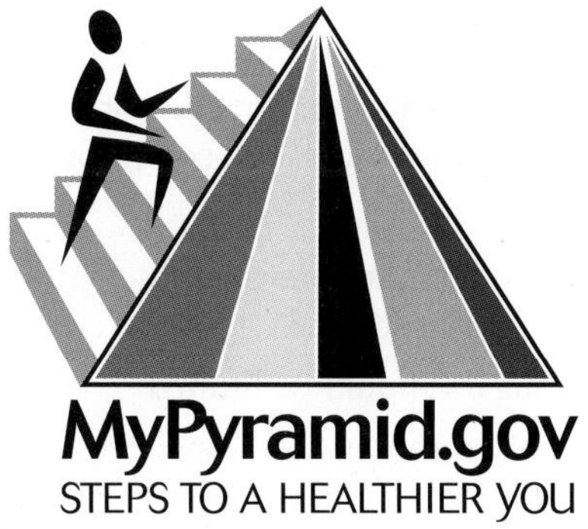

Figure 24-1 My Pyramid.

GENERAL USDA RECOMMENDATIONS

- Eat a variety of foods from each food group
- Combine healthy eating with physical activity
- Choose a diet low in saturated fat and cholesterol
- Eat plenty of grain products, fruit, and vegetables
- Note sodium content in food products and use in moderation
- Use alcoholic beverages in moderation

FOOD GROUPS IN ORDER OF LARGEST TO SMALLEST

1. Grains
2. Vegetables
3. Milk
4. Fruits
5. Meats and beans
6. Oils

COMMON THERAPEUTIC (SPECIAL) DIETS

- Pregnancy/lactating diet
  - Calorie intake as recommended by health care provider
  - Calcium, iron, vitamin C, and folic acid intake should increase
  - Weight gain as recommended by health care provider
- Clear liquid
  - Used in introducing foods back into diet (e.g., after illness or surgery and in preparation for specific procedures such as a colonoscopy)
  - Rule of thumb: clear liquids are those you can see through, such as apple juice, tea, clear broth, or noncaffeinated sodas
- Soft
  - Normal foods in mashed or pureed form
  - Accommodation for patients with difficulty chewing
- Bland
  - Nonirritating foods (e.g., most dairy products, hot cereals, mashed potatoes, grits)
  - Used in gastrointestinal tract disorders, such as various ulcer forms, ulcerative colitis, or gastritis
- Diabetic
  - Goal is to prevent abnormal fluctuations in insulin and blood glucose levels
  - Simple sugars should be limited
  - Intake of complex carbohydrates, protein, and unsaturated fats should increase
  - Calorie intake is tailored per patient
- Low (restricted) sodium
  - Used in hypertension, congestive heart failure, and other diseases that increase the body's normal fluid load
  - Educate patient to read sodium contents in food ingredient labels
- Low cholesterol (low fat)
  - Used in patients with high cholesterol, increased triglycerides, and cardiovascular disease
  - Limitation of fat calories to less than 20% of total daily caloric intake
- Low purine
  - Used in patients who have gout or the inability to metabolize uric acid
  - Limitation of purine-rich foods such as organ meats, red meat, asparagus, salmon, halibut
- Food intolerance
  - gluten free—avoid this protein contained in wheat, oats, barley and rye
  - lactose free—avoid or limit dairy products

ETHNIC CONSIDERATIONS

The demographics of the United States continue to change as diverse populations grow. Certain diseases prominent in specific races or cultures (e.g., hypertension in African Americans and diabetes in certain Native American tribes) are often controlled by diet. It is important for the patient educator to determine the dietary habits of the involved ethnic group. Every attempt should be made to maintain the foods of the specific culture with, perhaps, different methods of preparation—for example, baking instead of frying. The educator, who often is the medical assistant, must know the prescribed therapeutic diet and understand the fundamentals of nutrients. All health care workers are obligated to stay current as standards and guidelines change.

TERMS

Nutrition Review

The following list reviews the terms discussed in this chapter and other important terms you may see on the exam.

absorption the transfer of digested nutrients from the gastrointestinal system to the blood circulation

calorie unit of energy that produces heat

carbohydrates sugars and starches; the body's primary energy source

digestion physical and chemical changing of nutrients in the body to allow absorption

estimated energy requirement (EER) approximation of needed daily calories

fats (lipids) greasy material in nutrients; transport fat-soluble vitamins, insulate the body from the cold, and provide fatty acids
fiber nondigestible but edible portion of plants; necessary for the gastrointestinal elimination function
ingestion taking in of nutrients; eating and drinking
metabolism synthesizing of nutrients from the bloodstream, producing energy
nutrients components of food necessary for the body to perform physiologic functions
nutrition the process of taking food into the body and using it
obese 20% overweight for sex, height, and type of frame
proteins nutrients comprising amino acids (building blocks); build and heal body tissue
triglycerides component molecule of fat found in fatty foods; a combination of fatty acids and glycerol; high levels clog blood vessels, causing cardiovascular disease
vitamins organic substances found naturally in foods and needed in small amounts for metabolism and prevention of certain diseases

REVIEW QUESTIONS

All questions are relevant for the CMA (AAMA), RMA (AMT), and CMAS (AMT) exams.

1. The process of taking nutrients into the body is called:
   A. digestion.
   B. ingestion.
   C. absorption.
   D. metabolism.

Answer: **B**

Why: Ingestion is the process of introducing food and drink into the stomach. Digestion, absorption, and metabolism are part of the digestive process after the food enters the body.

Review: Yes ❑ No ❑

---

2. The cholesterol considered to be the "good" type is:
   A. triglycerides.
   B. high-density lipoprotein.
   C. low-density lipoprotein.
   D. saturated fat.
   E. unsaturated fat.

Answer: **B**

Why: High-density lipoproteins are considered the good cholesterol because they actually carry back to the liver cholesterol that has been deposited on arterial walls. Increased deposits on arterial walls can lead to blockage of arteries and result in a higher risk of heart disease or heart attack.

Review: Yes ❑ No ❑

---

3. The nutrient that primarily builds and heals body tissue is:
   A. carbohydrate.
   B. fat.
   C. protein.
   D. triglyceride.

Answer: **C**

Why: Protein is a nutrient comprising amino acids, the building blocks of the body. The amino acids help build up tissue and promote healing of damaged tissue.

Review: Yes ❑ No ❑

---

4. The vitamin that promotes red blood cell production is:
   A. vitamin A.
   B. vitamin C.
   C. vitamin D.
   D. vitamin K.
   E. vitamin B_{12}.

Answer: **E**

Why: Vitamin B_{12} is used to treat red blood cell deficiencies such as pernicious anemia. It promotes the production of red blood cells. Vitamin B_{12} is found in organ meats and dairy products.

Review: Yes ❑ No ❑

---

5. The organization that developed guidelines to assist people in making healthy food choices is the:
   A. FDA.
   B. USDA.
   C. CDC.
   D. AMA.

Answer: **B**

Why: The United States Department of Agriculture (USDA) developed the food pyramid that emphasizes food from the major food groups: (1) grains, (2) vegetables, (3) fruits, (4) milk, (5) meat and beans, and (6) oils. The FDA is the Food and Drug Administration, the CDC is the Centers for Disease Control and Prevention, and the AMA is the American Medical Association.

Review: Yes ❑ No ❑

6. A clear liquid diet includes the following EXCEPT:
   A. chicken broth.
   B. tea.
   C. milk.
   D. apple juice.
   E. water.

Answer: C

Why: Clear liquid means you can see through the liquid. Milk is not considered a clear liquid. A clear liquid diet is recommended for patients recovering from diarrhea or surgery.

Review: Yes ❑ No ❑

---

7. Metabolism is the process of:
   A. taking food into the body.
   B. physically changing nutrients to allow absorption.
   C. chemically changing nutrients in the body.
   D. using nutrients from the bloodstream to produce energy.

Answer: D

Why: Metabolism is the process by which nutrients are distributed into the blood and are used for growth and energy production.

Review: Yes ❑ No ❑

---

8. The fat-soluble vitamin that promotes blood clotting is:
   A. vitamin A.
   B. vitamin D.
   C. vitamin E.
   D. vitamin C.
   E. vitamin K.

Answer: E

Why: Vitamins A, D, E, and K are all fat-soluble vitamins, which means that they are stored in the body and can have a cumulative effect. Vitamin K has a chief function of production of prothrombin in the body. Prothrombin is one of the clotting factors.

Review: Yes ❑ No ❑

---

9. A person on a low-cholesterol diet should avoid which of the following food groups?
   A. Fruits
   B. Meats
   C. Vegetables
   D. Grains

Answer: B

Why: Cholesterol is found in animal products. This includes chicken and fish, although these tend to be lower in cholesterol than red meat. The human liver also naturally produces cholesterol. An increase in cholesterol is associated with an increased risk for heart disease and atherosclerosis (cholesterol plaque in the blood vessels).

Review: Yes ❑ No ❑

---

10. The mineral responsible for proper bone and tooth development is:
   A. iron.
   B. sodium.
   C. calcium.
   D. potassium.
   E. zinc.

Answer: C

Why: Calcium is primarily found in milk and milk products. It is also found in dark green leafy vegetables and promotes the formation of teeth and bones.

Review: Yes ❑ No ❑

---

11. Which of the following nutrients has the highest amount of calories per gram?
   A. Carbohydrate
   B. Fat
   C. Protein
   D. Fiber

Answer: B

Why: Carbohydrates and proteins have 4 calories per gram of food. Fat contains 9 calories per gram. Fiber is a nondigestible nutrient but one necessary for gastrointestinal elimination.

Review: Yes ❑ No ❑

12. A patient diagnosed with hypertension will usually benefit from a diet low in:
   A. sodium.
   B. calcium.
   C. iodine.
   D. iron.
   E. protein.

Answer: **A**

Why: Sodium is found in table salt and processed food. Sodium is responsible for maintaining fluid balance, so a diet low in sodium may help lower blood pressure by decreasing the amount of fluid retained by the body.

Review: Yes ❑ No ❑

---

13. Which of the following diets is recommended for a patient diagnosed with gout?
   A. Low salt
   B. Low carbohydrate
   C. Low purine
   D. Low fiber

Answer: **C**

Why: Gout is a condition associated with the inability to metabolize uric acid. If there is an excess of uric acid in the body, it is converted to sodium urate crystals that deposit in the joints. A common joint affected by the pain of gout is the great toe. Purine-rich foods are primarily organ meats such as liver and kidney.

Review: Yes ❑ No ❑

---

14. The substance necessary for hemoglobin to transport oxygen in the blood is:
   A. zinc.
   B. iodine.
   C. potassium.
   D. iron.
   E. calcium.

Answer: **D**

Why: Iron is found in organ meats and dark green leafy vegetables and is responsible for increasing the ability of the red blood cells to transport oxygen by providing hemoglobin. Iron injections are administered to help treat disorders including iron-deficiency anemia.

Review: Yes ❑ No ❑

---

15. The process by which nutrients leave the gastrointestinal system and enter the bloodstream is:
   A. ingestion.
   B. digestion.
   C. absorption.
   D. metabolism.

Answer: **C**

Why: Ingestion is the process of taking nutrients into the body. Digestion is the process of breaking down the nutrients for absorption into the bloodstream. Metabolism is the synthesizing of nutrients from the bloodstream, producing energy.

Review: Yes ❑ No ❑

---

16. An example of a saturated fat is:
   A. butter.
   B. olive oil.
   C. egg whites.
   D. walnuts.
   E. salmon.

Answer: **A**

Why: Saturated fat is a type of fat that is found in a solid state when at room temperature and is responsible for increasing blood cholesterol. Unsaturated fats are usually liquid at room temperature and are helpful in decreasing blood cholesterol. Olive oil is an example of an unsaturated fat. Egg whites are not fats but rather are proteins. Walnuts and salmon are proteins that contain unsaturated fat.

Review: Yes ❑ No ❑

17. A patient diagnosed with hypokalemia should increase the intake of:
A. copper.
B. potassium.
C. fluoride.
D. calcium.

Answer: **B**

Why: Hypokalemia is a condition in which an inadequate amount of potassium is found in the bloodstream. The treatment includes increasing the intake of potassium through certain foods or medication. Foods rich in potassium include fruits, especially bananas and citrus fruits.

Review: Yes ❑ No ❑

---

18. The mineral iodine is an essential substance for the proper function of which one of the following organs?
A. Kidneys
B. Adrenal glands
C. Thyroid gland
D. Liver

Answer: **C**

Why: The thyroid gland requires adequate amounts of iodine to function properly. A decrease in the function of the thyroid gland may result in development of a goiter, an enlargement of the thyroid gland.

Review: Yes ❑ No ❑

---

19. Night blindness can be caused by a deficiency of:
A. vitamin A.
B. vitamin B.
C. vitamin C.
D. vitamin D.

Answer: **A**

Why: Vitamin A is a fat-soluble vitamin that promotes good eyesight and may cause night blindness when deficient in the body. Vitamin A is found in milk and yellow vegetables.

Review: Yes ❑ No ❑

---

20. The diet recommended for the treatment of ulcers is:
A. low sodium.
B. soft.
C. clear liquid.
D. bland.
E. low cholesterol.

Answer: **D**

Why: A bland diet includes foods that are nonirritating, including dairy products, mashed potatoes, and hot cereals.

Review: Yes ❑ No ❑

---

21. A clear liquid diet is indicated for which of the following?
A. A patient with an ulcer
B. A patient with difficulty chewing
C. A patient with diarrhea
D. A patient who is limiting calories for weight loss

Answer: **C**

Why: A patient with diarrhea should initially limit intake to clear liquids and then gradually add foods back into the diet. A patient with an ulcer will usually benefit from a diet that is bland and nonirritating. A patient with difficulty chewing can usually eat soft foods but does not require only liquids. A patient who is limiting calories for weight loss should still eat balanced meals from all of the food groups; there is no indication for a clear liquid diet.

Review: Yes ❑ No ❑

22. A low-fat diet would be recommended to treat:
    A. hypertension.
    B. gallbladder disease.
    C. thyroid disease.
    D. gout.
    E. diabetes.

Answer: **B**

Why: The gallbladder is where bile is stored. Bile is necessary to break up fat particles that can be absorbed through the intestinal walls into the body. Patients with gallbladder disease will want to limit the intake of fat to decrease the need for bile. Most gallbladder disease is caused by obstruction of the bile ducts resulting from gallstones.

Review: Yes ❑ No ❑

---

23. Ascorbic acid is also known as vitamin:
    A. A.
    B. B.
    C. C.
    D. D.

Answer: **C**

Why: Ascorbic acid, also known as vitamin C, is a water-soluble vitamin present in citrus fruits, tomatoes, and green leafy vegetables. Vitamin C is essential for fighting bacterial infections and preventing scurvy. Scurvy is characterized by weakness, anemia, edema, soft bleeding gums with ulceration, and loosening of the teeth.

Review: Yes ❑ No ❑

---

24. Which of the following may be prevented with proper amounts of vitamin D in the diet?
    A. Diabetes
    B. Hemorrhage
    C. Blindness
    D. Heart disease
    E. Rickets

Answer: **E**

Why: Rickets is a condition characterized by weak bones. The disease usually is seen in infancy and childhood. The bones do not form properly because they are soft and pliable. Deformities may include bowlegs and knock-knees.

Review: Yes ❑ No ❑

---

25. Persons who need to limit their intake of iodine in the body will want to avoid:
    A. Milk
    B. Seafood
    C. Bananas
    D. Eggs

Answer: **B**

Why: Seafood, especially shellfish, is very high in iodine content. Some people are highly allergic to iodine and should avoid foods with iodine. Injected contrast media should also be avoided because of the high concentration of iodine.

Review: Yes ❑ No ❑

25

Pharmacology and Medication Administration

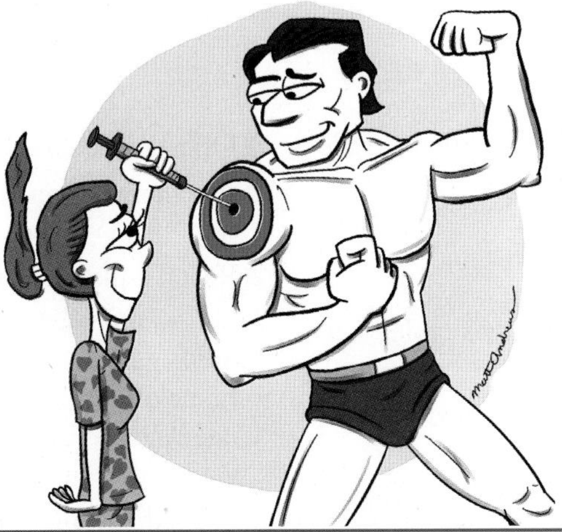

REVIEW TIP

The national exams contain medication dosage calculation problems. Know how to multiply and divide fractions and decimals. Practice solving problems without a calculator since you are not permitted to use one during the exam. The examiners usually provide scrap paper to work out the problem before listing the answer on the exam form. Practice problems follow the review terms in this chapter.

Pharmacology is the study of drugs. Two federal agencies regulate drugs and drug administration. The **Food and Drug Administration (FDA)** controls the drugs that are acceptable for use in the United States; the **Drug Enforcement Agency (DEA)** controls who may administer and use specific drugs. Both agencies hold enforcement powers, which may include imprisonment, fines, and revocation or suspension of professional licenses. Drugs are placed in five schedules for regulation and control, as described in Table 25-1. Visit RxList (www.rxlist.com) for a list of the 200 most current commonly used drugs.

ADMINISTRATION

MEDICAL DRUG USES

- Treatment—relieves symptoms of a disease or disorder (e.g., ibuprofen for fever and pain)
- Diagnosis—determine the presence of a specific disease by the body's reaction to specific drugs, such as Tensilon to aid in the diagnosis of myasthenia gravis
- Restoration—remove the cause of the disease or disorder (e.g., an antibiotic)
- Replacement—substitute chemical agents normally found in the body, such as hormone replacement therapy (HRT)
- Prevention—block or weaken certain diseases (e.g., immunizations for vaccine-preventable diseases); see Box 6-7, "Types of Immunity," and Box 6-8, "Common Vaccine-Preventable Diseases," in Chapter 6

COMMON DRUG TYPES

Drugs are named and grouped for their uses—for example, *antiemetics* are used to combat emesis (vomiting).

Table 25-1 **Drug Schedules**

Schedule	Use	Example
I	Illegal or restricted to research; dispensed with special permits; high potential for abuse	Heroin, marijuana
II	Medical use with precautions and limitations; dispensed with written prescription; high potential for abuse	Cocaine, morphine, Demerol, oxycodone, Ritalin
III	Medical use with precautions and limitations; dispensed with written prescription; moderate potential for abuse	Barbiturates, small doses of codeine in combination with other drugs (e.g., Tylenol with codeine)
IV	Medical use with precautions and limitations; dispensed with written or oral prescription; low potential for abuse	Valium
V	Medical use with purchase over the counter; very low potential for abuse	Benadryl, Robitussin

Table 25-2 lists common drug types and their trade names and uses.

COMMON DRUG ROUTES

- Buccal—placed between gum and cheek via tablet, gel, or spray
- Inhalation—inhaled into respiratory system via sprays, mists, masks (oxygen is considered a drug)
- Intradermal (ID)—injected into dermal layer of skin at 15° angle via fine (25–27) gauge short needle, producing a small wheal; forearm site is most common, as with a tuberculin skin test
- Intramuscular (IM)—injected into muscle at 90° angle via an 18- to 23-gauge long needle (1–3 inches); aspirate before injection to ensure that the needle is not in a blood vessel
  - Common IM sites
    - Deltoids (upper arms)
    - Gluteus medius (the ventrogluteal area of this muscle is now recommended over the dorsogluteal area)
    - Vastus lateralis (thighs)
  - Z-track—used for specific IM medications that irritate subcutaneous tissue (e.g., Imferon and Kenalog); the skin at the injection site is pulled to one side before injection; the medication is administered and skin released; prevents medication from seeping into subcutaneous layers
- Intravenous (IV)—injected into vein via 18- to 21-gauge needle ($1–1^1/_2$ inches)
- Ophthalmic—placed into eye via ointment or drops
- Oral—placed in the mouth and swallowed via tablet, capsule, liquid, gel (most common medication route)
- Otic—placed in ear via drops
- Parenteral—non-oral, usually refers to injected medication: IM, IV, subcutaneous, intradermal
- Rectal—placed in patient's rectum via suppository
- Subcutaneous (Sub-Q or subQ; S.C. or S.Q. no longer used, per The Joint Commission)—injected in fatty tissue under the skin at a 45° angle via 23- to 25-gauge needle ($^1/_2$–$^5/_8$ inches long); aspirate before injection to ensure that the needle is not in a blood vessel
  - Used for allergic extracts administered with tuberculin needle and syringe to avoid entering muscle, and for insulin administration
  - Common subcutaneous sites
    - Upper arms
    - Upper thighs
    - Upper medial back
    - Abdominal external obliques
- Sublingual—placed under the tongue via tablets or gels
- Topical—placed on skin or mucous membranes via ointments, creams, liquids, or sprays for direct treatment of skin or membranes
- Transdermal—placed on skin via medicated patch for medication to absorb through skin and enter bloodstream
- Urethral—placed into urethra and bladder via a urethral catheter
- Vaginal—placed into vagina via applicator of cream or via douche

Note: Implantable medication devices and eye-curing lens devices are also available; national exam question probability is extremely low for these routes.

Table 25-2 **Common Drug Types**

Drug Type	Common Use	Example
Analgesic	Lessens or relieves pain	Ibuprofen (Motrin) Acetaminophen (Tylenol)
Anesthetic (local)	"Deadens" an area to sensation, including pain	Lidocaine (Xylocaine)
Antacid	Neutralizes acid in gastrointestinal tract	Tums, Mylanta
Antibiotic	Eradicates or inhibits the growth of specific microbes	Penicillin, Augmentin
Anticoagulant	Prevents or decreases clotting	Heparin, Coumadin
Anticonvulsant	Prevents seizures	Dilantin, Tegretol
Antidepressant	Inhibits or decreases depression	Prozac, Cymbalta
Antidiarrheal	Inhibits or decreases diarrhea	Lomotil, Kaopectate
Antiemetic	Inhibits or decreases nausea	Compazine, Dramamine
Antihistamine	Inhibits or decreases symptoms of allergies	Benadryl, Claritin
Antihypertensive	Inhibits or controls high blood pressure	Aldomet, Lopressor
Anti-inflammatory	Inhibits or decreases inflammation	
■ Steroidal		Decadron
■ Nonsteroidal anti-inflammatory drug (NSAID)		Ibuprofen
Antipyretic	Decreases fever	Acetaminophen, ibuprofen
Antitussive	Inhibits or decreases cough	Codeine, Dimetapp
Bronchodilator	Dilates the bronchi	Albuterol
Decongestant	Decreases nasal congestion	Neo-Synephrine
Diuretic	Decreases body fluid by increasing urination	Lasix, Diuril
Immunization	Protects from specific communicable diseases	Hepatitis B, varicella,and polio vaccines

SYRINGES

Syringes are plastic or glass tube-like carriers used with an attached needle to administer substances into the body via injection.

- Insulin—small syringe with short, fine needle attached to administer insulin; measurements are in units (U) is another Joint Commision; 100 units = 1 mL; syringes are supplied with 100-unit (most common), 80-unit, or 40-unit capacities
- Tuberculin—small syringe with short, fine needle attached to administer Mantoux tuberculin skin test intradermally; measurements are in tenths of a millimeter (0.1 mL) with a 1-mL capacity; usual amount is 0.1 mL of purified protein derivative (PPD); test results should be read in 48 to 72 hours
- Cartridges—individual-dose glass tubes with needles that screw onto or slide into a dispenser designed for that cartridge

SEVEN "RIGHTS" OF DRUG ADMINISTRATION

These procedures must be carried out each time a drug is administered to avoid medication errors:

- Right patient—check the name on the physician's order and the medical record; ask the patient first and last name
- Right drug—check the drug label three times: when taking the drug container out (check drug expiration date at the same time), after placing the medication in the dispenser (e.g., syringe, medication cup), and before returning the drug container to storage
- Right route—check the route the physician ordered with the route you prepared (e.g., oral versus injectable)
- Right dose—check the dose on the physician's order with the dose prepared

- Right technique—ensure that the correct method is used throughout the procedure including positioning the patient and aseptic technique
- Right time—check when the medication is to be given (e.g., now, with meals)
- Right documentation—record the procedure in the patient's medical record on completion, noting date, time, drug, dose, route, site (if injectable, topical, or transdermal), results/tolerance, patient education, medical assistant signature, and title

SAFETY

When administering medication, safety and Occupational Safety and Health Administration (OSHA) guidelines apply:

- Prevent accidental needlesticks by using safety lock needles
- Discard needles and syringes immediately into biohazard containers
- Wear appropriate personal protective equipment (PPE)

DOSAGE CALCULATIONS

The majority of medical facilities maintain conversion charts to simplify medication dosage calculations when one unit (such as grams) must be changed to another unit (such as milligrams). In other instances, the amount of a medication ordered may be more or less than the medication on hand. The medical assistant is expected to determine the correct dosage. Table 25-3 contains the most common conversions used in dosage calculations.

METHODS

- Formula with like units—used when medication ordered is more than or less than the medication on hand (units are the same—for example, both milligrams). Box 25-1 shows the steps involved in calculating a dosage for like units.
- Conversion ratio—used when the units of medication on hand are different from the units ordered (e.g., milligrams are ordered, but the medication on hand is in grams). The conversion is done first, then the formula for the dosage. Box 25-2 shows the steps involved in calculating a dosage for unlike units.
- Body weight—used in instances in which medication dosage is more closely calculated for the individual patient (e.g., pediatrics); pounds are converted to kilograms. Box 25-3 shows the steps involved in calculating a dosage based on body weight.

Table 25-3 Common Conversions

Component	Equivalent
1 gram (G, Gm, g, gm)	1000 milligrams (mg) 5 grains (gr)
1 gr	60 mg
1 kilogram (kg)	2.2 pounds (lb) 1,000 Gm
1 milliliter (mL, ml)	15 drops (15 gtt) 1 cubic centimeter
1 teaspoon (tsp)	5 mL 60 gtt

- Body surface area—used to calculate pediatric medication doses; complicated formula rarely used in medical office.

PRESCIPTIONS

Prescriptions are written directions for therapeutic agents; the most common involve medications. Licensed physicians, licensed nurse practitioners with prescribing privileges, or properly credentialed physicians' assistants are the only persons authorized to write prescriptions. They provide a legal document, informing the pharmacist of the order to be filled. The medical assistant with a physician's order may administer drugs but may *never* prescribe drugs. The medical assistant and administrative medical specialist may call a prescription into a pharmacy as written by one of the above legal entities. This is not considered prescribing.

Dispensing is defined as preparing and distributing medication. Only pharmacists, physicians, and properly credentialed nurse practitioners and physicians' assistants may dispense drugs. The medical assistant and administrative medical specialist may not dispense drugs but may give a patient prepackaged drugs (e.g., samples as ordered by the physician). This is not considered dispensing.

PRESCRIPTION INFORMATION

Box 25-4 lists common abbreviations used on prescriptions.

- Physician name, address, phone number
- Date of prescription
- Patient name, address, and phone number
- Drug, dose, and form
- Number of doses to be dispensed
- Patient instructions
- Number of refills

Box 25-1

Dosage Calculation With Like Units

Problem 1: The physician ordered 800 mg ibuprofen po to be given now; the office stocks ibuprofen in 200 mg per tablet. How many tablets will you give?

Formula: $$\frac{\textbf{Dose ordered}}{\textbf{Dose on hand}} \times \frac{\textbf{Quantity}}{\textbf{1}} = \textbf{Amount desired}$$

(where "quantity" is the amount and form that contains the dose on hand)

Step 1: Set up formula.

$$\frac{800\text{ mg}}{200\text{ mg}} \times \frac{1\text{ tablet}}{1} = \text{number of tablets desired}$$

Step 2: Multiply 800 × 1 and 200 × 1.

$$\frac{800}{200} = 4\text{ tablets}$$

Answer: 4 tablets of 200 mg each are to be given.

Problem 2: The physician ordered 250 mg amoxicillin po to be given now; the office stocks amoxicillin 500 mg per tsp. How many teaspoons will you give?

Use the same formula as above:

$$\frac{250\text{ mg}}{500\text{ mg}} \times \frac{1\text{ tsp}}{1} = {}^{1}\!/_{2}\text{ or } 0.5\text{ tsp to be given}$$

- Physician signature
- DEA number

MEDICAL ASSISTANT RESPONSIBILITY TO AVOID DRUG ABUSE

- Security of prescription pads
- Protection of signature stamps and physician's DEA number

PERIPHERAL INTRAVENOUS THERAPY

Similar to radiography, involvement with IV therapy may or may not be in the medical assistant's scope of practice dependent on the state rules and regulations, the community standards, the medical assistant's training, and the medical practice's insurance carrier. The previous material in this chapter related to medication administration also pertains to IV therapy. The following are IV-related topics that may appear on the national exam. Table 25-4 lists common IV tubing by drip capacity.

INDICATIONS

- Rapid medication distribution and absorption
- Fluid volume replacement or maintenance
- Nutritional supplement
- Rapid access to vein
- Intolerance to medications via other routes

COMPLICATIONS

- Infiltration—the solution enters the tissue around the vein
- Extravasation—leakage of fluid from the vein into the surrounding tissue

Table 25-4 Selecting Common IV Tubing by Drip Capacity

Tubing	Drops	Use
Macrodrip	15 drops/mL	Standard adult infusion rates
Microdrip (minidrip)	60 drops/mL	Restricted or precise fluid delivery (e.g., certain medications or pediatrics)

Box 25-2

Dosage Calculation With Unlike Units

Problem: The physician ordered 0.4 Gm of ibuprofen po now; the office stocks ibuprofen 200 mg per tablet. How many tablets will you give?

Step 1: Because the units of the available dosage (mg) differ from the units of the ordered dosage (Gm), they must be converted. Grams are converted to milligrams using the following ratio:

$$\mathbf{1{,}000\ mg : 1\ Gm}$$

or

$$\mathbf{1{,}000\ mg = 1\ Gm}$$

Step 2: Set up the proportion to find the dosage using the above ratio, *x* (the unknown, in milligrams), and 0.4 Gm, which is the dose ordered:

$$1{,}000\ \text{mg} : 1\ \text{Gm} = x\ \text{mg} : 0.4\ \text{Gm}$$

or

$$1{,}000\ \text{mg} : 1\ \text{Gm} :: x\ \text{mg} : 0.4\ \text{Gm}$$

(*Hint:* Use like units for the first and third numbers and the second and fourth numbers.)

Step 3: The product of the first and fourth numbers equals the product of the second and third numbers: 400 mg $= x$ mg.

Step 4: Use the formula in Box 25-1:

$$\textbf{Formula: } \frac{\textbf{Dose ordered}}{\textbf{Dose on hand}} \times \frac{\textbf{Quantity}}{\textbf{1}} = \textbf{Amount desired}$$

$$\frac{400\ \text{mg}}{200\ \text{mg}} \times \frac{\text{tablet}}{1} = 2\ \text{tablets}$$

Answer: 2 tablets of 200 mg each are to be given.

- Infection—an illness caused by a microorganism; characterized by localized redness, swelling, and pain, fever, and other systemic symptoms

Box 25-3

Dosage Calculation With Body Weight

Problem: The physician ordered 15 mg Tylenol per kilogram (kg) of body weight. You weighed the child, who is 8 kg. How many milligrams of Tylenol will you give?

Formula: Dose ordered × Weight in kg = Dose to be given

Set up formula.

$15\ \text{mg} \times 8\ \text{kg} = 120\ \text{mg}$

Answer: 120 mg Tylenol is to be given.

- System(s) fluid overload—a result of too rapid or too much infusion of a solution
- Hematoma—discoloration and swelling in the tissue due to blood leaking from the vein
- Venous spasm—contraction of vein
- Thrombus—blood clot
- Thrombophlebitis—inflammation of the blood vessel
- Embolism—traveling clot, usually blood
- Air embolism—bolus of air, usually through IV tubing
- Nerve, tendon, ligament, or limb damage from initial venipuncture, infiltration, or infection
- Damaged IV catheter, which may cause harm at the side or break off and travel to vital organs

EXTREMITIES TO AVOID

- Legs
- Side of a radical mastectomy

Box 25-4

Common Prescription Abbreviations and Instructions

Time			
Once per day ("od" no longer used, per The Joint Commission)	bid: twice per day	tid: three times per day	qid: four times per day
q: every	Every day ("qd" no longer used, per The Joint Commission)	qh: every hour	q (2, 3, 4, etc.) h: every (2, 3, 4, etc.) hours
Select Administration Sites			
Right ear ("AD" no longer used, per The Joint Commission)	Left ear ("AS" no longer used, per The Joint Commission)	Both ears ("AU" no longer used, per The Joint Commission)	Right eye ("OD" no longer used, per The Joint Commission)
Left eye ("OS" no longer used, per The Joint Commission)	Both eyes ("OU" no longer used, per The Joint Commission)	po: by mouth	top: topically

Note: The Joint Commission eliminated a number of common abbreviations that resulted in medication errors.

- Side of cerebrovascular accident (CVA) or other paralysis
- Partial amputations, scars, or other deformities
- Shunts or grafts

Note: All OSHA and CDC guidelines for safety, asepsis, and biohazards in previous chapters apply to IV therapy. Review the sections "Fluid Balance" and "Cellular Movement of Substances" in Chapter 6.

TERMS

Pharmacology and Medication Administration Review

The following list reviews the terms discussed in this chapter as well as other important terms that you may see on the exam.

dispensing preparing and distributing medication

Drug Enforcement Agency (DEA) federal agency that controls who may administer and use specific drugs

electronic infusion device (EID) an electronic mechanism that regulates the amount and flow rate of intravenous solutions

extravasation the leakage of fluid from the vein into the surrounding tissue

Food and Drug Administration (FDA) federal agency that controls the drugs that are acceptable for use in the United States

infiltration IV solution enters the tissue around the vein

intramuscular (IM) injected into muscle at 90° angle via 18- to 23-gauge long needle

macrodrop a type of IV tubing that delivers approximately 15 drops of solution per milliliter

microdrop a type of IV tubing that delivers approximately 60 drops of solution per milliliter

parenteral substances administered by intramuscular, intradermal, intravenous, or subcutaneous routes

patient-controlled analgesia (PCA) an electronic infusion device that allows the patient to self-administer IV pain medication through an open IV line

pharmacology the study of drugs

piggybacked IV infusion a secondary IV line coupled to the primary infusion line through an injection port; the piggyback infusion solution must be hung above the primary infusion solution in order to run; IV antibiotics are often administered in this manner

prescriptions written directions for therapeutic agents; the most common involve medications

Rx most commonly found on prescription forms, meaning treatment or recipe

subcutaneous injected in fatty tissue under the skin at a 45° angle

syringes plastic or glass tube-like carriers used with an attached needle to administer substances into the body via injection

topical placed on skin or mucous membranes via ointments, creams, liquids, or sprays for direct treatment to skin or membranes

transdermal drug route in which medication is placed on skin via a patch for medication to absorb through skin and enter bloodstream

venoscope an illumination device used to assist in locating veins for venipuncture or IV therapy; the device directs cool light into subcutaneous tissue, which highlights the presence of a vein by causing it to appear as a dark line

Z-track a method of intramuscular (IM) medication administration used for specific IM medications that irritate subcutaneous tissue (e.g., Imferon, Kenalog); the skin is pulled to one side of the injection site before the injection; the medication is administered, and the skin is released; prevents medication from seeping into subcutaneous layers

PROBLEMS

MEDICATION DOSAGE CALCULATION

1. The physician orders 40 mg Depo-Medrol; 80 mg/mL is on hand. How many milliliters will you give? _________
2. The physician orders 750 mg Tagamet liquid; 1,500 mg/tsp is on hand. How many teaspoons will you give? _________
3. The physician ordered 75 mg of Seconal; 50 mg/mL is on hand. How many milliliters will you give? _________
4. The physician ordered 1,500 mg Duricef; 1 g/tablet is on hand. How many tablets will you give? _________
5. The physician orders 15 mg morphine sulfate; 1 gr/mL is on hand. How many milliliters will you give? _________
6. The physician ordered 10 units of regular insulin; 100 units/mL is on hand. How many millimeters will you give? _________
7. The physician ordered 5 mg Coumadin; 5 mg/tablet is on hand. How many tablets will you give? _________
8. The physician ordered 20 mg Tylenol/kg of body weight; on hand is 80 mg/tablet. The child weighs 12 kg. How many tablets will you give? _________
9. The physician ordered 20 mg Tylenol/kg of body weight; on hand is 80 mg/tablet. The child weighs 44 lb. How many tablets will you give? _________
10. The physician ordered 3,000 units of heparin; 5,000 units/mL is on hand. How many milliliters will you give? _________

Answers: (1) 0.5 mL, (2) 0.5 tsp, (3) 1.5 mL, (4) 1.5 tab, (5) 0.25 mL, (6) 0.1 mL, (7) 1 tab, (8) 3 tab, (9) 5 tab, (10) 0.6 mL

REVIEW QUESTIONS

All questions are relevant for the CMA (AAMA) and RMA (AMT) exams. Questions 1 through 15 are relevant for the CMAS (AMT) exam.

1. The agency that controls who may administer and use specific drugs is the:
   A. FDA.
   B. CDC.
   C. DEA.
   D. PDR.

Answer: **C**

Why: The Drug Enforcement Agency (DEA) is a federal branch of the Justice Department. Their responsibilities include overseeing the prescribing, refilling, and storing of controlled substances in the medical office. The FDA is the Food and Drug Administration, the CDC is the Centers for Disease Control and Prevention, and the PDR is the *Physician's Desk Reference*.

Review: Yes ❏ No ❏

---

2. Which of the following is not included in the "rights" of drug administration?
   A. Right drug
   B. Right physician
   C. Right patient
   D. Right route
   E. Right time

Answer: **B**

Why: The "rights" of drug administration are the procedures to be carried out each time a drug is administered to a patient to avoid medication errors. The "rights" include the right patient, drug, route, dose, technique, time, and documentation.

Review: Yes ❏ No ❏

---

3. Drugs that can be purchased over the counter are classified as schedule:
   A. I.
   B. II.
   C. IV.
   D. V.

Answer: **D**

Why: Drugs are placed in five schedules for regulation and control. Schedule I drugs are illegal or restricted to research. Schedule II and III drugs must be used with precautions and limitations and are dispensed with a written prescription. Schedule II drugs have a high potential for abuse, and Schedule III drugs have a moderate potential for abuse. Schedule IV drugs are dispensed with written or oral prescription and have a low potential for abuse.

Review: Yes ❏ No ❏

---

4. Parenteral administration of medication generally means that the medication is:
   A. administered through a suppository.
   B. injected.
   C. in liquid form to swallow.
   D. dissolved in and absorbed through the mouth
   E. placed under the tongue

Answer: **B**

Why: **Parenteral** is a term used to describe the administration of medication by injection so the medication does not pass through the gastrointestinal tract. This method includes intramuscular, subcutaneous, and intravenous routes.

Review: Yes ❏ No ❏

5. To convert grams to milligrams:
   A. divide by 100.
   B. divide by 1,000.
   C. multiply by 100.
   D. multiply by 1,000.

Answer: **D**

Why: Grams is a single unit of measure; *milli* is the prefix used for 1,000; 1,000 mg = 1 g.

Review: Yes ❑ No ❑

---

6. Information found on a prescription includes the following EXCEPT:
   A. patient instructions.
   B. number of doses to be dispensed.
   C. patient's date of birth.
   D. patient's name and address.
   E. number of refills.

Answer: **C**

Why: The patient's birth date is not included on a prescription. Most prescription forms are preprinted with the physician's name, address, phone number, and DEA number. The physician completes the prescription with the prescription date, drug requested, dose, drug form, and number of refills. There is also a space for the patient's name and address.

Review: Yes ❑ No ❑

---

7. Which of the following is an appropriate task for a medical assistant or administrative medical specialist?
   A. Call a drug renewal to a pharmacy
   B. Prescribe drugs
   C. Authorize reorder of drugs
   D. Dispense drugs

Answer: **A**

Why: A medical assistant or administrative medical specialist may call in a prescription for a drug that a physician has ordered for a patient. Only a physician can prescribe and authorize the reorder or refill of drugs. Dispensing drugs is only permitted by licensed pharmacists, physicians, or other credentialed medical personnel.

Review: Yes ❑ No ❑

---

8. The prescription directions "ii gtt q4h" mean:
   A. one drop every hour.
   B. one drop every four hours.
   C. two drops every hour.
   D. two drops every four hours.
   E. four drops every four hours.

Answer: **D**

Why: The abbreviation gtt means "drops." The Roman numeral ii means "two." "Every four hours" is abbreviated q4h.

Review: Yes ❑ No ❑

---

9. Which of the following classifications of medication is used to control high blood pressure?
   A. Antipyretic
   B. Antiemetic
   C. Antihypertensive
   D. Antihistamine

Answer: **C**

Why: The prefix *anti* means "to work against." Hypertension is the medical term for elevated or high blood pressure. Antipyretics are used to decrease fever, antiemetics to decrease nausea, and antihistamines to decrease symptoms of allergies.

Review: Yes ❑ No ❑

---

10. Of the following drugs, which one can be dispensed only with a written prescription?
   A. Valium
   B. Robitussin
   C. Tylenol
   D. Morphine
   E. Benadryl

Answer: **D**

Why: Morphine is classified as a Schedule II drug. Drugs in this category require a written prescription and are ordered with precautions and limitations. They have a high potential for abuse

Review: Yes ❑ No ❑

11. The method of administration of medication under the tongue is:
   A. topical.
   B. sublingual.
   C. parenteral.
   D. subcutaneous.

Answer: C

Why: Sublingual means "beneath the tongue." Nitroglycerin, used to treat angina, is an example of a medication administered sublingually. It is dissolved beneath the tongue and absorbed through the mucous membranes.

Review: Yes ❑ No ❑

---

12. The physician orders 300 mg of medication tid × 10 days. The medication is available in 150-mg capsules. How many capsules will the patient need to complete the course of therapy?
   A. 60
   B. 45
   C. 30
   D. 20
   E. 10

Answer: A

Why: The patient will need to take two capsules three times a day for 10 days. The total is 60 capsules for the entire course of therapy. The abbreviation tid means three times per day. To receive 300 mg of the medication with each dose, the patient will have to take two 150-mg capsules for each dose.

Review: Yes ❑ No ❑

---

13. The agency that controls the drugs that are acceptable for safe use and sale in the United States is the:
   A. DEA.
   B. AMA.
   C. FDA.
   D. CDC.

Answer: C

Why: The Food and Drug Administration (FDA) reviews drug applications and petitions for food additives and removes unsafe drugs from the sales market. The FDA also oversees the proper labeling of food, drugs, and cosmetics.

Review: Yes ❑ No ❑

---

14. The equivalent of 5 cubic centimeters is:
   A. 5 milligrams.
   B. 5 milliliters.
   C. 5 centimeters.
   D. 5 drops.
   E. 5 grams.

Answer: B

Why: The measurement of 1 cubic centimeter is the same as 1 milliliter. One cubic centimeter is a square cube 1 centimeter long by 1 centimeter wide by 1 centimeter high. One milliliter of fluid will equally fill 1 cubic centimeter of space; therefore, 5 cubic centimeters equals 5 milliliters.

Review: Yes ❑ No ❑

---

15. The physician orders 2.5 mg of Compazine, IM. Available is Compazine 5 mg/mL provided in a 10-mL multidose vial. How many milliliters will you give the patient?
   A. 0.1 mL
   B. 0.25 mL
   C. 0.5 mL
   D. 1.0 mL

Answer: C

Why: That the medication is provided in a 10-mL multidose vial is not important when performing the calculation. This information states the total number of milliliters in the container. If there are 5 milligrams of Compazine in 1 milliliter, then to give 2.5 mg, which is one-half of 5 mg, give one-half milliliter, or 0.5 mL.

Review: Yes ❑ No ❑

16. The classification of drugs that prevent or decrease clotting is:
    A. antiemetic.
    B. antipyretic.
    C. antineoplastic.
    D. antitussive.
    E. anticoagulant.

Answer: **E**

Why: Anticoagulants are used to prevent the formation of blood clots. Antiemetics are used to inhibit nausea. Antipyretics are used to decrease fever. Antineoplastics are indicated to slow the rate of tumor growth and delay metastasis (cancer). Antitussives are used to control coughing.

Review: Yes ❑ No ❑

---

17. The proper angle of the needle to the skin when administering an intramuscular injection is:
    A. 30°.
    B. 45°.
    C. 60°.
    D. 90°.

Answer: **D**

Why: The needle should be at a 90° angle to ensure that the beveled tip of the needle is placed within the muscle. If a lesser angle is used, the medication may be deposited within the subcutaneous or fatty layer of tissue.

Review: Yes ❑ No ❑

---

18. The muscle used for injection in the thigh is the:
    A. gluteus maximus.
    B. gluteus medius.
    C. vastus lateralis.
    D. rectus abdominis.
    E. rectus femoris.

Answer: **C**

Why: The vastus lateralis is the large (*vastus*) muscle on the side (*lateralis*, lateral) of the thigh. This is the preferred site for injections for infants.

Review: Yes ❑ No ❑

---

19. Which of the following is proper technique when administering a tuberculin skin test?
    A. Massage the injection site to lessen the pain of the procedure.
    B. Place a bandage over the injection site.
    C. After inserting the needle beneath the skin, aspirate to ensure the needle is not in a blood vessel.
    D. Leave the injection site uncovered.

Answer: **D**

Why: Massaging or covering the site may cause the medication to be pressed into the tissues or out of the wheal, and the results, if any, will be unreliable. Aspiration is not required for an intradermal injection.

Review: Yes ❑ No ❑

---

20. The physician orders ampicillin 0.5 Gm. Available is ampicillin 250 mg/mL. How many milliliters will you give the patient?
    A. 0.25 mL
    B. 0.5 mL
    C. 1 mL
    D. 1.5 mL
    E. 2 mL

Answer: **E**

Why: The first step to calculate the dose is to convert grams to milligrams. 0.5 Gm (grams) is equal to 500 mg (1 gram equals 1,000 milligrams). The dose ordered is 500 mg, and available is 250 mg in each milliliter. Two (2) milliliters of this medication contains 500 mg.

Review: Yes ❑ No ❑

---

21. A subcutaneous injection is injected into:
    A. muscle tissue.
    B. dermal tissue.
    C. fatty tissue.
    D. epidermal tissue.

Answer: **C**

Why: The subcutaneous tissue lies beneath the skin or dermis. It is the fatty layer. Medications injected in this tissue are absorbed slower than those given by the intramuscular method.

Review: Yes ❑ No ❑

22. A solution administered through the ID method is:
    A. Keflex.
    B. penicillin.
    C. hepatitis B vaccine.
    D. tuberculin solution.
    E. Imferon.

Answer: **D**

Why: ID is the abbreviation for intradermal. This is the injection method of placing a minute amount of solution just beneath the surface of the skin, within the dermis. Tuberculin solution is used to perform tuberculosis skin testing.

Review: Yes ❑ No ❑

---

23. Imferon, an iron preparation, is administered by which method?
    A. Subcutaneous
    B. Z-track
    C. Intravenous
    D. Sublingual

Answer: **B**

Why: Z-track is an intramuscular method of injection. Iron is a medication that will cause irritation and discoloration if deposited in the subcutaneous tissue. The Z-track method requires that the skin be pulled to one side before injection. After the injection is given, the skin is released, and there is no trailing or seeping of medication into the tissues.

Review: Yes ❑ No ❑

---

24. A subcutaneous injection is given using which technique?
    A. 90° angle, 21-gauge needle
    B. 15° angle, 25-gauge needle
    C. 60° angle, 21-gauge needle
    D. 45° angle, 25-gauge needle
    E. 30° 223-gauge needle

Answer: **D**

Why: The subcutaneous injection is administered into the fatty tissue. To avoid entering the muscle, a 45° angle is required. Solutions used for subcutaneous method are aqueous (watery), so they can be injected into the fatty tissue and absorbed slowly.

Review: Yes ❑ No ❑

---

25. The reason for aspirating before injecting a medication is to ensure that the:
    A. patient receives all the medication.
    B. injection will be deposited in the muscular tissue.
    C. needle is not in a blood vessel.
    D. injection will be less painful.

Answer: **C**

Why: Aspiration is the process of pulling back on the syringe plunger to ensure the needle is not positioned in a blood vessel. If blood appears in the syringe, the injection is discontinued and a new syringe is prepared. If the medication is injected into a blood vessel, the patient could have a serious adverse reaction to the medication.

Review: Yes ❑ No ❑

26

Emergency Preparedness

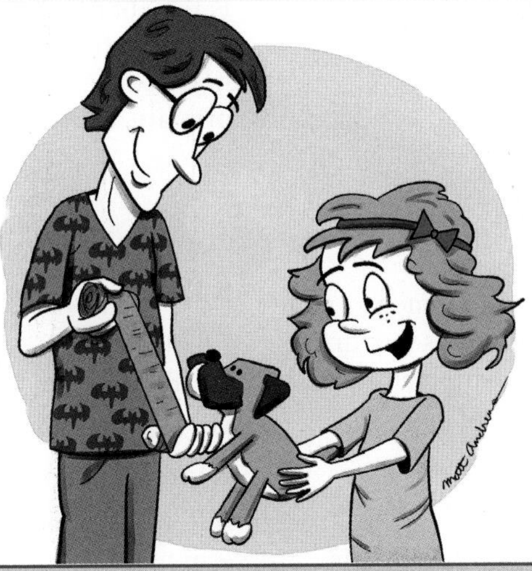

REVIEW TIP

After you complete the chapter, check your cardiopulmonary resuscitation (CPR) certification card and ensure it is current. If not, sign up for a course and bring a friend or relative. CPR is a separate certification, and the national exams contain only general questions.

The focus of this chapter is not to teach general first aid but to discuss emergency preparedness and provide an overview of recognizing and dealing with emergencies that may occur within the medical office or the community. Please note that the AAMA often refers to "emergency preparedness" as "protective practices."

Emergency preparedness or protective practices may be divided into three categories:

- The individual (patient, staff member, visitor)
- The medical office (emergency within the office such as fire or chemical exposure)
- The community (natural disaster, act of terrorism, horrific event such as a school fire)

THE INDIVIDUAL

Before proceeding, review the section on the Good Samaritan Act in Chapter 4, which discusses an individual's liability in emergency situations. No matter the location or the emergency, always ask the victim's permission before touching him or her, even though it is in the context of providing first aid. A **medical emergency** is the occurrence of a sudden injury or illness that requires immediate medical intervention. **First aid** is the immediate care rendered in an emergency until definitive or advanced care is available if needed. Being prepared is a major component in effectively dealing with emergencies that arise in the medical office. The medical office generally has guidelines, policies, and procedures for office emergencies and documentation. These should be reviewed and revised on a regular basis and followed when needed. Many of the elements of preparedness come under the roles of the medical assistant and medical administrative specialist.

ACTIVATION OF EMERGENCY MEDICAL SYSTEM (EMS)

- Dial 911 (in most areas)
- Know the correct number if there is no 911 system in the area (e.g., the emergency number for some rural areas may be the police or fire department)

- Know if an alternative to 911, such as 311, is available for less urgent situations
- Have readily available the numbers for poison control center, suicide hotlines, abuse shelters, emergency food banks, and other services that may be used in an emergency
- Know the capacity of the office telephone system (e.g., can you keep a patient on the line *and* activate EMS?)
- Know when your physicians and other medical staff are onsite

MEDICAL ASSISTANT AND MEDICAL ADMINISTRATIVE SPECIALIST ROLES IN EMERGENCIES

- Recognizing emergencies and responding
- Monitoring emergency supplies, equipment, and drug readiness (includes expiration dates on drugs and sterile packs; functioning of battery-operated equipment)
- Knowing the location of emergency supplies
- Restocking equipment after each use
- Maintaining up-to-date emergency phone numbers
- Keeping CPR and other first aid skills current
- Providing personal protection for self, patient, and other involved individuals
- Documenting the event and the first aid rendered
- Observing the environment for possible risks, such as frayed wiring or loose carpeting (risk management)

COMMON EMERGENCY EQUIPMENT AND SUPPLIES IN THE MEDICAL OFFICE

- Oxygen with nasal cannulas and various sizes of oxygen masks
- Various sizes of blood pressure cuffs
- Code cart containing cardiac monitor and defibrillator, emergency drugs, intravenous (IV) solutions with tubing and IV cannulas, tourniquets and tapes, bandage scissors, pen light, Ambu bag, airways, and intubation equipment per physician's preferences and training
- Automatic external defibrillator (AED)
- Personal protective equipment (PPE) (refer to Chapter 17)
- Materials for wound care: antiseptic solution, sterile dressings
- Cold packs
- Emergency childbirth delivery pack (for offices that practice obstetrics) with gloves, blankets, two Kelly clamps, cord clamp, scissors, nasal suction bulb, and plastic bag or container for placenta

RECOGNIZING EMERGENCIES

A four-pronged approach is used in recognizing medical emergencies and determining their seriousness. The first is the ability to determine an emergency exists; the second is to be sure the health care responder or others are not in danger. Health care personnel will then perform primary and secondary assessments.

SIGNS OF EMERGENCIES

- Respiratory distress
- Unconsciousness
- Hemorrhage
- Chest pain
- Wounds or penetrating objects
- Bone protrusions or deformities
- Skin burns
- High or low body temperatures
- Severe pain
- Abnormal skin color
- Abnormal behavior

SCENE MANAGEMENT

The guidelines here apply to the medical office in addition to other sites.

- Ensure dangers do not exist for responder (e.g., wet floor, "hot" wire)
- Remove hazard if this does not pose a danger to the responder
- Remove others in the vicinity of danger if appropriate
- Assign tasks; for example, have someone activate EMS while you are rendering first aid

PRIMARY ASSESSMENT AND TREATMENT PRIORITIES (ABCs)

- A—airway: check open airway using head-tilt/chin-lift method or jaw thrust (for suspected neck injuries) if needed

- B—breathing: ensure patient is breathing by looking for chest movement
- C—circulation: ensure patient has a pulse

SECONDARY ASSESSMENT, IF INDICATED

- Vital signs (pulse, respirations, blood pressure, temperature)
- Skin (color, temperature, degree of moisture)
- Head-to-toe observation and palpation for pain, abnormalities, and bleeding (usually done by physician, midlevel provider, or EMS personnel)
- Level of consciousness

COMMON EMERGENCIES

Common emergencies are listed, along with the first aid treatment generally administered by the medical assistant.

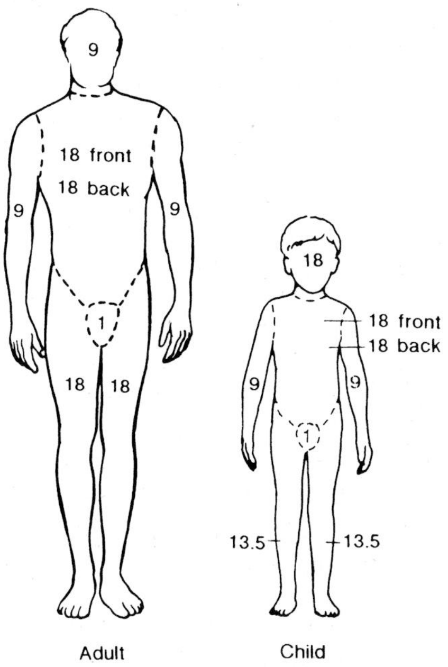

Figure 26-1 Rule of nines. (Reprinted with permission from Hosley JB, Jones SA, Molle-Matthews EA. Lippincott's Textbook for Medical Assistants. Philadelphia: Lippincott-Raven Publishers, 1997.)

BURNS

Burns are tissue damage caused by exposure to heat, chemicals, or electricity. The extent of burns is estimated using the **rule of nines**, in which each body part is considered 9% of the body: the affected parts are added to determine the percentage of body burned (Fig. 26-1).

- First degree (superficial)—involves epidermis; red appearance with minimal or no edema (such as sunburn)
  - Immerse in cool water or provide cool water compresses
  - Avoid ointments or other greasy substances (e.g., butter, which is a home remedy for some cultures)
- Second degree (partial thickness)—involves epidermis and part of dermis; blistered red appearance with edema
  - Immerse in cool (not cold) water or provide cool (not cold) compresses
  - Avoid ointments or other greasy substances
  - May apply dry, sterile dressing
- Third degree (full thickness)—involves epidermis, entire dermis, and often underlying tissues; pale white or charred appearance with broken skin and edema
  - Activate EMS
  - Check ABCs
  - Use sterile gloves and other PPE if indicated
  - Cover affected areas with sterile dressings soaked in sterile saline
  - Observe for shock

SHOCK

Shock is a life-threatening condition related to inadequate oxygen supply. It is often characterized by heavy blood loss; lowered blood pressure; weak, increased pulse; cool, clammy skin; increased respiratory rate; anxiety; and agitation. The most common types of shock are:

- Hypovolemic—shock resulting from hemorrhage (excessive bleeding)
  - Use PPE
  - Cover wound with sterile dressing (if possible) and apply direct pressure
  - Elevate bleeding area
  - Keep head lower than body (except in cases of head wounds)
  - Apply pressure to nearest pressure point (review Fig. 6-16, "Major arteries," in Chapter 6) between bleeding and heart if bleeding does not stop
  - Keep patient warm

- Anaphylactic (anaphylaxis)—shock caused by a severe allergic reaction that results in respiratory distress and, in some instances, cardiac arrest
  - Activate EMS
  - Check ABCs
  - Remove allergen if possible
  - Keep patient warm
- Septic—shock caused by an overwhelming infection affecting major body systems
  - Activate EMS
  - Check ABCs
- Cardiogenic—shock caused by impaired cardiac function; first aid is the same as for septic shock
- Neurogenic—shock caused by trauma or other insult (e.g., toxin) to the nervous system
  - Activate EMS
  - Check ABCs
  - Immobilize head for spinal injury
  - Keep patient warm
  - Prepare to assist with administration of antitoxin if known and available
- Insulin (see "Diabetic Emergencies")

DIABETIC EMERGENCIES

Box 26-1 contains a mnemonic to help differentiate between insulin shock and diabetic coma.

- Insulin shock—severe hypoglycemia in diabetic patients, characterized by rapid heart rate; cold, clammy skin; and confusion
  - Administer sugar (e.g., Insta-Glucose, a glucose gel rapidly absorbed through oral mucosa)
  - Keep patient quiet and at rest
- Diabetic coma—severe hyperglycemia in diabetic patients, characterized by rapid respirations; warm, dry skin; thirst; "fruity" breath (sometimes mistaken for alcohol); and confusion
  - Activate EMS
  - Prepare to bring the insulin and appropriate needle and syringe or administer insulin with the physician's order if within the scope of practice in your state

Box 26-1

Mnemonic to Help Differentiate Between Diabetic Coma and Insulin Shock

Hot and dry; sugar high (diabetic coma)
Cold and clammy; needs some candy (insulin shock)

MYOCARDIAL INFARCTION

Myocardial infarction (MI, heart attack) is necrosis of the cardiac muscle caused by blockage in the coronary artery. It is characterized by chest, left arm, or jaw pain; sweating; rapid respirations; and often nausea and vomiting.

- Activate EMS
- Check ABCs if needed
- Position code cart and AED
- Initiate cardiac monitor
- Take vital signs
- Keep patient calm
- Prepare to assist with administration of oxygen with physician's order

CEREBROVASCULAR ACCIDENT

A **cerebrovascular accident** (CVA, stroke) is the occlusion of a blood vessel or vessels in the brain or hemorrhage in the brain characterized by one or more of the following symptoms: weakness, paralysis of one or more areas, dysphasia or aphasia, and confusion.

- Activate EMS
- Check ABCs, if needed
- Take vital signs
- Keep patient calm
- Prepare to assist with administration of oxygen with physician's order

RESPIRATORY EMERGENCIES

Respiratory emergencies involve the impairment or absence of breathing.

- Respiratory arrest—total absence of breathing
  - Activate EMS
  - Check ABCs
  - Head-tilt/chin-lift maneuver
  - Support breathing by health care provider "breathing" for victim (CPR guidelines) or using an Ambu bag
  - Prepare for cardiac arrest (have code cart, emergency drugs, and cardiac monitor ready; begin chest compressions if pulse/heartbeat stops)
- Asthma—inflammatory lung disease characterized by difficulty breathing caused by airway obstruction
  - Check ABCs
  - Maintain sitting position if conscious

- Keep patient calm
- Assist patient with his or her inhaler if available
- Prepare to initiate small-volume nebulizer with physician order
- Monitor oxygen saturation by using a pulse oximeter

■ Hyperventilation—increased ventilation leading to decreased carbon dioxide, dizziness, and possible unconsciousness; usually stress induced
- Keep patient calm
- Seal paper bag over patient's mouth and nose
- Assist patient with taking slow, deep breaths into paper bag

■ Choking—laryngospasms, usually caused by obstruction of the airway with a foreign object, such as food
- Allow patient to cough
- Use Heimlich maneuver if coughing, speaking, or breathing ceases
  - Standing—get behind victim; rescuer's arms come around to below victim's xiphoid process; rescuer makes fist with dominant hand and administers inward and upward thrusts until foreign object is expelled
  - Lying—if patient loses consciousness, lower him or her to floor, check mouth for foreign objects and, if seen, sweep objects out with fingers; rescuer kneels beside patient, places closed dominant hand below xiphoid process, and administers inward and upward abdominal thrusts until foreign object is expelled

SEIZURES

A **seizure**, or **convulsion**, is an abnormal generalized series of involuntary muscle contraction and relaxation. There are many causes, including brain injury or high fever.

■ Activate EMS
■ Lower patient to floor
■ Protect from injury by furniture or other obstacles
■ Loosen tight clothing
■ Log roll patient if he or she is vomiting
■ Avoid restricting patient or putting *anything* in patient's mouth
■ Assist with breathing if necessary when seizure is over

SYNCOPE

Syncope, also called *fainting* or *swooning*, is transient unconsciousness, usually caused by a sudden decrease in blood pressure or oxygen.

■ Assist the patient in lying down or sitting with head to knees
■ Loosen tight clothing
■ Use ammonia capsule at least 6 inches from nose and avoiding eyes (office policy permitting)
■ Place cool cloth on forehead

COMMON INJURIES

■ Wounds
- Contusion (bruise)—a closed wound usually caused by blunt trauma
  - Apply ice pack or cold compress
  - Observe for increased swelling
- Abrasion—an open wound resulting from scraping off of skin layer(s) by trauma; may or may not produce bleeding
  - Cleanse with soap and water or antiseptic
  - Apply sterile dressing if needed
  - Determine patient's tetanus immunization status
- Avulsion—an open wound caused by forceful tearing away of skin from bony structure by trauma, sometimes leaving a skin flap and causing excessive bleeding
  - Replace skin flap if present
  - Treat the same as an abrasion
- Laceration—a jagged cut into the body tissue
  - Treat the same as an abrasion
  - May require sutures or Steri-Strips
- Puncture—an open wound caused by an object piercing the skin (first aid for bites and stings is the same as punctures and abrasions)
  - Treat the same as an abrasion
- Puncture with fixed penetrating object
  - Activate EMS
  - Leave object imbedded
  - Stabilize object to prevent movement
- Traumatic amputation—the removal of a body part by traumatic event
  - Treat the same as an avulsion
  - Wrap amputated part in sterile moist dressing and transport with patient (do not place on ice)

■ Fracture—broken bones; see Figure 6-10, "Types of fractures," in Chapter 6
- Open fracture—broken bone that protrudes through skin
  - Immobilize with a splint
  - Cover wound with sterile dressing
  - Arrange transport to hospital

- Closed fracture—broken bone without an open wound
  - Immobilize with a splint
  - Apply ice pack or cold compress
  - Elevate; sling may be used to elevate and support hand and lower arm; tie knot off to the side of the neck, avoiding spine

POISONINGS

A **poisoning** is the injection, respiration, or ingestion of a toxic substance (may be natural or chemical).

- Remove substance or victim from area of substance while protecting rescuer (PPE)
- Check ABCs
- Call poison control center for specific instructions
- Do not induce vomiting or administer ipecac unless instructed to do so

EXTREME TEMPERATURE EMERGENCIES

- Hyperthermia—abnormally high body temperature (e.g., heat exhaustion and heat stroke [most serious])
  - Remove from heat source
  - Check ABCs and activate EMS for heat stroke
  - Cool body with wet cloths
  - Slowly administer cool liquids if patient is alert
- Hypothermia—abnormally low body temperature
  - Check ABCs
  - Activate EMS
  - Remove any wet clothing
  - Warm with blankets
  - Slowly administer warm liquids if patient is alert (no alcoholic beverages)
- Frostbite—freezing of body parts; usually affects fingers, toes, ears, and nose
  - Gently wrap affected part in warm material, such as a blanket
  - Do not submerge in water or other liquid or rub
  - Transport to hospital

THE MEDICAL OFFICE

Risk management in Chapter 4 is also a part of medical office safety such as observing for frayed electrical cords. In addition to common hazards, the medical office is at risk for emergencies and safety hazards encompassing more than a single person such as fire or chemical or infectious disease exposures (refer to Chapter 17). The H1N1 influenza in 2009 was an example. Common Occupational Safety and Health Administration (OSHA) and state-specific emergency preparedness guidelines recommend that facilities have:

- An **exposure control plan** that describes personnel protective equipment (PPE) and other safety engineering devices and processes; it provides instructions of what an employee should do if an exposure occurs. The plan should be reviewed annually and contain:
  - Definitions such as biohazardous waste
  - Responsibilities
  - Availability of recommended immunizations
  - Availability and disposal mechanisms of PPE and safety engineering devices
  - Procedures to follow for prevention and exposures
  - Training guidelines
  - Record keeping and reporting
- Adequate PPE and safety engineering devices
- Contract for disposal of biohazardous material
- Material Safety Data Sheets (MSDS)
- Common safety features
  - Fire extinguishers; serviced annually; standard acronym for use
    - **P**—pull the pin
    - **A**—aim the nozzle at the base of the fire
    - **S**—squeeze the trigger while keeping the extinguisher upright
    - **S**—sweep the area using the nozzle and covering the fire with the extinguisher material
  - Proper labeling for safety equipment such as biohazardous waste material and eyewash stations (see Fig. 26-2)
  - Evacuation plan
    - Establish and post evacuation routes
    - Keep hallways and stairways unobstructed at all times
    - Move those closest to danger first
    - Initiate alarm
    - Move those requiring the most assistance last unless in immediate danger
    - Establish area to store mobility assistive devices such as wheelchairs
    - Establish the chain of command; specifically who is in charge
    - Avoid delaying to "grab" valuables
    - Designate responsibility for moving or shutting down flammable substances such as oxygen unless it places the person in danger

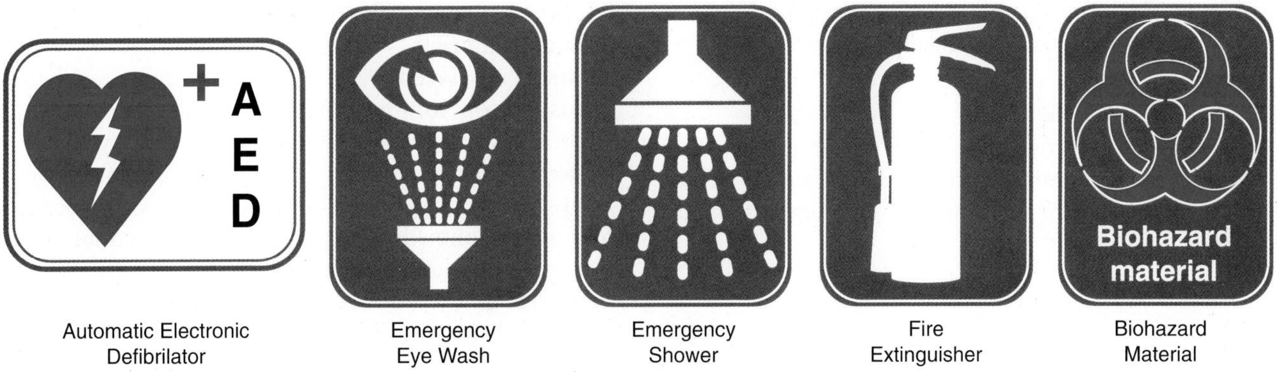

Figure 26-2 Examples of standard safety signs and symbols.

  - Designate a pre-established assembly place
  - Designate who leaves last and assures the facility is empty
  - Establish a means of accounting for all staff, patients, and visitors
  - Do not return until instructed by the appropriate emergency services personnel
  - Conduct evacuation drills (frequency of drills may be required by local authorities; for example, some cities require evacuation in high rise buildings quarterly)
- Clearly marked and lighted exits

THE COMMUNITY

Health care providers often feel a responsibility to the community in times of disaster; the "community" may be local, national or global. Many accrediting bodies such as The Joint Commission require emergency preparedness. This section addresses considerations for response to a local disaster. The medical assistant and medical administrative assistant may be involved in community emergency preparedness on two fronts: within the medical facility and directly within the community emergency preparedness system.

THE MEDICAL FACILITY RESPONSE

The medical facility may agree to take incoming **"walking wounded"** persons who have been triaged at a disaster command center, have minor injuries, and are capable of walking. This is dependent on the size and the affiliation of the facility such as a community health center or medical office adjacent to a hospital. It requires previous coordination and agreements with the local emergency preparedness authorities and the hospital or other facilities that provide a higher level of care. These agreements are updated at specified intervals. Generally, a medical office emergency preparedness committee is appointed. The committee develops and implements an emergency preparedness plan that, at a minimum, includes:

- Designation of roles such as triage officer, area coordinators, recorders, and runners
- Designation of medical office areas such as triage, holding, and treatment
- Readiness of emergency supplies such as PPE, dressings, splints, cots, and blankets; these should be stored and used only for disasters, not for general operation, and checked on a regular basis
- Preassembled "to go box" with pens, pads, tape, clips, vests or large name tags identifying staff roles, and emergency charts with specially designed emergency forms (to date, these forms are hardcopy, not electronic, and move with the patient)
- Staff training and drills (usually semi-annually and coordinated by the local emergency preparedness agency or hospital)
- Response call list for staff if a disaster occurs after hours
- Ancillary services and needs such as rapidly accessing more doses of tetanus toxoid, nearby child care for victims and staff, transport to a facility for higher level of care if needed
- Plan evaluation mechanism

INDIVIDUAL COMMITMENT

Health care providers, including medical assistants and medical administrative specialists, may volunteer, as individuals, with the local emergency preparedness authority or affiliates such as the local department of health to respond to a disaster or emergency. An example is pandemic flu requiring rapid mass immunization. For the individual volunteer this usually involves:

- Completing an application
- Verification of credentials and requirements (may include specific immunizations and fingerprinting or other clearance for working with vulnerable populations)
- Training (may be conducted online)

This community involvement is not covered by the Good Samaritan Act. The volunteer should check with the sponsoring agency to assure inclusion in their liability coverage.

TERMS

Emergency Preparedness Review

The following list reviews the terms discussed in this chapter and other important terms that you may see on the exam.

ABCs (airway, breathing, circulation) primary assessment in emergencies to determine whether the patient's airway is open, breathing is occurring, and blood is appropriately circulating

abrasion open wound resulting in scraping off of skin layer(s) by trauma; may or may not produce bleeding

anaphylaxis shock caused by a severe allergic reaction that results in respiratory distress and, in some instances, cardiac arrest

avulsion open wound caused by forceful tearing away of skin from bony structure by trauma, sometimes leaving a skin flap and causing excessive bleeding

burns tissue damage from exposure to heat, chemicals, or electricity

cardiopulmonary resuscitation (CPR) a standardized approach to providing first aid in a situation in which the victim is not breathing and the heart may have stopped beating

contusion (bruise) closed wound usually caused by blunt trauma

epistaxis nosebleed

exposure control plan plan that describes personnel protective equipment (PPE) and other safety engineering devices and processes; it provides instructions of what an employee should do if an exposure occurs

first aid the immediate care rendered in a medical emergency until definitive or advanced care is available

hemorrhage excessive bleeding that may result in hypovolemic shock

hyperglycemia abnormally high blood glucose level

hyperthermia abnormally high body temperature (e.g., heat exhaustion and heat stroke [most serious])

hypoglycemia abnormally low blood glucose level

hypothermia abnormally low body temperature

laceration straight or jagged cut into the body tissue

medical emergency the occurrence of a sudden injury or illness that requires immediate medical intervention

PASS pull, aim, squeeze, sweep; acronym for using a fire extinguisher

poisoning the injection, respiration, or ingestion of a toxic substance (may be natural or chemical)

rule of nines formula used to determine extent of the body burned; each body part is considered 9% of the body; the affected parts are added to determine the percentage of body burned

seizure convulsion generalized series of involuntary muscle contractions

shock life-threatening condition related to inadequate oxygen supply and often characterized by heavy blood loss; lowered blood pressure; weak, increased pulse; cool, clammy skin; increased respiratory rate; anxiety; and agitation

syncope transient unconsciousness, usually caused by a sudden decrease in blood pressure or oxygen; also called *fainting* or *swooning*

walking wounded persons in a disaster who have been triaged at a command center of the community disaster, have minor injuries, and are capable of walking.

REVIEW QUESTIONS

All questions are relevant for the CMA (AAMA), RMA (AMT), and CMAS (AMT) exam.

1. The type of shock caused by severe allergic reaction is:
   A. traumatic.
   B. septic.
   C. cardiogenic.
   D. anaphylactic.

Answer: **D**

Why: Anaphylactic shock is an immediate type of allergic reaction resulting from hypersensitivity to an antigen. Substances may include drugs, vaccines, certain foods, serum and allergen extracts, insect venom, or chemical products such as latex.

Review: Yes ❑ No ❑

---

2. The type of soft tissue injury that is a closed wound occurring from blunt trauma to the body is a(n):
   A. abrasion.
   B. avulsion.
   C. contusion.
   D. laceration.
   E. puncture.

Answer: **C**

Why: Abrasions, avulsions, lacerations, and punctures are all types of open wounds. A contusion is a closed wound that appears as a bruise on the skin. Blood collects under the skin and causes the discoloration.

Review: Yes ❑ No ❑

---

3. The type of fracture that is common in children and is a partial or incomplete break in the bone is:
   A. comminuted.
   B. greenstick.
   C. open.
   D. spiral.

Answer: **B**

Why: A greenstick fracture is named because the bone breaks like a green branch, only bending and causing a few of the fibers to separate. It is not an open or compound fracture. A spiral fracture is caused by the twisting of a bone.

Review: Yes ❑ No ❑

---

4. To control bleeding or hemorrhage, you should initially:
   A. place ice over the wound.
   B. apply direct pressure.
   C. apply a tourniquet above the injury.
   D. immobilize the body part.
   E. place the bleeding body part lower than the victim's heart.

Answer: **B**

Why: Application of direct pressure over the wound will stop hemorrhage in most cases. Use a tourniquet as a last resort if direct pressure does not stop the bleeding or if the wound is too large to apply direct pressure. If possible, the body part that is bleeding should be elevated higher than the victim's heart.

Review: Yes ❑ No ❑

---

5. The ABCs of CPR include management of:
   A. airway, breathing, circulation.
   B. assessment, breathing, compressions.
   C. alertness, bleeding, circulation.
   D. airway, bleeding, circulation.

Answer: **A**

Why: The ABCs of CPR include an assessment of the major systems of the body that can result in life-threatening situations. First, check the airway to make sure it is open and unobstructed. Second, if the airway is open, ensure that the victim is breathing. Third, determine that the victim's heart is pumping and proper circulation is taking place in the body. This is important to deliver oxygen to the vital body organs.

Review: Yes ❑ No ❑

6. The medical term used to describe a victim who has fainted is:
   A. epistaxis.
   B. shock.
   C. anaphylaxis.
   D. febrile.
   E. syncope.

Answer: **E**

Why: Syncope is usually caused by a sudden fall in blood pressure or loss of oxygen to the brain resulting in loss of consciousness.

Review: Yes ❑ No ❑

---

7. A stroke is also known as:
   A. CVD.
   B. CVA.
   C. CHF.
   D. COPD.

Answer: **B**

Why: The abbreviation CVA means cerebrovascular accident; this occurs when there is damage in the blood vessels in the brain blocking circulation to that part of the brain. Blockage can be caused by a thrombus (blood clot) or embolus (any other abnormal particle). CVD means cardiovascular disease, CHF means congestive heart failure, and COPD means chronic obstructive pulmonary disease.

Review: Yes ❑ No ❑

---

8. Another term for a heart attack is:
   A. cardiovascular disease.
   B. coronary artery disease.
   C. myocardial infarction.
   D. congestive heart failure.
   E. cardiogenic shock.

Answer: **C**

Why: Myocardial infarction means the myocardium, or heart muscle, has experienced damage because of blocked arteries. The blockage is usually the result of plaque buildup in the vessels.

Review: Yes ❑ No ❑

---

9. The treatment of third-degree burns includes:
   A. immersing body part in cold water.
   B. applying an ice pack to the affected part.
   C. removing any blisters that form.
   D. covering the victim and notifying EMS.

Answer: **D**

Why: Third-degree burns are the most invasive type of burn, involving the epidermis, the entire dermis, and sometimes subcutaneous tissue, muscle, and bone. Treatment includes covering the victim with a blanket to conserve warmth and transporting for further treatment, including management of shock.

Review: Yes ❑ No ❑

---

10. Treatment of a victim experiencing convulsions includes the following EXCEPT:
    A. placing the victim on the floor.
    B. providing privacy to the victim.
    C. clearing nearby objects.
    D. not restraining the victim.
    E. placing an airway in the mouth.

Answer: **E**

Why: Nothing should be placed in the victim's mouth during seizure activity. The object may break teeth or obstruct the airway.

Review: Yes ❑ No ❑

---

11. In some cases of poisoning, it is necessary to induce vomiting. The agent used is:
    A. iodine.
    B. ipecac.
    C. adrenalin.
    D. epinephrine.

Answer: **B**

Why: Syrup of ipecac is used to induce vomiting when the victim has ingested a poison that is noncorrosive. It is used because of the emetic (vomit-inducing) effect it has.

Review: Yes ❑ No ❑

12. The type of shock caused from bacterial infection is:
    A. anaphylactic.
    B. cardiogenic.
    C. psychogenic.
    D. septic.
    E. hypovolemic.

Answer: **D**

Why: Sepsis is a condition of something being dirty or unclean. Septic shock is caused from bacteria invading the body and causing a systemic infection, which leads to septicemia, or blood poisoning. The patient will ultimately go into shock.

Review: Yes ❑ No ❑

---

13. A victim experiencing a body temperature below 95°F is:
    A. hypothermic.
    B. hyperthermic.
    C. febrile.
    D. hypovolemic.

Answer: **A**

Why: Hypothermia is an abnormally low body temperature. The external environment can lead to hypothermia. Treatment of hypothermia is internal warming of the body.

Review: Yes ❑ No ❑

---

14. Which of the following is a sign or symptom of shock?
    A. Warm skin
    B. Slow pulse
    C. High blood pressure
    D. Pale skin
    E. Slow respiration

Answer: **D**

Why: Signs of shock include cool, clammy skin, low blood pressure, increased respiratory rate, and rapid pulse. The skin is pale and may appear cyanotic (a blue or purplish coloration) because of decreased oxygen of the blood.

Review: Yes ❑ No ❑

---

15. Characteristics of a first-degree burn include:
    A. blistered skin.
    B. charred skin.
    C. reddened skin.
    D. edema of the skin.

Answer: **C**

Why: First-degree burns are the least serious type of burn. Sunburn is an example of a first-degree burn. The skin is only reddened, with no blisters or broken skin.

Review: Yes ❑ No ❑

---

16. The type of soft tissue injury that causes a jagged wound that bleeds is a(n):
    A. abrasion.
    B. contusion.
    C. puncture.
    D. hematoma.
    E. laceration.

Answer: **E**

Why: A laceration results from tearing of tissues partly or completely. Lacerations are frequently caused by broken glass or metal objects.

Review: Yes ❑ No ❑

---

17. Diabetic coma is caused by:
    A. overproduction of insulin.
    B. low blood glucose level.
    C. lack of insulin.
    D. normal glucose with high insulin level.

Answer: **C**

Why: Diabetic coma results from a lack of insulin causing high blood glucose levels, which results in severe acidosis. A patient with low blood glucose could be in insulin shock, which is the opposite of diabetic coma.

Review: Yes ❑ No ❑

18. To control bleeding from a laceration of the palm of the hand, direct pressure should be placed over the:
    A. subclavian artery.
    B. brachial artery.
    C. medial artery.
    D. radial artery.
    E. cephalic artery.

Answer: **D**

Why: To control bleeding, direct pressure should be placed over the artery closest to the injury and between the injury and the heart.

Review: Yes ❑ No ❑

---

19. To transport a victim with a compound fracture, it is important to:
    A. apply a splint to the limb without repositioning the limb.
    B. straighten the limb and apply a splint.
    C. wrap the extremity with an elastic bandage.
    D. place the fractured bone in alignment and apply an elastic bandage.

Answer: **A**

Why: A compound fracture is a break in the bone with the bone protruding through broken skin. This type of fracture is to be managed without realigning, repositioning, or moving the fractured bone. Apply a splint to the limb in the position of the fracture and seek medical care.

Review: Yes ❑ No ❑

---

20. When applying a triangular sling to support an injured arm, it is important to do all the following EXCEPT:
    A. tie the sling at the neck off to the side of the spine to avoid nerve injury.
    B. elevate the hand slightly to promote better circulation in the hand.
    C. instruct the patient how to reapply the sling if removed.
    D. secure the sling at the elbow to better support the injured limb.
    E. position the hand lower than the level of the heart to avoid accumulation of fluid in the extremity.

Answer: **E**

Why: A triangular sling is used in first aid to immobilize an injured limb. If used to support an injured arm, the sling must be applied so the hand is slightly elevated to encourage good circulation and avoid accumulation of fluid in the extremity. If the hand is lower than the heart, edema can develop in the limb and cause further injury or pain.

Review: Yes ❑ No ❑

---

21. First aid treatment for a puncture wound with a fixed penetrating object includes the following EXCEPT:
    A. removing the object if it is still imbedded in the body.
    B. activating EMS.
    C. applying a sterile dressing around the puncture site.
    D. keeping the victim calm.

Answer: **A**

Why: It is important not to remove the imbedded object but to leave it, stabilize it, and transport the victim to an emergency medical facility for treatment. If the object is removed, further damage may occur to surrounding tissue. Hemorrhage may also be initiated if the object is removed and a blood vessel is opened.

Review: Yes ❑ No ❑

---

22. The type of wound that results from scraping off layer(s) of skin is a(n):
    A. bruise.
    B. laceration.
    C. avulsion.
    D. abrasion.
    E. contusion.

Answer: **D**

Why: An abrasion is described as a rubbing away of a surface. An example is a skinned knee.

Review: Yes ❑ No ❑

23. The emergency treatment for a conscious patient with hypoglycemia is to:
    A. monitor the patient and eventually he or she will recover after the body has produced more insulin.
    B. give the patient some form of sugar by mouth after you have notified and received instructions from the physician or EMS.
    C. give an insulin injection immediately.
    D. immediately transport the victim to his or her own physician's office for treatment.

Answer: **B**

Why: If the patient is conscious, you can give sugar by mouth, but you should always contact the physician or EMS for instructions for treatment. If a victim is unconscious, you will never give anything by mouth. If insulin is injected into a patient with a low blood sugar level (hypoglycemia), the blood sugar level will drop even lower. If it is necessary to transport the patient, use the closest emergency medical facility available, because the victim's medical provider may be too far away.

Review: Yes ❑ No ❑

---

24. Which of the following is a fracture of the radius bone at the wrist?
    A. Compound
    B. Closed
    C. Colles
    D. Greenstick
    E. Spiral

Answer: **C**

Why: A compound fracture occurs when the bone is broken and punctures through the skin. A closed fracture is a fracture of the bone without puncture of the skin. A greenstick is a partial or incomplete fracture of a bone, and a spiral fracture is caused from twisting of a bone. All of these fractures are not specific to a certain bone of the body, but a Colles fracture always involves the radial bone at the wrist.

Review: Yes ❑ No ❑

---

25. It is necessary to perform the Heimlich maneuver if:
    A. the victim is coughing.
    B. the victim says he or she is choking.
    C. the victim is conscious but cannot speak or cough.
    D. the victim becomes unconscious.

Answer: **C**

Why: The Heimlich maneuver is performed to dislodge an object that is obstructing the airway. It is performed when a person is conscious but cannot speak or cough. If he or she can speak or cough, there is an airway or at least a partial airway open and the object may dislodge by itself with enough coughing. The universal sign for choking is a person who is unable to talk or cough and is clutching his or her throat.

Review: Yes ❑ No ❑

---

26. The acronym PASS for using a fire extinguisher means:
    A. point, assess, squeeze, and squirt.
    B. pin, aim, squirt and, sweep.
    C. pull, aim, squeeze, and sweep.
    D. point, assess, squeeze, and sweep.
    E. pull, assert, squirt, and stop.

Answer: **C**

Why: Pull the pin, aim the extinguisher, squeeze the trigger, and sweep the fire is the process for using a fire extinguisher that is correct and has become a standard through common usage.

Review: Yes ❑ No ❑

---

27. Fire extinguishers should be serviced:
    A. monthly.
    B. quarterly.
    C. semi-annually.
    D. annually.

Answer: **D**

Why: Annually is the recommendation from the National Fire Protection Association unless in a "severe environment" such as a chemistry laboratory.

Review: Yes ❑ No ❑

28. Exposure control plan guidelines are recommended by:
    A. MSDS.
    B. OSHA.
    C. EEOC.
    D. ADA.
    E. HIPAA.

Answer: **B**

Why: OSHA is the Occupational Safety and Health Administration under which safety in the workplace falls. MSDS are material safety data sheets and provide information related to chemicals; EEOC is the Equal Employment Opportunity Commission and addresses discrimination in the workplace; the Americans with Disabilities Act (ADA) addresses equal accommodations for people with special needs and the Healthcare Insurance Portability and Accountability Act (HIPAA) involves confidentiality in health care.

Review: Yes ❑ No ❑

---

29. An element of evacuation of a facility is to:
    A. evacuate those closest to danger first.
    B. take valuables with you.
    C. avoid using wheelchairs or other mobility devices.
    D. return as often as possible to assist.

Answer: **A**

Why: To prevent the most harm you would evacuate those closest to the danger first. You should not take anything with you, and you would want to use mobility devices to assist with the evacuation of persons with mobility limitations. You should not return to a facility that is in the process of evacuation. You place yourself and emergency responders in danger.

Review: Yes ❑ No ❑

---

30. An exposure control plan would include:
    A. fire extinguisher servicing.
    B. the evacuation route.
    C. first aid for closed fractures.
    D. storage of mobility devices.
    E. recommended immunizations.

Answer: **E**

Why: The exposure control plan describes personnel protective equipment (PPE) and other safety engineering devices and processes. Recommended immunizations will protect an employee from specific bloodborne diseases and are included in the OSHA guidelines. Fire extinguisher servicing, mobility device storage, and an evacuation route are safety issues that do not fall under exposure control. First aid is not part of an exposure plan with the exception of how employees should protect themselves and others from the spread of pathogens.

Review: Yes ❑ No ❑

Unit 5

Exam Preparation

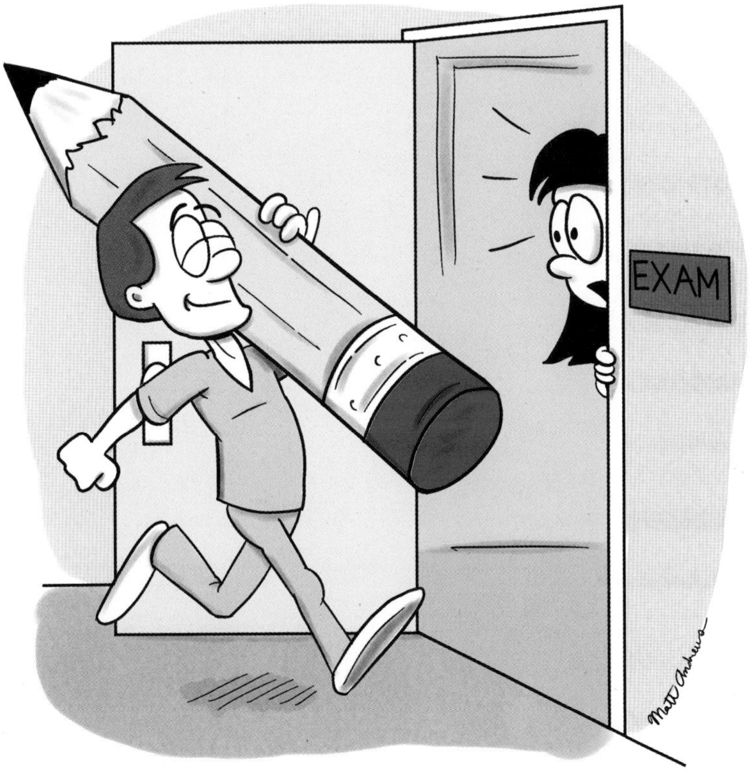

27 Certification Exam Day Advice

Here are a few simple strategies to help relieve the stress of exam day and increase your preparedness. Read them before taking the practice exam.

- Do not cram or study the night before.
- Do what works for you to get a good night's rest.
- Know the exact location of the exam site, including the room (do not guess; consider a trip to the site before exam day).
- Know the parking situation.
- Know the intensity of the traffic for the route and for the time of day of the exam and allow plenty of time to get there.
- Place your exam acceptance letter or permit, photo identification, and other instructions where you will not forget them.
- Wear layered clothes; exam rooms may be cold or hot regardless of the outside temperature.
- Eat a meal or snack that contains protein 30 to 60 minutes before the exam.

ADVICE FOR TAKING THE EXAM

- *Read* the exam instructions carefully; if you are taking the computerized version, know how to get back to answer questions you have not completed. DO NOT forget to submit the exam at the end.
- *Guess* if you do not know an answer. Neither the AAMA nor the AMT penalizes for guessing.
- *Review* the strategies for solving multiple choice questions found in Chapter 1.

Best wishes and remember the words of Sara Henderson, a writer and outpost manager in the Australian outback: "*All the strength you need to achieve anything is within you!*"

PRACTICE EXAM

This timed exam is your opportunity to take a practice exam within a specific period. This will help determine your readiness to sit for the actual exam. Follow these instructions carefully and then proceed with the exam.

1. There are 100 questions and you have 1 hour to complete the practice exam. Set a timer or have someone time the exam for you. Be honest and stop the exam when the hour is completed. Unanswered questions are counted as wrong answers.
2. Use the answer sheet provided. You may photocopy the sheet so you can retake the exam.
3. Do not look at the answer key until you have completed the exam; then compare your answers with the answer key.
4. Choose a quiet, comfortable place to take the exam. Make sure others are aware that you are taking the practice exam so they will not interrupt you.

PRACTICE EXAM–CMA (AAMA)

1. Pathogens that thrive in the absence of oxygen are called:
   A. antitoxins.
   B. anaerobes.
   C. spores.
   D. aerobes.
   E. deoxygenators.

2. A communicable disease that does not have to be reported to the county health department is:
   A. tuberculosis.
   B. streptococcus.
   C. rubella.
   D. syphilis.
   E. rabies.

3. The term **esophagogastritis** means inflammation of the:
   A. larynx and pharynx.
   B. stomach and small intestine.
   C. small intestine and stomach.
   D. esophagus and stomach.
   E. esophagus and small intestine.

4. The structure in the body that lays over the larynx like a lid and prevents food from entering the trachea is the:
   A. pharynx.
   B. uvula.
   C. epiglottis.
   D. glottis.
   E. esophagus.

5. Proper interaction with pediatric patients includes the following EXCEPT:
   A. allowing them to handle safe medical equipment to see that it will not harm them.
   B. using words the child will understand to describe the procedure.
   C. telling a child that a procedure will not hurt at all.
   D. talking in the same tone and volume as you would use with an adult.
   E. positioning yourself at the same level when speaking to the child.

6. A urine test that compares the weight of urine to that of distilled water is:
   A. specific gravity.
   B. clarity.
   C. sedimentation rate.
   D. pH.
   E. ketone analysis.

7. A patient is noncompliant if he or she:
   A. follows the instructions exactly as they were provided.
   B. does not progress as quickly as expected to the treatment plan.
   C. refuses to follow prescribed orders.
   D. has a reaction to prescribed medication.
   E. asks his or her family to participate in the plan.

8. A telephone call that the medical assistant can handle is:
   A. authorizing a prescription refill in the absence of the physician.
   B. advising a patient who is complaining of chest pain after taking new medication.
   C. taking results from a referring physician about a patient's abnormal electrocardiogram results.
   D. a hospital admitting clerk with the room number for a newly admitted patient.
   E. ordering exams for a hospitalized patient.

9. If a certain number of patients are scheduled to come in for an appointment at the beginning of the same clock hour, this is:
   A. modified wave scheduling.
   B. wave scheduling.
   C. block scheduling.
   D. group scheduling.
   E. tidal wave scheduling.

10. When alphabetically filing, which of the following is last?
    A. John A. Hall
    B. John A. Hale
    C. John A. Haley
    D. John A. Halee
    E. John A. Halley

11. The salutation of a letter is placed:
    A. two lines below the inside address.
    B. two lines below the signature line.
    C. before the inside address.
    D. after the complimentary closing.
    E. before the date of the letter.

12. Medical expenses resulting from a back injury while at work are submitted to:
    A. Medicare.
    B. HMO.
    C. Workers' compensation.
    D. employee's health insurance.
    E. Blue Cross/Blue Shield.

13. A ledger is also used as the patient's:
    A. receipt.
    B. charge slip.
    C. statement.
    D. posting.
    E. claim.

14. The book containing procedure and service codes performed by doctors and medical personnel is the:
    A. International Classification of Diseases.
    B. Current Procedural Terminology.
    C. Physician's Desk Reference.
    D. Insurance Payment Manual.
    E. AMA Journal.

15. Ringworm is an example of a disease caused by:
    A. bacteria.
    B. fungus.
    C. virus.
    D. parasite.
    E. yeast.

16. The faint tapping sounds heard as the blood pressure cuff initially deflates are recorded as the:
    A. pulse pressure.
    B. diastolic pressure.
    C. rhythm pressure.
    D. systolic pressure.
    E. apical pressure.

17. A forceps is an instrument used to:
    A. grasp tissue.
    B. retract tissue.
    C. cut tissue.
    D. suture tissue.
    E. clamp a blood vessel.

18. The ECG lead that measures the difference in electrical potential between the right arm and left arm is:
    A. lead II.
    B. lead I.
    C. aVR.
    D. aVF.
    E. V6.

19. Medicare Part B does not cover:
    A. doctor's office visits.
    B. diagnostic laboratory services.
    C. hospital charges.
    D. x-rays in an outpatient facility.
    E. durable medical equipment.

20. The vacuum tube used to collect blood so the blood will clot in the tube is:
    A. red.
    B. lavender.
    C. gray.
    D. green.
    E. blue.

21. An intravenous pyelogram is used to examine the:
    A. liver and gallbladder.
    B. stomach and large intestine.
    C. kidneys and bladder.
    D. colon and ileum.
    E. kidneys and pelvis.

22. Passive exercise means that the patient:
    A. does not move the body part without assistance.
    B. can move the joints freely.
    C. has full range of motion.
    D. cannot move the joints freely.
    E. uses weights when exercising.

23. When nutrients are initially taken into the body, it is called:
    A. digestion.
    B. ingestion.
    C. absorption.
    D. metabolism.
    E. salivation.

24. The muscle used for an injection located in the thigh is the:
    A. gluteus medius.
    B. gluteus maximus.
    C. rectus femoris.
    D. vastus lateralis.
    E. gastrocnemius.

25. Emergency treatment for third-degree burns is:
    A. immersing the body part in cold water.
    B. applying an ice pack to the affected part.
    C. removing any blisters that form.
    D. covering the victim and notifying EMS.
    E. applying an antibiotic ointment.

26. A patient's implied consent usually covers:
    A. organ donation.
    B. biopsy.
    C. blood transfusion.
    D. appendectomy.
    E. electrocardiogram.

27. The medical term that means "within a vessel" is:
    A. intercellular.
    B. interarterial.
    C. intravascular.
    D. intravalvular.
    E. intervascular.

28. An organ located in the left upper quadrant is the:
    A. thymus.
    B. spleen.
    C. appendix.
    D. liver.
    E. gallbladder.

29. Which of the following is an example of nonverbal communication?
    A. Clarification
    B. Feedback
    C. Body language
    D. Messages
    E. E-mail

30. A patient who is sight impaired would benefit from patient educational training materials that are produced as:
    A. Braille materials.
    B. videotapes.
    C. posters.
    D. pamphlets.
    E. brochures.

31. When the medical assistant is dealing with a difficult caller on the phone, he or she should first:
    A. ask the physician to handle the call.
    B. forward the call to the office manager.
    C. tell the caller you will hang up if he or she continues to be difficult.
    D. determine the problem and the appropriate staff that can help.
    E. alert another staff member to witness the call.

32. The abbreviation used in an appointment book to indicate a patient is coming in to see the physician about a medical problem already treated is:
    A. F/U.
    B. CPX.
    C. NP.
    D. BE.
    E. NS.

33. An outguide used in filing is a:
    A. file that is no longer in use.
    B. file of a patient who is not a patient in the office any longer.
    C. guide to alphabetizing file.
    D. folder inserted in the file to hold the place of a file in use.
    E. tickler to remind the staff of something missing from that file.

34. The inside address of a professional letter includes the:
    A. address of the sending physician.
    B. recipient's address written with abbreviation to save space.
    C. physician's residence address printed at the left margin.
    D. recipient's address written without abbreviations.
    E. recipient's insurance company address.

35. The person covered by a benefits plan is the:
    A. administrator.
    B. carrier.
    C. employee.
    D. insured.
    E. payer.

36. The listing of charges for a medical practice is the:
    A. coding chart.
    B. customary charges.
    C. value scale.
    D. value unit.
    E. fee schedule.

37. The withholding from an employee's paycheck for Social Security and Medicare is required under which law?
    A. FICA
    B. FCC
    C. HCFA
    D. IRA
    E. FUTA

38. A yeast infection that causes vaginitis is:
    A. *Candida*.
    B. staphylococci.
    C. *Trichomonas*.
    D. tinea.
    E. scabies.

39. A respiration rate that falls within the average adult range is:
    A. 10 per minute.
    B. 20 per minute.
    C. 25 per minute.
    D. 30 per minute.
    E. below 10 per minute.

40. Proper technique to ensure package sterility includes using:
    A. a sterile package with only a small tear.
    B. sterile packages up to 30 days after the expiration date.
    C. a dry, undamaged sterile package.
    D. sterile gloves to transport sterile packages.
    E. a sterile pack still damp from the autoclave.

41. AC interference in an ECG tracing means:
    A. the patient is having a muscle tremor.
    B. there is a loose electrode connection.
    C. there is electrical interference in the room.
    D. the electrodes are too tight on the patient.
    E. the power to the machine is off.

42. The clear liquid portion of whole blood is:
    A. serum.
    B. thrombin.
    C. hemoglobin.
    D. fibrinogen.
    E. plasma.

43. To convert milligrams to grams:
    A. divide by 100.
    B. divide by 1,000.
    C. multiply by 100.
    D. multiply by 1,000.
    E. subtract the numerator from the denominator.

44. Diabetic coma is due to:
    A. overproduction of insulin.
    B. low blood glucose level.
    C. lack of insulin.
    D. normal glucose with high insulin level.
    E. increased metabolism of glucose.

45. An arthrogram is the radiographic visualization of:
    A. a joint.
    B. a blood vessel.
    C. the gallbladder.
    D. the spinal column.
    E. an artery.

46. Diathermy is an example of an agent that incorporates the use of:
    A. paraffin wax.
    B. cold water.
    C. ultraviolet light.
    D. deep heat.
    E. hot water.

47. Which of the following conditions would benefit from a low-purine diet?
    A. Gout
    B. Obesity
    C. High blood pressure
    D. Constipation
    E. Coronary artery disease

48. Antihypertensive medications are associated with the treatment of:
    A. fever.
    B. vomiting.
    C. high blood pressure.
    D. allergies.
    E. gout.

49. A laceration appears as a:
    A. scrape on the skin.
    B. bruise.
    C. jagged cut.
    D. swelling on the skin.
    E. hematoma.

50. *Res ipsa loquitur* is a Latin term that means which of the following?
    A. Let the buyer beware.
    B. The thing speaks for itself.
    C. The employer is responsible for the employee.
    D. The patient is always first.
    E. The physician is responsible.

51. The medical term meaning "inflammation of the bone" is:
    A. arthritis.
    B. bursitis.
    C. chondritis.
    D. osteitis.
    E. tendonitis.

52. The superior vena cava is the:
   A. vein that carries blood from the lower extremities to the aorta.
   B. artery that carries blood between the heart and lungs.
   C. vein that carries blood between the heart and lungs.
   D. artery that carries blood from the aorta to the kidneys.
   E. vein that carries blood from the upper body back to the heart.

53. Basic communication requires a message and:
   A. sender and receiver.
   B. feedback and body language.
   C. clarification and feedback.
   D. receiver and body language.
   E. a decoder.

54. The term **facsimile** refers to:
   A. fax.
   B. photocopy.
   C. e-mail.
   D. voice mail.
   E. Internet.

55. A matrix is a(n):
   A. form of billing.
   B. appointment book schedule with blocked out periods of time.
   C. form used for insurance filing.
   D. timed laboratory test.
   E. document used for patient billing.

56. The most common method used to chart the patient's medical record is:
   A. CPT.
   B. SOMR.
   C. SOAP.
   D. HCFA.
   E. ICD.

57. The salutation of a letter is the:
   A. closing.
   B. reference line.
   C. enclosure.
   D. greeting.
   E. purpose for writing.

58. Coordination of benefits means:
   A. the amount of money paid by the patient for medical services before the insurance pays.
   B. one insurance plan will work with other insurance plans to determine how much each plan pays.
   C. there is a flat fee paid for each service.
   D. there is a deductible required by the patient before payment from the insurance is made.
   E. each insurance company will pay an equal amount of the patient's bill.

59. ICD-9 codes that identify medical problems for reasons other than illness or injury are known as:
   A. E codes.
   B. M codes.
   C. CPT codes.
   D. V codes.
   E. neoplasms.

60. When a bank uses the term NSF, it means that:
   A. the check is voided and not to be used.
   B. the account is a newly opened account.
   C. there is not enough money to cover the amount of the check.
   D. the bank will issue a cashier's check in the amount of the check.
   E. the bank must wait 1 week before depositing the check.

61. The proper time and temperature for sterilizing instruments is:
   A. 30 minutes at 150°F.
   B. 45 minutes at 250°F.
   C. 60 minutes at 150°F.
   D. 30 minutes at 250°F.
   E. 20 minutes at 150°F.

62. The Fowler's position is used for:
   A. female pelvic exam.
   B. exam of the abdomen.
   C. patient with difficulty breathing.
   D. sigmoidoscopy.
   E. exam of the spine.

63. The abbreviation OU is no longer in use. Instead of using OU, which of the following should be written?
   A. Both eyes
   B. Right ear
   C. Both ears
   D. Left eye
   E. Optical unit

64. Which of the following is the finer or smaller suture?
A. 2-0
B. 4-0
C. 0-0
D. 10-0
E. 1-0

65. The V1 ECG lead is located:
A. between the fourth and fifth intercostal space.
B. over the left nipple.
C. between the second and third intercostal space.
D. at the fourth intercostal space to the right of the sternum.
E. at the fourth intercostal space to the left of the sternum.

66. Which of the following is a proper site for a capillary puncture?
A. Tip of ring finger
B. Heel of an adult
C. Tip of index finger
D. Tip of little finger
E. Earlobe of an infant

67. The abbreviation used to indicate that a patient should be fasting for an exam is:
A. NPO.
B. AC.
C. PC.
D. NOS.
E. CBC.

68. KUB is an x-ray examination of the:
A. heart and lungs.
B. spinal column.
C. liver and gallbladder.
D. abdomen.
E. urinary system.

69. Cold applied to part of the body causes the effect of:
A. vasoconstriction.
B. vasodilation.
C. increased blood flow to the body part.
D. increased blood pressure to the area.
E. muscle rigor.

70. A patient with arteriosclerosis would benefit from which of the following diets?
A. Low salt
B. Low carbohydrate
C. Low protein
D. Low cholesterol
E. High protein

71. The first action to control bleeding or hemorrhage is to:
A. place ice over the wound.
B. apply direct pressure.
C. apply a tourniquet above the injury.
D. immobilize the body part.
E. elevate the head.

72. The term **enteritis** means inflammation of the:
A. colon.
B. small intestine.
C. stomach.
D. esophagus.
E. gallbladder.

73. An example of active immunity is:
A. maternal antibodies passed through the uterus to the baby.
B. immunization with antibodies.
C. maternal antibodies acquired by the baby from breast milk.
D. producing antibodies as a result of having a disease.
E. avoiding an infected person.

74. When a person refuses to acknowledge the loss of a loved one, this type of behavior is:
A. sympathy.
B. mourning.
C. denial.
D. depression.
E. withdrawal.

75. The computer device that displays the written data is the:
A. disk drive.
B. monitor.
C. hard drive.
D. floppy disk.
E. software.

76. When the doctor is late and not yet at the office, the medical assistant should:
A. offer waiting patients an opportunity to reschedule.
B. cancel all remaining appointments for the day.
C. reschedule all the patients for another day.
D. offer to refer the patients to another physician's practice.
E. close the office and notify the answering service.

77. The "O" in the SOAP method of charting includes the:
A. blood pressure reading.
B. opinion of a family member.
C. symptoms the patient states.
D. prior complaints from the patient.
E. patient's demographics.

78. To retain insurance coverage, the individual must pay the cost of the insurance, which is the:
A. premium.
B. copayment.
C. coinsurance.
D. deductible.
E. reimbursement.

79. CPT is an abbreviation of the reference manual used for:
A. ordering laboratory tests.
B. billing insurance companies for procedures.
C. reporting diseases to the CDC.
D. selecting the fees for each exam.
E. providing the diagnosis on a claim.

80. The best way to ensure that patients pay for services is to:
A. ask patients where they would like the bill mailed.
B. give a copy of the bill to patients when they leave the office.
C. confirm the name of the patient's insurance company.
D. accept checks only, not credit cards.
E. ask for payment of services at the time of the office visit.

81. Acquired immunodeficiency syndrome is caused by:
A. yeast.
B. fungi.
C. bacteria.
D. a virus.
E. a parasite.

82. The pulse point located on the top of the foot is the:
A. femoral.
B. dorsalis pedis.
C. temporal.
D. popliteal.
E. ulnar.

83. An instrument required on a suture tray is a:
A. dilator.
B. scalpel.
C. retractor.
D. needle holder.
E. stapler remover.

84. The ECG grounding lead is attached to the:
A. RA.
B. LA.
C. RL.
D. LL.
E. AV.

85. A urine specimen that is collected after eating is called:
A. clean catch.
B. random.
C. voided.
D. postprandial.
E. timed.

86. A myelogram is an x-ray examination of the:
A. spinal cord.
B. brain.
C. muscles.
D. heart.
E. abdomen.

87. A physician orders amoxicillin 1 Gm to be divided into 4 equal doses. Available is amoxicillin 250 mg/5 mL. How many milliliters will the patient receive for each dose?
A. 0.5 mL
B. 1 mL
C. 5 mL
D. 10 mL
E. 2 mL

88. Anaphylaxis refers to a:
A. nose bleed.
B. type of shock.
C. hemorrhage disorder.
D. congenital disorder.
E. heart attack.

89. Dyspepsia refers to:
A. difficulty speaking.
B. difficult digestion.
C. difficulty breathing.
D. abnormal pain.
E. difficulty swallowing.

90. The perineum is the:
A. lining of the abdomen.
B. covering of the spinal cord.
C. floor of the pelvis.
D. outside lining of the lungs.
E. lining of the heart.

91. *Respondeat superior* refers to:
A. a subpoena.
B. a physician's responsibility for the actions of his staff.
C. something for something, a favor for a favor.
D. responding to your superiors.
E. the thing speaks for itself.

92. The proper angle of the needle to the skin when administering a subcutaneous injection is:
A. 10°.
B. 15°.
C. 45°.
D. 75°.
E. 90°.

93. Which of the following is not considered for use on the skin for cleansing?
A. Acetone
B. Povidone-iodine
C. Betadine
D. Alcohol
E. Hibiclens

94. Which of the following instruments is used to evaluate lung capacity?
A. Audiometer
B. Goniometer
C. Sphygmomanometer
D. Spirometer
E. Doppler

95. The process by which nutrients transfer from the gastrointestinal system into the blood is referred to as:
A. ingestion.
B. digestion.
C. absorption.
D. metabolism.
E. mastication.

96. The classification of drugs used to relieve pain is:
A. antidepressant.
B. analgesic.
C. antibiotic.
D. antidote.
E. antihypertensive.

97. The device used to check vision is a(n):
A. otoscope.
B. ophthalmoscope.
C. Snellen chart.
D. tuning fork.
E. flashlight.

98. A wound that results from scraping the skin is a(n):
A. laceration.
B. avulsion.
C. contusion.
D. evisceration.
E. abrasion.

99. When several tubes of blood are to be drawn, which is drawn first?
A. Anticoagulant tubes
B. Blood culture tubes
C. Tubes with no additive
D. Heparinized tubes
E. EDTA tubes

100. The parenteral method of administration of medication means that the drug is:
A. rubbed on the skin.
B. inserted rectally.
C. swallowed.
D. dissolved in the mouth.
E. injected.

ANSWERS TO PRACTICE EXAM—CMA (AAMA)

1. B
2. B
3. D
4. C
5. C
6. A
7. C
8. D
9. B
10. E
11. A
12. C
13. C
14. B
15. B
16. D
17. A
18. B
19. C
20. A
21. C
22. A
23. B
24. D
25. D
26. E
27. C
28. B
29. C
30. A
31. D
32. A
33. D
34. D
35. D
36. E
37. A
38. A
39. B
40. C
41. C
42. E
43. B
44. C
45. A
46. D
47. A
48. C
49. C
50. B
51. D
52. E
53. A
54. A
55. B
56. C
57. D
58. B
59. D
60. C
61. D
62. C
63. A
64. D
65. D
66. A
67. A
68. E
69. A
70. D
71. B
72. B
73. D
74. C
75. B
76. A
77. A
78. A
79. B
80. E
81. D
82. B
83. D
84. C
85. D
86. A
87. C
88. B
89. B
90. C
91. B
92. C
93. A
94. D
95. C
96. B
97. C
98. E
99. B
100. E

PRACTICE EXAM–RMA (AMT)

1. Pathogens that thrive in the absence of oxygen are called:
   A. antitoxins.
   B. anaerobes.
   C. spores.
   D. aerobes.

2. A communicable disease that does not have to be reported to the county health department is:
   A. tuberculosis.
   B. streptococcus.
   C. rubella.
   D. syphilis.

3. The term **esophagogastritis** means inflammation of the:
   A. larynx and pharynx.
   B. stomach and small intestine.
   C. small intestine and stomach.
   D. esophagus and stomach.

4. The structure in the body that lays over the larynx like a lid and prevents food from entering the trachea is the:
   A. pharynx.
   B. uvula.
   C. epiglottis.
   D. glottis.

5. Proper interaction with pediatric patients includes the following EXCEPT:
   A. allowing them to handle safe medical equipment to see that it will not harm them.
   B. using words the child will understand to describe the procedure.
   C. telling a child that a procedure will not hurt at all.
   D. talking in the same tone and volume as you would use with an adult.

6. A urine test that compares the weight of urine to that of distilled water is:
   A. specific gravity.
   B. clarity.
   C. sedimentation rate.
   D. pH.

7. A patient is noncompliant if he or she:
   A. follows the instructions exactly as they were provided.
   B. does not progress as quickly as expected to the treatment plan.
   C. refuses to follow prescribed orders.
   D. has a reaction to prescribed medication.

8. A telephone call that the medical assistant can handle is:
   A. authorizing a prescription refill in the absence of the physician.
   B. advising a patient who is complaining of chest pain after taking new medication.
   C. taking results from a referring physician about a patient's abnormal electrocardiogram results.
   D. a hospital admitting clerk with the room number for a newly admitted patient.

9. If a certain number of patients are scheduled to come in for an appointment at the beginning of the same clock hour, this is:
   A. modified wave scheduling.
   B. wave scheduling.
   C. block scheduling.
   D. group scheduling.

10. When alphabetically filing, which of the following is last?
    A. John A. Hall
    B. John A. Hale
    C. John A. Halley
    D. John A. Halee

11. The salutation of a letter is placed:
    A. two lines below the inside address.
    B. two lines below the signature line.
    C. before the inside address.
    D. after the complimentary closing.

12. Medical expenses resulting from a back injury while at work are submitted to:
    A. Medicare.
    B. HMO.
    C. Workers' compensation.
    D. employee's health insurance.

13. A ledger is also used as the patient's:
    A. receipt.
    B. charge slip.
    C. statement.
    D. posting.

14. The book containing procedure and service codes performed by doctors and medical personnel is the:
    A. International Classification of Diseases.
    B. Current Procedural Terminology.
    C. Physician's Desk Reference.
    D. Insurance Payment Manual.

15. Ringworm is an example of a disease caused by:
    A. bacteria.
    B. fungus.
    C. virus.
    D. parasite.

16. The faint tapping sounds heard as the blood pressure cuff initially deflates are recorded as the:
    A. pulse pressure.
    B. diastolic pressure.
    C. rhythm pressure.
    D. systolic pressure.

17. A forceps is an instrument used to:
    A. grasp tissue.
    B. retract tissue.
    C. cut tissue.
    D. suture tissue.

18. The ECG lead that measures the difference in electrical potential between the right arm and left arm is:
    A. lead II.
    B. lead I.
    C. aVR.
    D. aVF.

19. Medicare Part B does not cover:
    A. doctor's office visits.
    B. diagnostic laboratory services.
    C. hospital charges.
    D. x-rays in an outpatient facility.

20. The vacuum tube used to collect blood so the blood will clot in the tube is:
    A. red.
    B. lavender.
    C. gray.
    D. green.

21. An intravenous pyelogram is used to examine the:
    A. liver and gallbladder.
    B. stomach and large intestine.
    C. kidneys and bladder.
    D. colon and ileum.

22. Passive exercise means that the patient:
    A. does not move the body part without assistance.
    B. can move the joints freely.
    C. has full range of motion.
    D. cannot move the joints freely.

23. When nutrients are initially taken into the body, it is called:
    A. digestion.
    B. ingestion.
    C. absorption.
    D. metabolism.

24. The muscle used for an injection located in the thigh is the:
    A. gluteus medius.
    B. gluteus maximus.
    C. rectus femoris.
    D. vastus lateralis.

25. Emergency treatment for third-degree burns is:
    A. immersing the body part in cold water.
    B. applying an ice pack to the affected part.
    C. removing any blisters that form.
    D. covering the victim and notifying EMS.

26. A patient's implied consent usually covers:
    A. organ donation.
    B. electrocardiogram.
    C. blood transfusion.
    D. appendectomy.

27. The medical term that means "within a vessel" is:
    A. intercellular.
    B. interarterial.
    C. intravascular.
    D. intravalvular.

28. An organ located in the left upper quadrant is the:
    A. thymus.
    B. spleen.
    C. appendix.
    D. liver.

29. Which of the following is an example of nonverbal communication?
    A. Clarification
    B. Feedback
    C. Body language
    D. Messages

30. A patient who is sight impaired would benefit from patient educational training materials that are produced as:
    A. Braille materials.
    B. videotapes.
    C. posters.
    D. pamphlets.

31. When the medical assistant is dealing with a difficult caller on the phone, he or she should first:
A. ask the physician to handle the call.
B. forward the call to the office manager.
C. tell the caller you will hang up if he or she continues to be difficult.
D. determine the problem and the appropriate staff that can help.

32. The abbreviation used in an appointment book to indicate a patient is coming in to see the physician about a medical problem already treated is:
A. F/U.
B. CPX.
C. NP.
D. BE.

33. An outguide used in filing is a:
A. file that is no longer in use.
B. file of a patient that is not a patient in the office any longer.
C. guide to alphabetizing file.
D. folder inserted in the file to hold the place of a file in use.

34. The inside address of a professional letter includes the:
A. address of the sending physician.
B. recipient's address written with abbreviation to save space.
C. physician's residence address printed at the left margin.
D. recipient's address written without abbreviations.

35. The person covered by a benefits plan is the:
A. administrator.
B. carrier.
C. employee.
D. insured.

36. The listing of charges for a medical practice is the:
A. fee schedule.
B. customary charges.
C. value scale.
D. value unit.

37. The withholding from an employee's paycheck for Social Security and Medicare is required under which law?
A. FICA
B. FCC
C. HCFA
D. IRA

38. A yeast infection that causes vaginitis is:
A. *Candida.*
B. staphylococci.
C. *Trichomonas.*
D. tinea.

39. A respiration rate that falls within the average adult range is:
A. 10 per minute.
B. 20 per minute.
C. 25 per minute.
D. 30 per minute.

40. Proper technique to ensure package sterility includes using:
A. a sterile package with only a small tear.
B. sterile packages up to 30 days after the expiration date.
C. a dry, undamaged sterile package.
D. sterile gloves to transport sterile packages.

41. AC interference in an ECG tracing means:
A. the patient is having a muscle tremor.
B. there is a loose electrode connection.
C. there is electrical interference in the room.
D. the electrodes are too tight on the patient.

42. The clear liquid portion of whole blood is:
A. serum.
B. thrombin.
C. hemoglobin.
D. plasma.

43. To convert milligrams to grams:
A. divide by 100.
B. divide by 1,000.
C. multiply by 100.
D. multiply by 1,000.

44. Diabetic coma is due to:
A. overproduction of insulin.
B. low blood glucose level.
C. lack of insulin.
D. normal glucose with high insulin level.

45. An arthrogram is the radiographic visualization of:
A. a joint.
B. a blood vessel.
C. the gallbladder.
D. the spinal column.

46. Diathermy is an example of an agent that incorporates the use of:
A. paraffin wax.
B. cold water.
C. ultraviolet light.
D. deep heat.

47. Which of the following conditions would benefit from a low-purine diet?
A. Gout
B. Obesity
C. High blood pressure
D. Constipation

48. Antihypertensive medications are associated with the treatment of:
A. fever.
B. vomiting.
C. high blood pressure.
D. allergies.

49. A laceration appears as a:
A. scrape on the skin.
B. bruise.
C. jagged cut.
D. swelling on the skin.

50. *Res ipsa loquitur* is a Latin term that means which of the following?
A. Let the buyer beware.
B. The thing speaks for itself.
C. The employer is responsible for the employee.
D. The patient is always first.

51. The medical term meaning "inflammation of the bone" is:
A. arthritis.
B. bursitis.
C. chondritis.
D. osteitis.

52. The superior vena cava is the:
A. vein that carries blood from the lower extremities to the aorta.
B. artery that carries blood between the heart and lungs.
C. vein that carries blood from the upper body back to the heart.
D. vein that carries blood between the heart and lungs.

53. Basic communication requires a message and:
A. sender and receiver.
B. feedback and body language.
C. clarification and feedback.
D. receiver and body language.

54. The term **facsimile** refers to:
A. fax.
B. photocopy.
C. e-mail.
D. voice mail.

55. A matrix is a(n):
A. form of billing.
B. appointment book schedule with blocked out periods of time.
C. form used for insurance filing.
D. timed laboratory test.

56. The most common method used to chart the patient's medical record is:
A. CPT.
B. SOMR.
C. SOAP.
D. HCFA.

57. The salutation of a letter is the:
A. closing.
B. reference line.
C. enclosure.
D. greeting.

58. Coordination of benefits means:
A. the amount of money paid by the patient for medical services before the insurance pays.
B. one insurance plan will work with other insurance plans to determine how much each plan pays.
C. each insurance company will pay an equal amount of the patient's bill.
D. there is a deductible required by the patient before payment from the insurance is made.

59. ICD-9 codes that identify medical problems for reasons other than illness or injury are known as:
A. E codes.
B. M codes.
C. CPT codes.
D. V codes.

60. When a bank uses the term NSF, it means that:
A. the check is voided and not to be used.
B. the account is a newly opened account.
C. there is not enough money to cover the amount of the check.
D. the bank will issue a cashier's check in the amount of the check.

61. The proper time and temperature for sterilizing instruments is:
    A. 30 minutes at 150°F.
    B. 45 minutes at 250°F.
    C. 60 minutes at 150°F.
    D. 30 minutes at 250°F.

62. The Fowler's position is used for:
    A. female pelvic exam.
    B. exam of the abdomen.
    C. patient with difficulty breathing.
    D. sigmoidoscopy.

63. The abbreviation OU is no longer in use. Instead of using OU, which of the following should be written?
    A. Both eyes
    B. Right ear
    C. Both ears
    D. Left eye

64. Which of the following is the finer or smaller suture?
    A. 2-0
    B. 4-0
    C. 0-0
    D. 10-0

65. The V1 ECG lead is located:
    A. between the fourth and fifth intercostal space.
    B. at the fourth intercostal space to the left of the sternum.
    C. between the second and third intercostal space.
    D. at the fourth intercostal space to the right of the sternum.

66. Which of the following is a proper site for a capillary puncture?
    A. Tip of ring finger
    B. Heel of an adult
    C. Tip of index finger
    D. Tip of little finger

67. The abbreviation used to indicate that a patient should be fasting for an exam is:
    A. NPO.
    B. AC.
    C. PC.
    D. NOS.

68. KUB is an x-ray examination of the:
    A. urinary system.
    B. spinal column.
    C. liver and gallbladder.
    D. abdomen.

69. Cold applied to part of the body causes the effect of:
    A. vasoconstriction.
    B. vasodilation.
    C. increased blood flow to the body part.
    D. increased blood pressure to the area.

70. A patient with arteriosclerosis would benefit from which of the following diets?
    A. Low salt
    B. Low carbohydrate
    C. Low protein
    D. Low cholesterol

71. The first action to control bleeding or hemorrhage is to:
    A. place ice over the wound.
    B. apply direct pressure.
    C. apply a tourniquet above the injury.
    D. immobilize the body part.

72. The term **enteritis** means inflammation of the:
    A. colon.
    B. small intestine.
    C. stomach.
    D. esophagus.

73. An example of active immunity is:
    A. maternal antibodies passed through the uterus to the baby.
    B. immunization with antibodies.
    C. maternal antibodies acquired by the baby from breast milk.
    D. producing antibodies as a result of having a disease.

74. When a person refuses to acknowledge the loss of a loved one, this type of behavior is:
    A. sympathy.
    B. mourning.
    C. denial.
    D. depression.

75. The computer device that displays the written data is the:
    A. disk drive.
    B. monitor.
    C. hard drive.
    D. floppy disk.

76. When the doctor is late and not yet at the office, the medical assistant should:
    A. offer waiting patients an opportunity to reschedule.
    B. cancel all remaining appointments for the day.
    C. reschedule all the patients for another day.
    D. offer to refer the patients to another physician's practice.

77. The "O" in the SOAP method of charting includes the:
A. blood pressure reading.
B. opinion of a family member.
C. symptoms the patient states.
D. prior complaints from the patient.

78. To retain insurance coverage, the individual must pay the cost of the insurance, which is the:
A. premium.
B. copayment.
C. coinsurance.
D. deductible.

79. CPT is an abbreviation of the reference manual used for:
A. ordering laboratory tests.
B. billing insurance companies for procedures.
C. reporting diseases to the CDC.
D. selecting the fees for each exam.

80. The best way to ensure that patients pay for services is to:
A. ask patients where they would like the bill mailed.
B. ask for payment of services at the time of the office visit.
C. confirm the name of the patient's insurance company.
D. accept checks only, not credit cards.

81. Acquired immunodeficiency syndrome is caused by:
A. yeast.
B. fungi.
C. bacteria.
D. a virus.

82. The pulse point located on the top of the foot is the:
A. femoral.
B. dorsalis pedis.
C. temporal.
D. popliteal.

83. An instrument required on a suture tray is a:
A. dilator.
B. scalpel.
C. retractor.
D. needle holder.

84. The ECG grounding lead is attached to the:
A. RA.
B. LA.
C. RL.
D. LL.

85. A urine specimen that is collected after eating is called:
A. clean catch.
B. random.
C. voided.
D. postprandial.

86. A myelogram is an x-ray examination of the:
A. spinal cord.
B. brain.
C. muscles.
D. heart.

87. A physician orders amoxicillin 1 Gm to be divided into 4 equal doses. Available is amoxicillin 250 mg/5 mL. How many milliliters will the patient receive for each dose?
A. 0.5 mL
B. 1 mL
C. 5 mL
D. 10 mL

88. Anaphylaxis refers to a:
A. nose bleed.
B. type of shock.
C. hemorrhage disorder.
D. congenital disorder.

89. Dyspepsia refers to:
A. difficulty speaking.
B. difficult digestion.
C. difficulty breathing.
D. abnormal pain.

90. The perineum is the:
A. lining of the abdomen.
B. covering of the spinal cord.
C. floor of the pelvis.
D. outside lining of the lungs.

91. *Respondeat superior* refers to:
A. a subpoena.
B. a physician's responsibility for the actions of his staff.
C. something for something, a favor for a favor.
D. responding to your superiors.

92. The proper angle of the needle to the skin when administering a subcutaneous injection is:
A. 10°.
B. 15°.
C. 45°.
D. 75°.

93. Which of the following is not considered for use on the skin for cleansing?
A. Acetone
B. Povidone-iodine
C. Betadine
D. Alcohol

94. Which of the following instruments is used to evaluate lung capacity?
A. Audiometer
B. Goniometer
C. Sphygmomanometer
D. Spirometer

95. The process by which nutrients transfer from the gastrointestinal system into the blood is referred to as:
A. ingestion.
B. digestion.
C. absorption.
D. metabolism.

96. The classification of drugs used to relieve pain is:
A. antidepressant.
B. analgesic.
C. antibiotic.
D. antidote.

97. The device used to check vision is a(n):
A. otoscope.
B. ophthalmoscope.
C. Snellen chart.
D. tuning fork.

98. A wound that results from scraping the skin is a(n):
A. laceration.
B. avulsion.
C. contusion.
D. abrasion.

99. When several tubes of blood are to be drawn, which is drawn first?
A. Anticoagulant tubes
B. Blood culture tubes
C. Tubes with no additive
D. Heparinized tubes

100. The parenteral method of administration of medication means that the drug is:
A. rubbed on the skin.
B. inserted rectally.
C. swallowed.
D. injected.

ANSWERS TO PRACTICE EXAM—RMA (AMT)

1. B
2. B
3. D
4. C
5. C
6. A
7. C
8. D
9. B
10. C
11. A
12. C
13. C
14. B
15. B
16. D
17. A
18. B
19. C
20. A
21. C
22. A
23. B
24. D
25. D
26. B
27. C
28. B
29. C
30. A
31. D
32. A
33. D
34. D
35. D
36. A
37. A
38. A
39. B
40. C
41. C
42. D
43. B
44. C
45. A
46. D
47. A
48. C
49. C
50. B
51. D
52. C
53. A
54. A
55. B
56. C
57. D
58. B
59. D
60. C
61. D
62. C
63. A
64. D
65. D
66. A
67. A
68. A
69. A
70. D
71. B
72. B
73. D
74. C
75. B
76. A
77. A
78. A
79. B
80. B
81. D
82. B
83. D
84. C
85. D
86. A
87. C
88. B
89. B
90. C
91. B
92. C
93. A
94. D
95. C
96. B
97. C
98. D
99. B
100. D

PRACTICE EXAM–CMAS (AMT)

1. Pathogens that thrive in the absence of oxygen are called:
   A. antitoxins.
   B. anaerobes.
   C. spores.
   D. aerobes.

2. A communicable disease that does not have to be reported to the county health department is:
   A. tuberculosis.
   B. streptococcus.
   C. rubella.
   D. syphilis.

3. The term **esophagogastritis** means inflammation of the:
   A. larynx and pharynx.
   B. stomach and small intestine.
   C. small intestine and stomach.
   D. esophagus and stomach.

4. The structure in the body that lays over the larynx like a lid and prevents food from entering the trachea is the:
   A. pharynx.
   B. uvula.
   C. epiglottis.
   D. glottis.

5. Proper interaction with pediatric patients includes the following EXCEPT:
   A. allowing them to handle safe medical equipment to see that it will not harm them.
   B. using words the child will understand to describe the procedure.
   C. telling a child that a procedure will not hurt at all.
   D. talking in the same tone and volume as you would use with an adult.

6. A urine test that compares the weight of urine to that of distilled water is:
   A. specific gravity.
   B. clarity.
   C. sedimentation rate.
   D. pH.

7. A patient is noncompliant if he or she:
   A. follows the instructions exactly as they were provided.
   B. does not progress as quickly as expected to the treatment plan.
   C. refuses to follow prescribed orders.
   D. has a reaction to prescribed medication.

8. A telephone call that the medical assistant can handle is:
   A. authorizing a prescription refill in the absence of the physician.
   B. advising a patient who is complaining of chest pain after taking new medication.
   C. taking results from a referring physician about a patient's abnormal electrocardiogram results.
   D. a hospital admitting clerk with the room number for a newly admitted patient.

9. If a certain number of patients are scheduled to come in for an appointment at the beginning of the same clock hour, this is:
   A. modified wave scheduling.
   B. wave scheduling.
   C. block scheduling.
   D. group scheduling.

10. When alphabetically filing, which of the following is last?
    A. John A. Hall
    B. John A. Hale
    C. John A. Halley
    D. John A. Halee

11. The salutation of a letter is placed:
    A. two lines below the inside address.
    B. two lines below the signature line.
    C. before the inside address.
    D. after the complimentary closing.

12. Medical expenses resulting from a back injury while at work are submitted to:
    A. Medicare.
    B. HMO.
    C Workers' compensation.
    D. employee's health insurance.

13. A ledger is also used as the patient's:
    A. receipt.
    B. charge slip.
    C. statement.
    D. posting.

14. The book containing procedure and service codes performed by doctors and medical personnel is the:
    A. International Classification of Diseases.
    B. Current Procedural Terminology.
    C. Physician's Desk Reference.
    D. Insurance Payment Manual.

15. Ringworm is an example of a disease caused by:
    A. bacteria.
    B. fungus.
    C. virus.
    D. parasite.

16. The faint tapping sounds heard as the blood pressure cuff initially deflates are recorded as the:
    A. pulse pressure.
    B. diastolic pressure.
    C. rhythm pressure.
    D. systolic pressure.

17. A forceps is an instrument used to:
    A. grasp tissue.
    B. retract tissue.
    C. cut tissue.
    D. suture tissue.

18. An evacuation plan requires:
    A. keeping hallways unobstructed at all times.
    B. maintaining MSDS.
    C. using a fire extinguisher.
    D. returning to the building to help others.

19. Medicare Part B does not cover:
    A. doctor's office visits.
    B. diagnostic laboratory services.
    C. hospital charges.
    D. x-rays in an outpatient facility.

20. PASS is an acronym for:
    A. using a fire extinguisher.
    B. keeping hallways unobstructed at all times.
    C. maintaining MSDS.
    D. returning to the building during an evacuation to help others.

21. An intravenous pyelogram is used to examine the:
    A. liver and gallbladder.
    B. stomach and large intestine.
    C. kidneys and bladder.
    D. colon and ileum.

22. Passive exercise means that the patient:
    A. does not move the body part without assistance.
    B. can move the joints freely.
    C. has full range of motion.
    D. cannot move the joints freely.

23. When nutrients are initially taken into the body, it is called:
    A. digestion.
    B. ingestion.
    C. absorption.
    D. metabolism.

24. The term that demonstrates how each rank is accountable to those directly superior is called:
    A. the agenda.
    B. autocratic management style.
    C. participatory management.
    D. the chain of command.

25. Emergency treatment for third-degree burns is:
    A. immersing the body part in cold water.
    B. applying an ice pack to the affected part.
    C. removing any blisters that form.
    D. covering the victim and notifying EMS.

26. A patient's implied consent usually covers:
    A. organ donation.
    B. electrocardiogram.
    C. blood transfusion.
    D. appendectomy.

27. The medical term that means "within a vessel" is:
    A. intercellular.
    B. interarterial.
    C. intravascular.
    D. intravalvular.

28. An organ located in the left upper quadrant is the:
    A. thymus.
    B. spleen.
    C. appendix.
    D. liver.

29. Which of the following is an example of nonverbal communication?
    A. Clarification
    B. Feedback
    C. Body language
    D. Messages

30. A patient who is sight impaired would benefit from patient educational training materials that are produced as:
    A. Braille materials.
    B. videotapes.
    C. posters.
    D. pamphlets.

31. When the medical assistant is dealing with a difficult caller on the phone, he or she should first:
    A. ask the physician to handle the call.
    B. forward the call to the office manager.
    C. tell the caller you will hang up if he or she continues to be difficult.
    D. determine the problem and the appropriate staff that can help.

32. The abbreviation used in an appointment book to indicate a patient is coming in to see the physician about a medical problem already treated is:
    A. F/U.
    B. CPX.
    C. NP.
    D. BE.

33. An outguide used in filing is a:
    A. file that is no longer in use.
    B. file of a patient that is not a patient in the office any longer.
    C. guide to alphabetizing file.
    D. folder inserted in the file to hold the place of a file in use.

34. The inside address of a professional letter includes the:
    A. address of the sending physician.
    B. recipient's address written with abbreviation to save space.
    C. physician's residence address printed at the left margin.
    D. recipient's address written without abbreviations.

35. The person covered by a benefits plan is the:
    A. administrator.
    B. carrier.
    C. employee.
    D. insured.

36. The listing of charges for a medical practice is the:
    A. fee schedule.
    B. customary charges.
    C. value scale.
    D. value unit.

37. The withholding from an employee's paycheck for Social Security and Medicare is required under which law?
    A. FICA
    B. FCC
    C. HCFA
    D. IRA

38. A yeast infection that causes vaginitis is:
    A. *Candida*.
    B. staphylococci.
    C. *Trichomonas*.
    D. tinea.

39. A respiration rate that falls within the average adult range is:
    A. 10 per minute.
    B. 20 per minute.
    C. 25 per minute.
    D. 30 per minute.

40. A plan that describes personnel protective equipment (PPE) and other safety engineering devices and processes and provides instructions of what an employee should do if a related incident occurs is called:
    A. risk management.
    B. quality assurance.
    C. exposure control.
    D. aseptic technique.

41. The schedule of travel and events with arrival and departure times and other specifics such as contact numbers is called a(n):
    A. agenda.
    B. budget.
    C. itinerary.
    D. conference.

42. The first aid for frostbite is to:
    A. vigorously rub the affected body part.
    B. immerse the affected body part in water.
    C. gently wrap the affected body part in warm material.
    D. instruct the person to move around to increase circulation.

43. Facilities management includes all the following EXCEPT:
    A. hiring and firing disposable waste contractors.
    B. negotiating contracts with insurance companies.
    C. maintaining carpeting, elevators, and other structures.
    D. complying with the Americans with Disabilities Act.

44. Diabetic coma is due to:
    A. overproduction of insulin.
    B. low blood glucose level.
    C. lack of insulin.
    D. normal glucose with high insulin level.

45. An arthrogram is the radiographic visualization of:
    A. a joint.
    B. a blood vessel.
    C. the gallbladder.
    D. the spinal column.

46. Diathermy is an example of an agent that incorporates the use of:
   A. paraffin wax.
   B. cold water.
   C. ultraviolet light.
   D. deep heat.

47. Which of the following conditions would benefit from a low-purine diet?
   A. Gout
   B. Obesity
   C. High blood pressure
   D. Constipation

48. Antihypertensive medications are associated with the treatment of:
   A. fever.
   B. vomiting.
   C. high blood pressure.
   D. allergies.

49. A laceration appears as a:
   A. scrape on the skin.
   B. bruise.
   C. jagged cut.
   D. swelling on the skin.

50. *Res ipsa loquitur* is a Latin term that means which of the following?
   A. Let the buyer beware.
   B. The thing speaks for itself.
   C. The employer is responsible for the employee.
   D. The patient is always first.

51. The medical term meaning "inflammation of the bone" is:
   A. arthritis.
   B. bursitis.
   C. chondritis.
   D. osteitis.

52. The superior vena cava is the:
   A. vein that carries blood from the lower extremities to the aorta.
   B. artery that carries blood between the heart and lungs.
   C. vein that carries blood from the upper body back to the heart.
   D. vein that carries blood between the heart and lungs.

53. Basic communication requires a message and:
   A. sender and receiver.
   B. feedback and body language.
   C. clarification and feedback.
   D. receiver and body language.

54. The term **facsimile** refers to:
   A. fax.
   B. photocopy.
   C. e-mail.
   D. voice mail.

55. A matrix is a(n):
   A. form of billing.
   B. appointment book schedule with blocked out periods of time.
   C. form used for insurance filing.
   D. timed laboratory test.

56. The most common method used to chart the patient's medical record is:
   A. CPT.
   B. SOMR.
   C. SOAP.
   D. HCFA.

57. The salutation of a letter is the:
   A. closing.
   B. reference line.
   C. enclosure.
   D. greeting.

58. Coordination of benefits means:
   A. the amount of money paid by the patient for medical services before the insurance pays.
   B. one insurance plan will work with other insurance plans to determine how much each plan pays.
   C. each insurance company will pay an equal amount of the patient's bill.
   D. there is a deductible required by the patient before payment from the insurance is made.

59. ICD-9 codes that identify medical problems for reasons other than illness or injury are known as:
   A. E codes.
   B. M codes.
   C. CPT codes.
   D. V codes.

60. When a bank uses the term NSF, it means that:
    A. the check is voided and not to be used.
    B. the account is a newly opened account.
    C. there is not enough money to cover the amount of the check.
    D. the bank will issue a cashier's check in the amount of the check.

61. Supplies that are stored and maintained for emergencies in the medical office are:
    A. available for daily use.
    B. used and replaced on a routine basis.
    C. often kept off site to better utilize space.
    D. unintended for routine use.

62. The Fowler's position is used for:
    A. female pelvic exam.
    B. exam of the abdomen.
    C. patient with difficulty breathing.
    D. sigmoidoscopy.

63. The abbreviation OU is no longer in use. Instead of using OU, which of the following should be written?
    A. Both eyes
    B. Right ear
    C. Both ears
    D. Left eye

64. A fire extinguisher should be serviced at least:
    A. daily.
    B. monthly.
    C. every 6 months.
    D. annually.

65. The role of the practice manager generally includes all the following EXCEPT:
    A. negotiating insurance contracts.
    B. evaluating personnel.
    C. reviewing policies and procedures.
    D. developing treatment protocols.

66. An exposure control plan should be reviewed at least:
    A. annually.
    B. monthly.
    C. every 6 months.
    D. quarterly.

67. The abbreviation used to indicate that a patient should be fasting for an exam is:
    A. NPO.
    B. AC.
    C. PC.
    D. NOS.

68. KUB is an x-ray examination of the:
    A. urinary system.
    B. spinal column.
    C. liver and gallbladder.
    D. abdomen.

69. Another term for participatory management is:
    A. democratic management.
    B. autocratic management.
    C. laissez faire management.
    D. bureaucratic management.

70. A patient with arteriosclerosis would benefit from which of the following diets?
    A. Low salt
    B. Low carbohydrate
    C. Low protein
    D. Low cholesterol

71. The first action to control bleeding or hemorrhage is to:
    A. place ice over the wound.
    B. apply direct pressure.
    C. apply a tourniquet above the injury.
    D. immobilize the body part.

72. The term **enteritis** means inflammation of the:
    A. colon.
    B. small intestine.
    C. stomach.
    D. esophagus.

73. An example of active immunity is:
    A. maternal antibodies passed through the uterus to the baby.
    B. immunization with antibodies.
    C. maternal antibodies acquired by the baby from breast milk.
    D. producing antibodies as a result of having a disease.

74. When the person refuses to acknowledge the loss of a loved one, the type of behavior is:
    A. sympathy.
    B. mourning.
    C. denial.
    D. depression.

75. The computer device that displays the written data is the:
    A. disk drive.
    B. monitor.
    C. hard drive.
    D. floppy disk.

76. When the doctor is late and not yet at the office, the medical assistant should:
 A. offer waiting patients an opportunity to reschedule.
 B. cancel all remaining appointments for the day.
 C. reschedule all the patients for another day.
 D. offer to refer the patients to another physician's practice.

77. The "O" in the SOAP method of charting includes the:
 A. blood pressure reading.
 B. opinion of a family member.
 C. symptoms the patient states.
 D. prior complaints from the patient.

78. To retain insurance coverage, the individual must pay the cost of the insurance, which is the:
 A. premium.
 B. copayment.
 C. coinsurance.
 D. deductible.

79. CPT is an abbreviation of the reference manual used for:
 A. ordering laboratory tests.
 B. billing insurance companies for procedures.
 C. reporting diseases to the CDC.
 D. selecting the fees for each exam.

80. The best way to ensure that patients pay for services is to:
 A. ask patients where they would like the bill mailed.
 B. ask for payment of services at the time of the office visit.
 C. confirm the name of the patient's insurance company.
 D. accept checks only, not credit cards.

81. Acquired immunodeficiency syndrome is caused by:
 A. yeast.
 B. fungi.
 C. bacteria.
 D. a virus.

82. The pulse point located on the top of the foot is the:
 A. femoral.
 B. dorsalis pedis.
 C. temporal.
 D. popliteal.

83. Ensuring a system is in place to review and report results of all diagnostic tests is an example of:
 A. exposure control.
 B. incident reporting.
 C. facility management.
 D. risk management.

84. Another term for an occurrence report is a(n):
 A. subpoena.
 B. civil suit.
 C. torte.
 D. incident report.

85. When the physician improperly terminates his or her contract with the patient, this is called:
 A. patient abandonment.
 B. breach of confidentiality.
 C. noncompliance.
 D. reciprocity.

86. A myelogram is an x-ray examination of the:
 A. spinal cord.
 B. brain.
 C. muscles.
 D. heart.

87. The term used when an outside entity examines the practice's medical records to ensure accuracy, completeness, and sequence of the documents is:
 A. medical records management.
 B. accreditation.
 C. audit.
 D. aging analysis.

88. Anaphylaxis refers to a:
 A. nose bleed.
 B. type of shock.
 C. hemorrhage disorder.
 D. congenital disorder.

89. Dyspepsia refers to:
 A. difficulty speaking.
 B. difficult digestion.
 C. difficulty breathing.
 D. abnormal pain.

90. The perineum is the:
 A. lining of the abdomen.
 B. covering of the spinal cord.
 C. floor of the pelvis.
 D. outside lining of the lungs.

91. *Respondeat superior* refers to:
   A. a subpoena.
   B. a physician's responsibility for the actions of his staff.
   C. something for something, a favor for a favor.
   D. responding to your superiors.

92. Management of the electronic health record does not require:
   A. archiving.
   B. retrieving.
   C. conditioning.
   D. security.

93. The medical record provides all the following EXCEPT a:
   A. resource for public education.
   B. legal document.
   C. tool for quality monitoring.
   D. method for continuity of care.

94. The telecommunications device for the deaf is what type of communication?
   A. Closed
   B. Body language
   C. Verbal
   D. Nonverbal

95. The process by which nutrients transfer from the gastrointestinal system into the blood is referred to as:
   A. ingestion.
   B. digestion.
   C. absorption.
   D. metabolism.

96. The classification of drugs used to relieve pain is:
   A. antidepressant.
   B. analgesic.
   C. antibiotic.
   D. antidote.

97. The device used to check vision is a(n):
   A. otoscope.
   B. ophthalmoscope.
   C. Snellen chart.
   D. tuning fork.

98. A wound that results from scraping the skin is a(n):
   A. laceration.
   B. avulsion.
   C. contusion.
   D. abrasion.

99. In the medical office, the electronic medical record will decrease the need for:
   A. security.
   B. transcription.
   C. a release of information form.
   D. staff.

100. Retention of medical records for minors is generally:
   A. 7–10 years.
   B. 7–10 years after reaching 18 years old.
   C. 7–10 years after becoming an emancipated minor.
   D. 7–10 years after the age of majority.

ANSWERS TO PRACTICE EXAM—CMAS (AMT)

1. B
2. B
3. D
4. C
5. C
6. A
7. C
8. D
9. B
10. C
11. A
12. C
13. C
14. B
15. B
16. D
17. A
18. A
19. C
20. A
21. C
22. A
23. C
24. D
25. D
26. B
27. C
28. B
29. C
30. A
31. D
32. A
33. D
34. D
35. D
36. A
37. A
38. A
39. B
40. C
41. C
42. C
43. B
44. C
45. A
46. D
47. A
48. C
49. C
50. B
51. D
52. C
53. A
54. A
55. B
56. C
57. D
58. B
59. D
60. C
61. D
62. C
63. A
64. D
65. D
66. A
67. A
68. A
69. A
70. D
71. B
72. B
73. D
74. C
75. B
76. A
77. A
78. A
79. B
80. B
81. D
82. B
83. D
84. D
85. A
86. A
87. C
88. B
89. B
90. C
91. B
92. C
93. A
94. C
95. C
96. B
97. C
98. D
99. B
100. D

ANSWER SHEET

1. Ⓐ Ⓑ Ⓒ Ⓓ Ⓔ	26. Ⓐ Ⓑ Ⓒ Ⓓ Ⓔ	51. Ⓐ Ⓑ Ⓒ Ⓓ Ⓔ	76. Ⓐ Ⓑ Ⓒ Ⓓ Ⓔ
2. Ⓐ Ⓑ Ⓒ Ⓓ Ⓔ	27. Ⓐ Ⓑ Ⓒ Ⓓ Ⓔ	52. Ⓐ Ⓑ Ⓒ Ⓓ Ⓔ	77. Ⓐ Ⓑ Ⓒ Ⓓ Ⓔ
3. Ⓐ Ⓑ Ⓒ Ⓓ Ⓔ	28. Ⓐ Ⓑ Ⓒ Ⓓ Ⓔ	53. Ⓐ Ⓑ Ⓒ Ⓓ Ⓔ	78. Ⓐ Ⓑ Ⓒ Ⓓ Ⓔ
4. Ⓐ Ⓑ Ⓒ Ⓓ Ⓔ	29. Ⓐ Ⓑ Ⓒ Ⓓ Ⓔ	54. Ⓐ Ⓑ Ⓒ Ⓓ Ⓔ	79. Ⓐ Ⓑ Ⓒ Ⓓ Ⓔ
5. Ⓐ Ⓑ Ⓒ Ⓓ Ⓔ	30. Ⓐ Ⓑ Ⓒ Ⓓ Ⓔ	55. Ⓐ Ⓑ Ⓒ Ⓓ Ⓔ	80. Ⓐ Ⓑ Ⓒ Ⓓ Ⓔ
6. Ⓐ Ⓑ Ⓒ Ⓓ Ⓔ	31. Ⓐ Ⓑ Ⓒ Ⓓ Ⓔ	56. Ⓐ Ⓑ Ⓒ Ⓓ Ⓔ	81. Ⓐ Ⓑ Ⓒ Ⓓ Ⓔ
7. Ⓐ Ⓑ Ⓒ Ⓓ Ⓔ	32. Ⓐ Ⓑ Ⓒ Ⓓ Ⓔ	57. Ⓐ Ⓑ Ⓒ Ⓓ Ⓔ	82. Ⓐ Ⓑ Ⓒ Ⓓ Ⓔ
8. Ⓐ Ⓑ Ⓒ Ⓓ Ⓔ	33. Ⓐ Ⓑ Ⓒ Ⓓ Ⓔ	58. Ⓐ Ⓑ Ⓒ Ⓓ Ⓔ	83. Ⓐ Ⓑ Ⓒ Ⓓ Ⓔ
9. Ⓐ Ⓑ Ⓒ Ⓓ Ⓔ	34. Ⓐ Ⓑ Ⓒ Ⓓ Ⓔ	59. Ⓐ Ⓑ Ⓒ Ⓓ Ⓔ	84. Ⓐ Ⓑ Ⓒ Ⓓ Ⓔ
10. Ⓐ Ⓑ Ⓒ Ⓓ Ⓔ	35. Ⓐ Ⓑ Ⓒ Ⓓ Ⓔ	60. Ⓐ Ⓑ Ⓒ Ⓓ Ⓔ	85. Ⓐ Ⓑ Ⓒ Ⓓ Ⓔ
11. Ⓐ Ⓑ Ⓒ Ⓓ Ⓔ	36. Ⓐ Ⓑ Ⓒ Ⓓ Ⓔ	61. Ⓐ Ⓑ Ⓒ Ⓓ Ⓔ	86. Ⓐ Ⓑ Ⓒ Ⓓ Ⓔ
12. Ⓐ Ⓑ Ⓒ Ⓓ Ⓔ	37. Ⓐ Ⓑ Ⓒ Ⓓ Ⓔ	62. Ⓐ Ⓑ Ⓒ Ⓓ Ⓔ	87. Ⓐ Ⓑ Ⓒ Ⓓ Ⓔ
13. Ⓐ Ⓑ Ⓒ Ⓓ Ⓔ	38. Ⓐ Ⓑ Ⓒ Ⓓ Ⓔ	63. Ⓐ Ⓑ Ⓒ Ⓓ Ⓔ	88. Ⓐ Ⓑ Ⓒ Ⓓ Ⓔ
14. Ⓐ Ⓑ Ⓒ Ⓓ Ⓔ	39. Ⓐ Ⓑ Ⓒ Ⓓ Ⓔ	64. Ⓐ Ⓑ Ⓒ Ⓓ Ⓔ	89. Ⓐ Ⓑ Ⓒ Ⓓ Ⓔ
15. Ⓐ Ⓑ Ⓒ Ⓓ Ⓔ	40. Ⓐ Ⓑ Ⓒ Ⓓ Ⓔ	65. Ⓐ Ⓑ Ⓒ Ⓓ Ⓔ	90. Ⓐ Ⓑ Ⓒ Ⓓ Ⓔ
16. Ⓐ Ⓑ Ⓒ Ⓓ Ⓔ	41. Ⓐ Ⓑ Ⓒ Ⓓ Ⓔ	66. Ⓐ Ⓑ Ⓒ Ⓓ Ⓔ	91. Ⓐ Ⓑ Ⓒ Ⓓ Ⓔ
17. Ⓐ Ⓑ Ⓒ Ⓓ Ⓔ	42. Ⓐ Ⓑ Ⓒ Ⓓ Ⓔ	67. Ⓐ Ⓑ Ⓒ Ⓓ Ⓔ	92. Ⓐ Ⓑ Ⓒ Ⓓ Ⓔ
18. Ⓐ Ⓑ Ⓒ Ⓓ Ⓔ	43. Ⓐ Ⓑ Ⓒ Ⓓ Ⓔ	68. Ⓐ Ⓑ Ⓒ Ⓓ Ⓔ	93. Ⓐ Ⓑ Ⓒ Ⓓ Ⓔ
19. Ⓐ Ⓑ Ⓒ Ⓓ Ⓔ	44. Ⓐ Ⓑ Ⓒ Ⓓ Ⓔ	69. Ⓐ Ⓑ Ⓒ Ⓓ Ⓔ	94. Ⓐ Ⓑ Ⓒ Ⓓ Ⓔ
20. Ⓐ Ⓑ Ⓒ Ⓓ Ⓔ	45. Ⓐ Ⓑ Ⓒ Ⓓ Ⓔ	70. Ⓐ Ⓑ Ⓒ Ⓓ Ⓔ	95. Ⓐ Ⓑ Ⓒ Ⓓ Ⓔ
21. Ⓐ Ⓑ Ⓒ Ⓓ Ⓔ	46. Ⓐ Ⓑ Ⓒ Ⓓ Ⓔ	71. Ⓐ Ⓑ Ⓒ Ⓓ Ⓔ	96. Ⓐ Ⓑ Ⓒ Ⓓ Ⓔ
22. Ⓐ Ⓑ Ⓒ Ⓓ Ⓔ	47. Ⓐ Ⓑ Ⓒ Ⓓ Ⓔ	72. Ⓐ Ⓑ Ⓒ Ⓓ Ⓔ	97. Ⓐ Ⓑ Ⓒ Ⓓ Ⓔ
23. Ⓐ Ⓑ Ⓒ Ⓓ Ⓔ	48. Ⓐ Ⓑ Ⓒ Ⓓ Ⓔ	73. Ⓐ Ⓑ Ⓒ Ⓓ Ⓔ	98. Ⓐ Ⓑ Ⓒ Ⓓ Ⓔ
24. Ⓐ Ⓑ Ⓒ Ⓓ Ⓔ	49. Ⓐ Ⓑ Ⓒ Ⓓ Ⓔ	74. Ⓐ Ⓑ Ⓒ Ⓓ Ⓔ	99. Ⓐ Ⓑ Ⓒ Ⓓ Ⓔ
25. Ⓐ Ⓑ Ⓒ Ⓓ Ⓔ	50. Ⓐ Ⓑ Ⓒ Ⓓ Ⓔ	75. Ⓐ Ⓑ Ⓒ Ⓓ Ⓔ	100. Ⓐ Ⓑ Ⓒ Ⓓ Ⓔ

INDEX

Note: Page numbers followed by *b*, *f* and *t* indicate boxed text, figures and tables respectively

N

W

X

Z

Study Calendar

SUNDAY	MONDAY	TUESDAY	WEDNESDAY	THURSDAY	FRIDAY	SATURDAY

Study Calendar

SUNDAY	MONDAY	TUESDAY	WEDNESDAY	THURSDAY	FRIDAY	SATURDAY

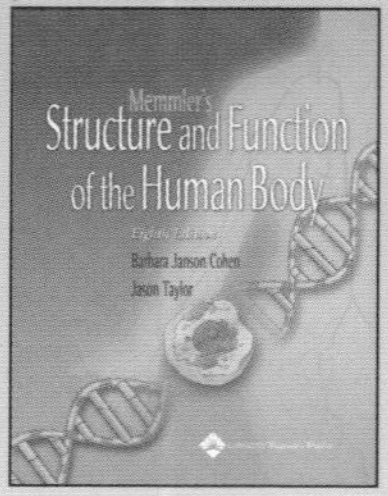

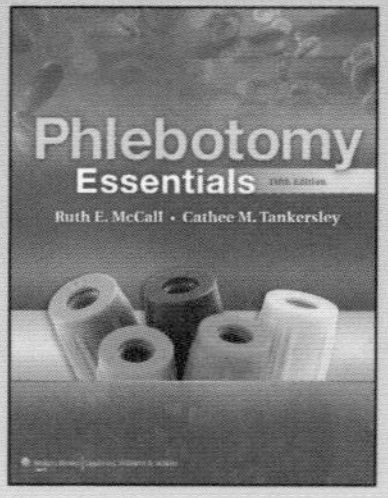

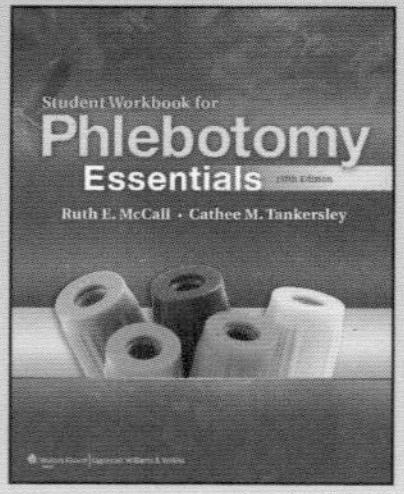

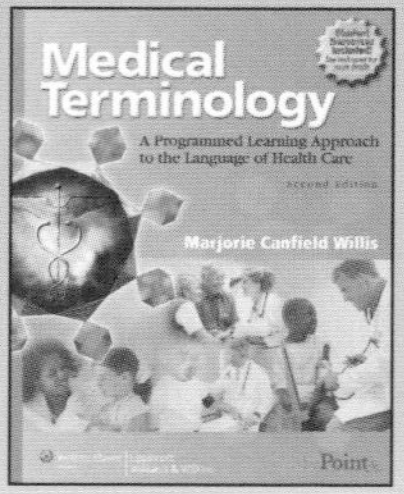

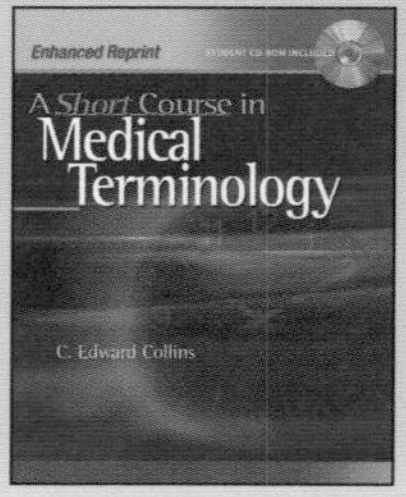

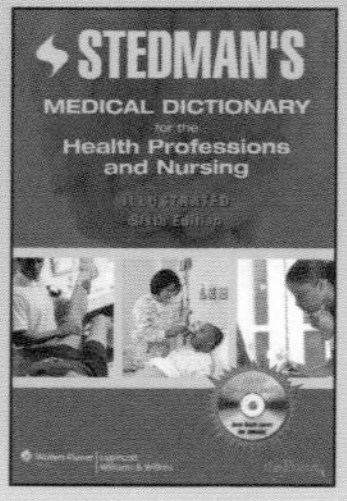

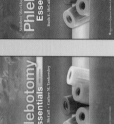